CARDIAC VALVE REPLACEMENT

CARDIAC VALVE REPLACEMENT

CURRENT STATUS

PROCEEDINGS OF THE FOURTH INTERNATIONAL SYMPOSIUM
ON THE ST. JUDE MEDICAL® VALVE,
MARCH 11–14, 1984

JACK M. MATLOFF, EDITOR

MARTINUS NIJHOFF PUBLISHING
A MEMBER OF THE KLUWER ACADEMIC PUBLISHERS GROUP
BOSTON   DORDRECHT   LANCASTER

Distributors for North America:
Kluwer Academic Publishers
190 Old Derby Street
Hingham, MA 02043

Distributors for all other countries:
Kluwer Academic Publishers Group
Distribution Centre
P.O. Box 322
3300 AH Dordrecht
The Netherlands

Library of Congress Cataloging in Publication Data

International Symposium on the St. Jude Medical
    Valve (4th : 1984 : Montego Bay, Jamaica)
    Cardiac valve replacement.

    Includes bibliographies.
    1. Heart valve prosthesis—Congresses.   I. Matloff,
Jack M.   II. Title.   III. Title: St. Jude Medical
Valve. [DNLM: 1. Heart Valve Prosthesis—
congresses. W3 IN924NU 4th 1984c / WG 169 I608 1984c]
RD598.I54   1984   617'.412   85-5059
ISBN 0-89838-722-1

CONTENTS

REGISTERED TRADEMARKS USED IN THIS BOOK

BJÖRK-SHILEY®—Shiley Corporation
CARPENTIER-EDWARDS®—American Edwards Laboratories
COUMADIN®—The DuPont Corporation
DACRON®—The DuPont Corporation
DELRIN®—The DuPont Corporation
HANCOCK®—Vascor, Inc.
IONESCU-SHILEY®—Shiley Corporation
KEFLIN®—Eli Lilly and Company
LILLEHEI-KASTER®—Medical Incorporated
MEADOX-COOLEY®—Meadox Medicals, Inc.
MEDTRONIC HALL™—Blood Systems, Inc.
OMNISCIENCE®—Medical Incorporated
PERSANTINE®—Boehringer Ingelheim
SILASTIC®—Dow Corning
ST. JUDE MEDICAL®—St. Jude Medical, Inc.
STARR-EDWARDS®—American Edwards Laboratories
STELLITE®—Cabot Corporation
SWAN-GANZ®—Edwards Laboratories
TEFLON®—DuPont Corporation

CONTRIBUTING AUTHORS

Oscar Baeza, M.D.
Passaic General Hospital
Passaic, NJ 07055
Address for correspondence:
350 Boulevard
Passaic, NJ 07055

Eugene M. Baudet
Dept. of Cardiovascular Surgery
Hopital Cardiologique
Avenue de Magellan
33604 Bordeaux
France

Stuart L. Boe, M.D.
Suite 609
3661 South Miami Avenue
Miami, FL 33133

A. Michael Borkon, M.D.
Division of Cardiac Surgery
The Johns Hopkins Hospital
600 North Wolfe Street
Baltimore, MD 21205

Lawrence H. Cohn, M.D.
Brigham & Women's Hospital
75 Francis Street
Boston, MA 02115

Denton A. Cooley, M.D.
P.O. Box 20345
Texas Heart Institute of
St. Luke's Episcopal and
Texas Children's Hospitals
Houston, Texas 77225

Fred A. Crawford, Jr., M.D.
The Medical University of
South Carolina
171 Ashley Avenue
Charleston, SC 29425

George J. D'Angelo, M.D.
Hamot Medical Center
Erie, PA
Address for correspondence:
104 East Second Street
Erie, PA 16507

Donald B. Doty, M.D.
LDS Hospital
Primary Children's Medical Center
Salt Lake City, UT
Address for correspondence:
324 - 10th Avenue
Salt Lake City, UT 84103

J. Michael Duncan, M.D.
Texas Heart Institute
P.O. Box 20345
Houston, TX 77225

Prof. Henri Dupon, M.D.
35, rue Paul Bert
44035 Nantes
France

R. Leighton Fisk, M.D.
Phoenix Foundation for
Cardiovascular Research,
St. Luke's Hospital Heart-Lung Center
525 North 18th Street
Suite 5
Phoenix, AZ 85006

Isaac Gielchinsky, M.D.
Dept. of Cardiothoracic Surgery
Newark Beth Israel Medical Center
201 Lyons Avenue
Newark, NJ 17112

Lorenzo Gonzalez-Lavin, M.D.
Chairman, Department of Surgery
Deborah Heart and Lung Center
Browns Mills, NJ 08015

Richard J. Gray, M.D.
Cedars Sinai Medical Center
8700 Beverly Blvd.
Los Angeles, CA 90048

Prof. Andreas Hoffmann, M.D.
Lange Gasse 78
4052 Basel
Switzerland

Dieter Horstkotte, M.D.
Department of Medicine B
University Hospital Duesseldorf
Moorenstr. 5
4000 Duesseldorf
West Germany

E. Hjelms, M.D.
Department of Cardiothoracic Surgery
Rigshospitalet
University of Copenhagen
Blegdamsvej 9,
DK-2100
Copenhagen, Denmark

W. R. Eric Jamieson, M.D.
University of British Columbia
Vancouver, B.C.
Canada
Address for correspondence:
750 West Broadway
Vancouver, B.C. V5Z 1HL
Canada

Jean-Louis LeClerc, M.D.
University Hospital Brugmann
Cardiac Surgery
808 route de Lennik
1070 Brussels
Belgium

William G. Lindsay, M.D.
Cardiac Surgical Assoc.
2545 Chicago Avenue
Suite 730
Minneapolis, MN 55404

Joseph LoCicero, III, M.D.
Northwestern University
Div. of Cardiothoracic Surgery
Ward Building 9-105
303 East Chicago Avenue
Chicago, IL 60611

John W. Mack, M.D.
Clinical Associate Professor
University of Texas Health Sciences Center
San Antonio, TX
Address for correspondence:
13702 Wilderness Point
San Antonio, TX 78231

Christopher T. Maloney, M.D.
Southwest Cardio-Thoracic
Surgery, Ltd.
5200 East Grant Road
Suite 200-A
Tucson, AZ 85712

Jack M. Matloff, M.D.
Cedars Sinai Medical Center
8700 Beverly Blvd.
Los Angeles, CA 90048

Eldred D. Mundth, M.D.
The Hahnemann Medical College
and Hospital
230 North Broad Street
Suite 6328
Philadelphia, PA 19102

Demetre M. Nicoloff, M.D.
Cardiac Surgical Assoc., P.A.
2545 Chicago Avenue
Suite 730
Minneapolis, MN 55404

James R. Pluth, M.D.
Mayo Clinic
200 - 1st Street S.W.
W6-B
Rochester, MN 55901

Shahbudin Rahimtoola, M.D.
Professor of Medicine
Chief, Section of Cardiology
University of Southern California
2025 Zonal Avenue
Los Angeles, CA 90033

Robert M. Sade, M.D.
The Medical University of
South Carolina
Div. of Cardiothoracic Surgery
171 Ashley Avenue
Charleston, SC 29025

Lester R. Sauvage, M.D.
528 - 18th Avenue
Seattle, WA 98122

Francis Wellens, M.D.
Hopital Erasme
808, Route de Lennik
1070 Bruxelles
Belgium

DEDICATION

Cardiac Valve Replacement: Current Status is dedicated to all those patients and their families who have had cardiac valve replacement surgery. Their story has been one of personal courage because they decided to accept such therapy when a precise definition of their future with one valve substitute or another was not clear. This courageous decision was initiated with the first implantations of the Harken and STARR-EDWARDS® caged-ball valves in 1960 and has continued to exist as each new valve substitute has been implanted, because laboratory testing of such devices, no matter how sophisticated the *in vitro* or animal test, has never been able to precisely define the device performance characteristics in humans. In this sense, the ultimate determination of each valve's clinical record has only been defined during its clinical use in patients. Thus, each patient who undergoes valve replacement owes a debt to those who previously had such surgical therapy; each repays that debt by contributing to the learning experience that makes the valve safer and easier for those who benefit later.

All of us—patients, their families, cardiologists and cardiac surgeons—therefore should recognize the contributions of Mary Richardson and her pioneering surgeon, Dwight E. Harken, M.D. They shared this initial experience with total aortic valve excision and replacement in the anatomic position in February 1960 at the Peter Bent Bingham Hospital in Boston.

With regard to the experience with the ST. JUDE MEDICAL® valve, 2 patients are deserving of particular note for their special contributions. Mrs. Helen Heikkinen underwent the first ST. JUDE MEDICAL valve replacement in October 1977. She has to be recognized for her courage in accepting the recommendation for this valve's initial use, at a time when there were other valves available, with well-defined clinical track records. She continues to be well and establishes the standard for durability of the valve.

Henry Jaffe also must be recognized for his exquisite understanding of this process of shared patient responsibility. Because of his sensitivity for this sequence and his innate intellectual curiosity, he and his wife, Florence have personally funded more clinical investigations of the ST. JUDE MEDICAL valve than any other individual or agency, to my knowledge.

While the medical contributions to this symposium are identified, all of us must also acknowledge the contributions of the uncited coauthors, our patients. On behalf of my colleagues, we thank you.

Jack M. Matloff

Cardiac Valve Replacement: Current Status is the proceedings of the Fourth International Symposium on the ST. JUDE MEDICAL® valve. The first three symposia on this topic were held primarily for designated investigators involved in clinical trials of the ST. JUDE MEDICAL valve. The last meeting, chaired by Michael E. DeBakey, M.D., was held in November 1982 [1], immediately before the valve was released for general clinical use in the United States by the Food and Drug Administration. These proceedings then are the first comprehensive compilation of clinical data since that time; and they include, particularly in the discussions, the experience of physicians other than the original clinical investigators.

Over the past 5 years the character of these symposia has changed. Whereas the first two dealt almost entirely with the ST. JUDE MEDICAL valve, the last two have evolved into a more generic cardiac valvular surgery meeting, focusing primarily on valve replacement rather than valve repair [2]. Thus, these proceedings contain a wide spectrum of topics, including a keynote presentation on criteria for selection of cardiac valve substitutes in 1984, complications of cardiac valve replacement and their treatment, a review of the current status of cardiac valve substitutes other than the ST. JUDE MEDICAL valve and a consideration of cardiac valve replacement in special circumstances. Among these special circumstances are four presentations on pediatric use of the ST. JUDE MEDICAL valve. Finally, there are three presentations by groups who have had experience with BJÖRK-SHILEY® spherical, HANCOCK® porcine, IONESCU-SHILEY® pericardial and ST. JUDE MEDICAL valves and who attempt to define their comparative results. That these presentations are from a number of groups around the world establishes this as a truly international symposium and reflects the fact that the ST. JUDE MEDICAL valve has become the most widely used cardiac prosthesis in the world.

Chapters that constitute each of the sections are followed by the recorded discussions that took place after each session of the symposium. For these, I am indebted to the moderators who chaired the various sections; they are Lawrence H. Cohn, Dieter Horstkotte, Donald B. Doty, Eugene M. Baudet, Demetre M. Nicoloff, Shahbudin Rahimtoola and Richard J. Gray. These discussions have been included in an attempt to make these proceedings a current progress report. The medical literature is replete with somewhat dated abstracts and articles in a format that does not allow for a ready opportunity to resolve the multiplicity of opinions. I have felt these discussions should be included because they are an interaction between the presenters and other participants, are an attempt to share their experiences, and are an attempt to resolve apparent and real differences and to generally learn from each other. I, therefore, would like to thank each of the discussants for their participation as well.

It is apparent from this forum that there is not an international, national or even local standard of terminology for valvular heart surgery. While editing this volume I have tried to achieve some degree of standardization in the terminology. Thus, *valve repair* and *valve replacement with substitutes* are used in this volume to reflect the two basic methods of valvular heart surgery. Unfortunately, there is no term for the issue of whether a valve is deserving of surgical intervention. This decision has become one of the most difficult issues of valvular heart surgery to resolve, especially when so many patients are now studied for considerations other than valvular and are found to have varying degrees of concomitant *valvular* or *prosthetic dysfunction*. The term *bioprosthesis* is used in this volume to include those valves fabricated from tissue or biological components; and the term *prosthesis* includes all mechanical valves fabricated from materials other than tissue. *Mobile element* refers to functional components whether they are tissue leaflets, mechanical leaflets, poppets, occluders, balls or discs. I have also tried to standardize the reporting of mortalities as *operative* or *less than 30 days* if a patient was discharged from the hospital and *late* if mortality occurred more than 30 days after surgery and after discharge. In the same manner, thromboembolism, thrombotic occlusions and valve-related events (dysfunction, hemolysis and infection) are reported as *percent (%) per patient year of follow-up* when possible.

I would be remiss if I did not thank St. Jude Medical on behalf of all who attended the symposium that was the basis of this volume. Even though St. Jude Medical sponsored this symposium, they did not and do not desire that this book be a testimonial to any valve substitute, including their own. Rather, it was their intention that this be a forum for initiating exchanges about the valve-related topics presented. To their credit, they did not, in any way, intrude on the choice of topics discussed, the choice of papers presented or the scientific organization of the symposium. If there is a bias projected, it is an unintended reflection of my thoughts about valvular heart surgery. Given the widespread use of the ST. JUDE MEDI-CAL valve and its seemingly increasing popularity, I have felt that there has been a disparity between its use reflected at this symposium and what has been presented previously in the medical literature. My choices, therefore, are an attempt to correct this disparity.

Finally, I want to thank all of the presenters for their efforts. They are the individuals who are responsible for whatever this volume may or may not be. In particular, I would like to thank Denton Cooley, M.D. for his active participation. Of all of the illustrious trainees of Alfred Blalock, M.D. at the Johns Hopkins Hospital, none has attained as much in clinical cardiac surgery as Dr. Cooley. He personally has performed more cardiac surgery than anyone else ever has and probably ever will in the future. From this experience, he has distilled the essence of cardiac surgery—constantly innovating, introducing, revising and improving existing procedures, to become the virtuoso technician and consummate teacher that he is. Even more amazingly, he has done this in the three major areas of cardiac surgery: congenital heart disease, coronary heart disease and valvular heart disease. In the keynote presentation, "Cardiac Valvular Surgery, 1984—Criteria for Selection of Cardiac Valve Substitutes," by Dr. Cooley established the outline for the presentations that follow.

Jack M. Matloff, M.D.

REFERENCES

1. DeBakey ME (ed): *Advances in Cardiac Valves: Clinical Perspectives.* New York, Yorke Medical Books, 1983.
2. Oury J: *Recent Progress in Mitral Valve Disease.* Kent, England, Butterworths, Sevenoaks, 1984.

KEYNOTE ADDRESS: CARDIAC VALVULAR SURGERY, 1984— CRITERIA FOR SELECTION OF CARDIAC VALVE SUBSTITUTES

DENTON A. COOLEY

Thirty years have elapsed since the introduction of the first artificial heart valves. Since that time, many improvements have been made in the design and fabrication of prosthetic valves, but the perfect valve remains elusive. Although much has been learned, more remains to be clarified.

The earliest valvular substitute was the Hufnagel valve, which was introduced into the descending thoracic aorta in 1952 [1]. Early investigators were confused, however, by the misconception that the prosthetic valve should closely resemble the human anatomy. Attempts to apply this concept in the early years of replacement met with limited success. The valves of Hufnagel, McGoon, Bahnson, and others came to an abrupt end when thrombosis, fracture and disruption occurred.

In the early 1960s, Harken [2] and Starr [3] devised caged-ball prostheses that aroused objections from advocates of the anatomic design concept (figure 1). This caged-ball design had been in use a long time and, in fact, was illustrated in 1858 by a request for a bottle stopper patent [4]. The Harken and STARR-EDWARDS® valves were placed in the normal anatomic position, or the subcoronary and mitral annular positions, respectively. The STARR-EDWARDS valve design is still practical, although a number of design modifications and improvements have been made since the early models. These included a method of "curing" the silicone ball in 1965 that eliminated the "ball variance" problem and an extension of the cloth covering of the sewing ring to reach the inlet orifice to lessen the incidence of thromboembolic events [5,6]. The primary disadvantage of the

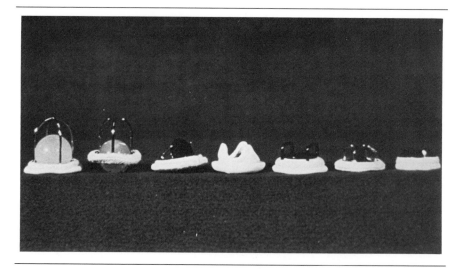

Figure 1. Valves used during the past two decades. Left to right, Starr-Edwards, Smeloff-Cutter, Lillehei-Kaster, Hancock porcine bioprosthesis, Beall Surgitool, Cooley-Cutter, and St. Jude Medical.

STARR-EDWARDS valve is its high profile, which is a liability in patients with a small left ventricle or small aortic root. Under such circumstances, the ball may be partially obstructing. The bulky cage also makes it technically difficult to implant the valve in a small aortic anulus.

As it became obvious that the caged-ball prosthesis would not be totally satisfactory, attention was turned to valves with low profile designs employing discs [7]. The LILLEHEI-KASTER® disc valve (currently the OMNISCIENCE® valve) survived unchanged from its introduction in 1969 until 1977 when the titanium components were replaced by a housing made of pyrolytic carbon, a much more durable material. The base of the valve was made thinner, and the thickness of the disk was reduced (figure 2). The disc is now suspended by a system of ridges in the base that make the original struts unnecessary [8,9].

The BJÖRK-SHILEY® cageless tilting disc valve was first introduced clinically in 1969 [10,11]. The original valve design incorporated a free-floating DEL-RIN® disc occluder, suspended in a stellite cage that was covered with a TE-FLON® ring. The valve has undergone several design changes since. In 1971, the DELRIN disc, which had a rather high coefficient of expansion, was changed to pyrolytic carbon. The opening angle of the original mitral valve was increased from 50° to 60°, as in the aortic model, to achieve better hemodynamic function; changes in the sewing ring were made to allow for variations in the suture technique to seat the valve [12]. The most recent modification has been the introduction of a convexo-concave model in an attempt to decrease thromboembolic complications [13] (figure 3). The new design allows the carbon disc to pivot

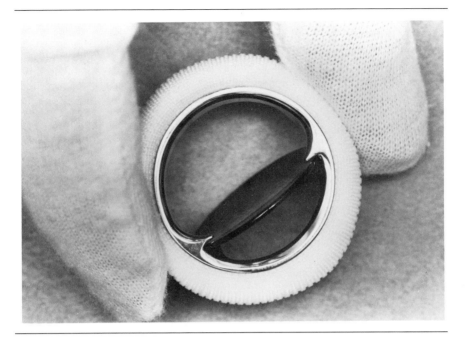

Figure 2. Omniscience disc valve.

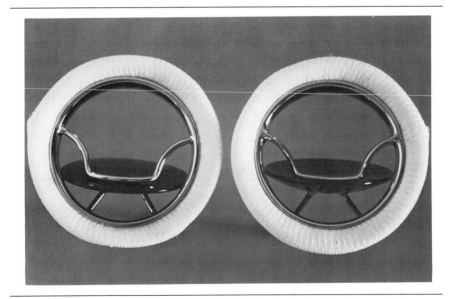

Figure 3. Björk-Shiley convex-concave disc valve.

2.5 mm downstream during opening, to allow for a *washing* effect at the pivot points and increase flow through the minor orifice.

Also during the 1960s, valve replacement with biologic tissue was tried, including formaldehyde-treated porcine xenografts, stented and unstented fascia lata, freeze-dried homografts, pulmonary valve autografts and various chemical treatments to stented and unstented homografts. Many of these valves sounded perfect, but most deteriorated rapidly. Ionescu, however, persevered and developed a pericardial valve, cured with glutaraldehyde, which is still in use today [14,15].

Besides the IONESCU-SHILEY® valve, the two other bioprostheses commercially available today are the HANCOCK® porcine xenograft and the CARPENTIER-EDWARDS® porcine xenograft. Both are preserved with glutaraldehyde and mounted on cloth-covered flexible stents [16,17] (figures 4 and 5). Both valves are silent, do not cause hemolysis and are relatively free of thromboembolic complications [18,19]. The main disadvantages of the bioprostheses are restricted hemodynamic performance and durability. The original HANCOCK valve, which had a muscle bar across the noncoronary leaflet, was partially obstructive [20,21]. In an attempt to rectify this hemodynamic problem, Hancock developed a modified orifice valve. Although the hemodynamic characteristics of this new valve are better, transvalvular gradients in the smaller valve sizes are still higher than those found with some mechanical valves. A new HANCOCK bovine pericardial valve (figure 6) is currently under clinical investigation.

The IONESCU-SHILEY valve is made from bovine pericardium treated with

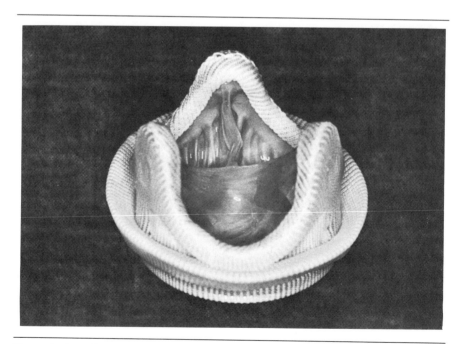

Figure 4. Hancock porcine bioprosthesis.

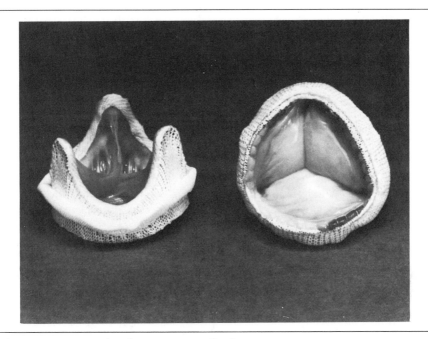

Figure 5. Carpentier-Edwards porcine xenograft valve.

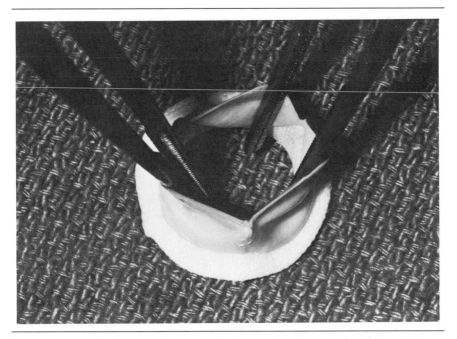

Figure 6. Hancock bovine pericardial bioprosthesis currently undergoing clinical investigation.

glutaraldehyde [22] (figure 7). Each of the valve leaflets is cut and sutured on a cloth-covered titanium frame. Hydraulic characteristics are good since there is no muscle bar at the base of any leaflet and a very low flow gradient across the valve [23]. A lower profile design is currently undergoing evaluation (figure 8). The IONESCU-SHILEY valve has been used in 2680 patients since 1978 at the Texas Heart Institute. Although the rate of valve failure in this series was 1.76% per patient-year, the failure rate is time-related and increases after five years. We are concerned that the failure rate of this group may be unacceptably high in the future [24–26].

The 1970s also saw the development of additional tilting disc valves, including the ST. JUDE MEDICAL® valve (figure 9). It is our current valve of choice in all patients, unless long-term anticoagulation is contraindicated [27]. The ST. JUDE MEDICAL valve is a low-profile, bileaflet, central-flow prosthesis made entirely of pyrolytic carbon [28,29]. The valve has an excellent sewing ring, fabricated of velour-knitted DACRON® fabric. The valve has a wide opening angle with low resistance to forward flow, and the low profile makes the valve very satisfactory in both the mitral and aortic positions as well as in the tricuspid anulus. It is easy to insert, even in a small anulus [30]. We began using the ST. JUDE MEDICAL valve in 1978. In a follow-up of 615 patients, we have not found any instances of valve dysfunction and few instances of systemic embolism [31]. Its low profile is a distinct advantage.

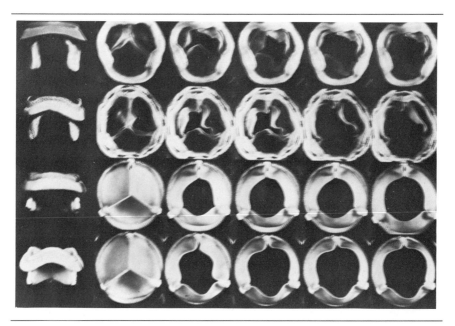

Figure 7. Valve prostheses in mock circulation showing differing degrees of opening and obstruction to forward flow. The largest orifice is found in the Ionescu-Shiley valve (bottom row).

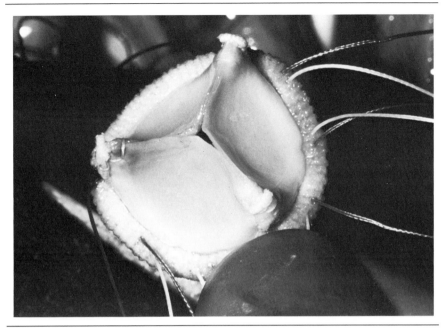

Figure 8. Recently modified low profile Ionescu–Shiley valve prosthesis.

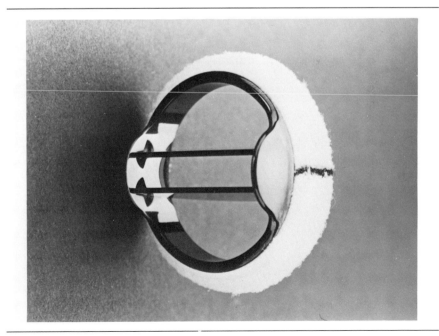

Figure 9. St. Jude Medical tilting disc valve.

COMPLICATIONS

Complications from the use of prosthetic valves have been frequent and have fallen into several categories: 1) thromboembolism; 2) hemolysis; 3) hemodynamics, obstruction and regurgitation; and 4) material failure. Associated complications include infection and the possibility of a foreign body in the bloodstream. At this time, whether one valve is more prone to infection than another, either early or late, is difficult to ascertain. Thrombosis and embolism are less prevalent in the aortic position. There is a much higher incidence of thromboembolic complications in mechanical valves, and thromboemboli can occur despite anticoagulation (figure 10). Hemolysis has been a well-known complication of prosthetic valves. The small-sized, totally cloth-covered caged-ball aortic valve prostheses almost uniformly led to hemolysis, which is not always evident clinically. However, it can almost always be detected by studying the serum enzymes (lactose dehydrogenase [LDH] and serum haptoglobin levels). Such complications led us to abandon the fabric-covered valves. Regardless of design, all valves with a fabric sewing ring will cause hemolysis if a paravalvular leak develops. Thus, even an ideal valve must be sutured accurately and securely in the valve anulus.

Selection and preparation of materials for valve components did not seem difficult in the early years because inert, durable materials that caused minimal tissue irritation and blood damage were available. It seemed that valve occluders

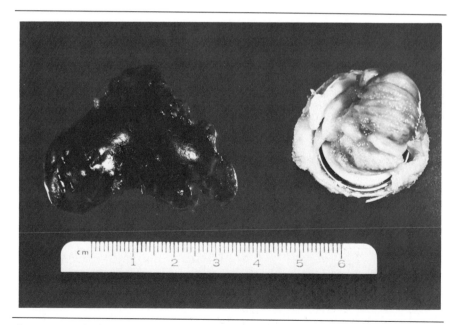

Figure 10. Björk-Shiley valve removed 10 years after implantation in the mitral valve position. The patient had discontinued anticoagulation three months prior to entering the hospital. A dense, rubbery thrombus is shown on the right. A more recent left atrial thrombus that was floating free above the valve is shown on the left.

made of SILASTIC® would last almost indefinitely. However, a slight flaw in the curing and processing of Silastic caused the occluders to deteriorate when exposed to the enzymes and fatty acids in the blood. As a result, swelling, fracture and occasional dislodgement and embolization of the poppet into the circulation occurred [32,33] (figure 11). SILASTIC was not the only material that failed. TEFLON occluders used in the Beall and Wada valves also deteriorated, sometimes with fatal consequences. Fascia lata and dura mater were both destroyed very quickly [34,35,36]. As noted earlier, covering surfaces with cloth to encourage ingrowth of tissue proved unsatisfactory [37]. Metal wear or fatigue was also a problem.

Obviously, more durable materials were needed; and new designs were tried using glutaraldehyde-treated tissue and pyrolytic carbon components. Tissue valves, however, thicken with age and are subject to calcification, especially in young children [38,39] (figure 12). Although glutaraldehyde prolongs the life of a tissue valve, it will eventually undergo degeneration and possible leaflet disruption [40,41] (figure 13). It would seem reasonable, then, to use tissue valves only when anticoagulants are contraindicated. Surfaces of pyrolytic carbon seem most encouraging from the standpoint of wear and the nonthrombogenic nature of this material. Optimum healing is obtained with this material. Apparently, the negatively charged pyrolytic carbon inhibits the overgrowth of fibrous tissue.

Peripheral versus central flow is still an issue in design of prosthetic heart valves. Advantages of the full orifice principle in reducing the flow pressure gradient are obvious, but the self-washing action is another distinct advantage.

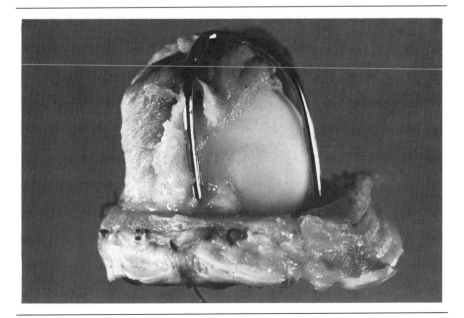

Figure 11. Starr-Edwards prosthesis with swollen poppet.

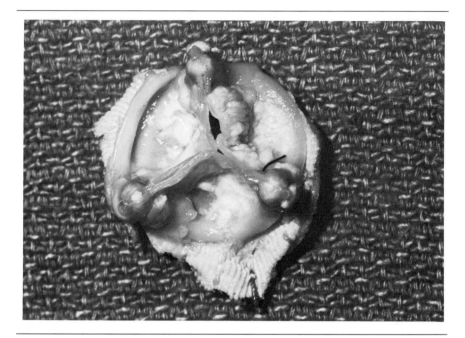

Figure 12. Ionescu-Shiley valve three years after implantation in the mitral position in a 67-year-old patient. Note the calcification and stenosis.

CONCLUSION

As is obvious from the foregoing discussion, an ideal valve prosthesis still eludes us. Tissue valves offer freedom from anticoagulation for most patients, a low incidence of thromboembolism, and acceptable hemodynamic function. However, durability and reliability remain problems. At our present 5-year follow-up on the IONESCU-SHILEY bovine pericardial valve, the valve appears to be performing satisfactorily with regard to thromboembolism, paravalvular leak, endocarditis and hemodynamics. Because of accelerated calcification rates, however, there is no question that use of this valve should be avoided in children and adults under 30 years of age and perhaps even under 50 years of age. It is, however, of great concern that the number of valves with leaflet disruption has increased and seems to be time-related, with a mean occurrence rate of 37 to 58 months and a late occurrence in the aortic position of 50 to 58 months. When leaflet disruption is added to calcification, even in older patients, an unacceptably high failure rate may occur on longer follow-up. Because of this, we presently reserve use of bioprosthetic valves for elderly patients with possible anticoagulation problems and patients with small anuli, where a bioprosthetic valve with good effective-orifice area and hemodynamics is essential.

We currently prefer to use the ST. JUDE MEDICAL valve in all patients under the age of 65 who have a good life expectancy and have no medical contraindica-

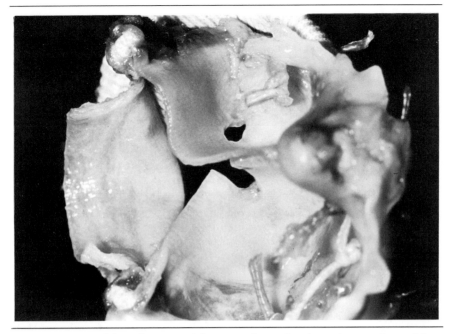

Figure 13. Ionescu-Shiley valve removed five years after aortic valve replacement in an adult shows leaflet disruption and a laceration in the cusp.

tions to long-term anticoagulation. The record reveals that the ST. JUDE MEDI-CAL valve represents a state-of-the-art level of excellence. When the results are analyzed for mechanical failure, valve thrombosis, thromboembolic complications and prosthetic infection, the record is indeed impressive. In our hands, it has given the lowest incidence of complications.

We must remember, however, that not all valvular diseases require valve replacement. Pure mitral stenosis is a lesion which can respond very well to mitral valvotomy for 10-year periods. Mitral valve replacement is seldom indicated in childhood mitral regurgitation. Moreover, valve surgery should probably be withheld until hemodynamic studies indicate a physiologic need for this procedure.

The knowledge learned through clinical experience with prosthetic valves during the past three decades should help us steer a more intelligent course in the future. Continued critical analyses of each valve in use today should produce a valve superior to those presently available.

REFERENCES

1. Hufnagel CA, Harvey WP: The surgical correction of aortic insufficiency. Bull Georgetown U Med Cent 1953; 6:60.
2. Harken DE, Soroff HS, Taylor WJ, et al: Partial and complete prostheses in aortic insufficiency. J Thorac Cardiovasc Surg 1960; 40:744–762.

3. Starr A, Edwards ML: Mitral replacement: Clinical experience with a ball-valve prosthesis. Ann Surg 1961; 154:726–740.
4. Williams JB: US Patent No 19323, February 9, 1858.
5. Starr A, Pierie WR, Raible DA, et al: Cardiac valve replacement: Experience with the durability of silicone rubber. Circulation 1966; 33 (Suppl 1):115–123.
6. Starr A, Grunkemeier GL, Lambert LE: Aortic valve replacement: A ten-year follow-up on noncloth-covered vs. cloth-covered caged-ball prostheses. Circulation 1977; 56(3) (Part II): Abstracts 133–139.
7. Lillehei CW, Kaster RL, Coleman M, et al: Heart-valve replacement with Lillehei-Kaster pivoting disk prosthesis. NY State Med J 1974; 74:1426–1438.
8. Lillehei CW: Heart valve replacement with the pivoting disc prosthesis: Appraisal of results and description of a new all-carbon model. J Assoc Advance Med Instr 1977; 11:85–94.
9. Nitter-Hauge S, Hall KV, Froysaker T, et al: Aortic valve replacement, one year results with Lillehei-Kaster and Björk-Shiley disc prostheses: A comparative clinical study. Am Heart J 1974; 88:23.
10. Björk VO: A new tilting disc valve prosthesis. Scand J Thorac Cardiovasc Surg 1969; 3:1–10.
11. Björk VO: The central-flow tilting disc valve prosthesis (Björk-Shiley) for mitral valve replacement. Scand J Thorac Cardiovoasc Surg 1970; 4:15–23.
12. Björk VO, Henze A: Ten years' experience with the Björk-Shiley tilting disc valve. J Thorac Cardiovasc Surg 1979; 78:331–342.
13. Aberg B, Henze A: Comparison between the in-vitro flow dynamics of the standard and the convexo-concave Bjork-Shiley tilting disc valve prosthesis. Scand J Thorac Cardiovasc Surg 1979; 13:177–189.
14. Ionescu MI, Pakrashi BC, Holden MP, et al: Results of aortic valve replacement with frame-supported fascia lata and pericardial grafts. J Thorac Cardiovasc Surg 1972; 64:340–353.
15. Ionescu MI, Tandon AP, Mary DAS, et al: Heart valve replacement with the Ionescu-Shiley pericardial xenograft. J Thorac Cardiovasc Surg 1977; 73:31–42.
16. Reis RL, Hancock WD, Yarbrough JW, et al: The flexible stent: A new concept in the fabrication of tissue valve prostheses. J Thorac Cardiovasc Surg 1971; 62:683–689.
17. Carpentier A, Dubost A: From xenograft to bioprosthesis: Evolution of concepts and techniques of valvular xenografts, in Ionescu MI, Ross DN, Wooler GH (eds): Biological Tissue in Heart Valve Replacement. London, Butterworths, 1971, pp 515–541.
18. Stinson EB, Griepp RB, Oyer PE, et al: Long-term experience with porcine aortic valve xenografts. J Thorac Cardiovasc Surg 1977; 73:54–63.
19. Oyer PE, Stinson EB, Reitz BA, et al: Long-term evaluation of the porcine xenograft bioprosthesis. J Thorac Cardiovasc Surg 1979; 78:343–350.
20. Kaiser GA, Hancock WD, Lukban SB, et al: Clinical use of a new design stented xenograft heart valve prosthesis. Surg Forum 1969; 20:137–138.
21. Lurie AJ, Miller RR, Maxwell K, et al: Postoperative hemodynamic assessment of the glutaraldehyde-preserved porcine heterograft in the aortic and mitral positions. Circulation 1976; 53–54 (Suppl II):II-148.
22. Ionescu MI, Tandon AP: The Ionescu-Shiley pericardial xenograft heart valve, in Ionescu MI (ed). Tissue Heart Valves. London, Butterworths, 1979, pp 201–252.
23. Ionescu MI, Tandon AP, Saunders NR, et al: Clinical durability of the pericardial xenograft valve: 11 years' experience, in Cohn LH, Gallucci V (eds). Cardiac Bioprostheses. New York, Yorke Medical Books, 1982, pp 42–60.
24. Ott DA, Coelho AT, Cooley DA, et al: Ionescu-Shiley pericardial xenograft valve: Hemodynamic evaluation and early clinical follow-up of 326 patients. Cardiovasc Dis, Bull Texas Heart Inst 1980; 7:137–148.
25. Reul GJ, Cooley DA, Duncan JM, et al: Valve failure with the Ionescu-Shiley bovine pericardial bioprosthesis: Analysis of 2,680 patients. J Vasc Surg 1985; 2:192–204.
26. Gabbay S, Bortolotti U, Wasserman F, et al: Fatigue-induced failure of the Ionescu-Shiley pericardial xenograft in the mitral position. J Thorac Cardiovasc Surg 1984; 87:836–844.
27. Duncan JM, Cooley DA, Livesay JJ, et al: The St. Jude Medical valve: Early clinical results in 253 patients. Texas Heart Institute Journal 1983; 10:11–16.
28. Emery RW, Nicoloff DM: St. Jude Medical cardiac valve prosthesis: In-vitro studies. J Thorac Cardiovasc Surg 1979; 78:269–276.

29. Nicoloff DM, Emery RW, Arom KV, et al: Clinical and hemodynamic results with the St. Jude Medical cardiac valve prosthesis. J Thorac Cardiovasc Surg 1981; 82:674–683.
30. Wortham DC, Tri TB, Bowen TE: Hemodynamic evaluation of the St. Jude Medical valve prosthesis in the small aortic annulus. J Thorac Cardiovasc Surg 1981; 81:615–620.
31. Duncan JM, Cooley DA, Reul GJ, et al: Experience with the St. Jude Medical valve and the Ionescu-Shiley bovine pericardial valve at the Texas Heart Institute in Matloff JM (ed). *Cardiac Valve Replacement: Current Status.* Boston, Martinus Nijhoff Publishers, 1985, pp 233–245.
32. Hylen JC, Hodam RP, Klester FE: Changes in the durability of silicone rubber in ball-valve prostheses. Ann Thorac Surg 1972; 13:324–329.
33. Leatherman LL, Leachman RD, McConn RG, et al: Malfunction of mitral ball-valve prostheses due to swollen poppet. J Thorac Cardiovasc Surg 1969; 57:160–163.
34. Olsen EGJ, Al-Janabi N, Salamao CS, et al: Fascia lata valves: A clinicopathological study. Thorax 1975; 30:528–534.
35. Highison GJ, Allen DJ, Didio LJA, et al: Ultrastructural morphology of dura mater aortic allografts after 44–73 months of implantation in humans. J Submicrosc Cytol 1980; 12:165–187.
36. Liotta D, Messmer BJ, Hallman GL, et al: Prosthetic and fascia lata valves: Hydrodynamics and clinical results. Trans Amer Soc Artif Intern Organs 1970; 16:244–251.
37. Wukasch DC, Sandiford FM, Reul GJ, et al: Complications of cloth-covered prosthetic valves: Results with a new mitral prosthesis. J Thorac Cardiovasc Surg 1975; 69:107–116.
38. Barnhart GT, Jones M, Ishihara T, et al: Degeneration and calcification of bioprosthetic cardiac valves. Am J Pathol 1982; 106:136–139.
39. Walker WE, Duncan JM, Frazier OH, et al: Early experience with the Ionescu-Shiley pericardial xenograft valve: Accelerated calcification in children. J Thorac Cardiovasc Surg 1983; 86: 570–575.
40. Broom ND: Fatigue-induced damage in glutaraldehyde-preserved heart valve tissue. J Thorac Cardiovasc Surg 1978; 76:202–211.
41. Ferrans VJ, Spray TL, Billingham ME, et al: Structural changes in glutaraldehyde-treated porcine heterografts used as substitute cardiac valves. Am J Cardiol 1978; 41:1159–1184.

I. COMPLICATIONS OF CARDIAC VALVE REPLACEMENTS AND THEIR TREATMENT

1. FOLLOWING THE PATIENT WITH PROSTHETIC HEART VALVES

SHAHBUDIN RAHIMTOOLA

When following a patient with a prosthetic valve, there are two important prophylactic measures the physician must keep in mind. First, prosthetic valve endocarditis is one of the most lethal complications of prosthetic valves. Hence, the antibiotic regimen recommended by the American Heart Association for prophylaxis against infective endocarditis is of vital importance. Second, even though the incidence of rheumatic carditis has decreased in the United States, after valve replacement the patient is not free of the risk of recurrent rheumatic carditis and antibiotic therapy for prophylaxis against this complication also is important.

Preoperatively the physician needs to know which valves are affected and the severity of each valve lesion, the status of left ventricular function, alterations in hemodynamics, the extent and severity of associated coronary artery disease, the status of the pulmonary vascular bed and right ventricular function.

During the operative period these elements must be documented: which valve was replaced and why; what valve substitute was implanted (model, size) and why; whether the patient has multivalvular disease and what was done to the other valves and why; whether coronary bypass was performed and if not, why; details of the procedures used for myocardial protection during surgery; and whether there was any perioperative myocardial infarction or damage.

Follow-up should occur in three stages: the first few weeks after valve replacement; the sixth week postoperative visit; and routine follow-up at 6 to 12 month intervals after surgery.

In the first few weeks the physician is concerned with heart failure, arrhythmias, cardiac tamponade, postcardiotomy syndrome and postperfusion syndrome. A patient with postcardiotomy syndrome may present in cardiac tamponade a few weeks after valve replacement. A single pericardial tap will frequently relieve that patient of the risk of death.

The sixth week postoperative visit should include an assessment of New York Heart Association (NYHA) Classification from the history, physical examination, electrocardiogram, chest x-ray, blood count, lactate dehydrogenase (LDH), electrolytes, etc. When deciding which tests to order, the physician must determine the questions to be answered and then select tests that will best answer those questions.

At 6 weeks, 6 months and the annual follow-up, the physician needs to assess the effects of valve replacement on the patient's NYHA class, left ventricular function, the reason for performing valve replacement, and the presence of complications.

COMPLICATIONS

Clearly the complications of prosthetic valve surgery include operative mortality; perioperative myocardial infarction; prosthetic endocarditis; prosthetic dehiscence; prosthetic dysfunction from structural failure, thrombosis or hemolysis; and prosthetic obstruction due to structural failure, thrombosis, prosthetic endocarditis, prosthetic dehiscence or thromboemboli. Other complications are prosthetic regurgitation, peripheral thromboembolism, hemorrhage with anticoagulation therapy, valve prosthesis/patient mismatch, the need for reoperative valve replacement and late mortality, including sudden death.

Recent data from the University of Alabama [1] demonstrate the most frequent incidence of prosthetic endocarditis is within the first 2 months or up to 6 months after valve replacement. However, even after that high-risk period, the risk of prosthetic endocarditis remains. Starr's data [2] out to 20 years of follow-up indicate no patient is ever free of the risk of prosthetic endocarditis. Data from the University of Alabama [3] show that surgical treatment of prosthetic endocarditis by reoperation results in a 50% reduction of mortality, even though with surgical treatment the operative mortality is high.

Early and aggressive therapy for heart failure is needed for patients who unfortunately develop prosthetic endocarditis. An outline of management for these patients would include immediate admission to an intensive cardiac care unit, hemodynamic monitoring, digitalis, diuretics, antibiotics and vasodilators. Our drug of choice in the early treatment of regurgitant lesions and heart failure is nitroprusside. If the patient has mild heart failure, the physician must quickly determine if it can be controlled or if the prosthesis should be replaced. If the patient has prosthetic endocarditis or valve regurgitation and the physician is unsure about heart failure, the pulmonary artery wedge pressure and cardiac output must be measured with use of a balloon floatation catheter.

Indications for prosthesis replacement are heart failure, infections uncontrolled by antibiotics, fungal endocarditis and staphylococcal infections of the aortic and/or mitral valve. Some staphylococcal infections, especially those affecting the tricuspid valve, can be controlled with medical therapy. In my experience, gram negative bacillary infections usually require prosthesis replacement.

THROMBOEMBOLISM

Edmunds' review of the literature [4] has shown that the incidence of thromboembolism in *aortic valve replacement* with either mechanical or bioprostheses is about 2% per patient-year. However, less than 10% of patients with bioprostheses need anticoagulant therapy. In *mitral valve replacement* the rate of thromboembolism is about 4% per patient-year for mechanical and bioprosthetic valves.

THROMBOSIS

Kirklan's data [5] show the actuarial incidence of sudden prosthetic thrombosis for the BJÖRK-SHILEY® valve in the aortic position to be 3% (2% to 5%) per patient-year at 4 years, and for the mitral position, 13% (5% to 27%) per patient-year. Eighty percent of these patients died.

BIOPROSTHETIC FAILURE

Data from Stanford University [6] show an incidence of failure with use of the HANCOCK® bioprosthesis at 5 years after surgery to be 0.2% per patient-year in adults and 9.8% per patient-year in children under 15 years of age. Actuarially determined freedom from failure at 5 years was 95.4% for adult aortic patients and 90.9% for adult mitrals at 6 years post-op. The critical period for primary tissue failure was after the fifth year when the freedom probability drops sharply by 4.4%.

Many patients with bioprostheses will have hemodynamic evidence of valve failure without other symptoms of valve dysfunction. Echocardiography, including Doppler echocardiography, was useful to us in detecting dysfunction in the IONESCU-SHILEY® valve. What we do not know is the sensitivity, specificity and predictive accuracy of these noninvasive techniques in detecting valve dysfunction. In my personal experience they have limited value in detecting dysfunction in mechanical prostheses but hold promise for detecting dysfunction in bioprostheses.

LATE MORTALITY

Starr's data [2] examining patients who had initial valve surgery in the 1960s and 1970s show the major cause of late mortality is cardiac in origin. Approximately 50% of deaths were due to heart failure. Prosthesis-related problems only account for 25% of late deaths.

If we are to reduce late mortality, we need to focus on left ventricular function and cardiac function. A patient may have had left ventricular dysfunction before surgery and either that left ventricular dysfunction did not improve or improved less than ideally after valve replacement. Another cause of late mortality may be perioperative myocardial damage. As illustrative cases, I will cite two examples.

A 20-year-old patient, 18 months after valve replacement demonstrated an increased heart size and went from Class II to Class III or IV. His calculated ejection fraction dropped from 69% preoperatively to 19% postoperatively. This was attributable to perioperative myocardial damage associated with gross Q wave development and ST segment changes immediately after surgery. He died unexpectedly, presumably of an arrhythmia.

Another patient in his 50s had mitral stenosis and mitral regurgitation with a left ventricular ejection fraction of 59%. He underwent mitral valve replacement 7 months later and remained in NYHA Class III. Postoperatively his calculated ejection fraction dropped considerably to 28%. With intensive medical therapy his functional Class moved to II within the next 3 years and his calculated ejection fraction improved to 37%. His heart size significantly improved and pulmonary venous congestion disappeared, due to diuretics. However, ventricular function was not normal. In such a situation, if we rely solely on x-ray for judging ventricular function, we run the risk of being misled, since with intensive medical therapy the lungs can appear clearer and the heart size smaller. Objective measurements of left ventricular function are critical to understanding what is happening in any patient who does not do well after valve replacement.

CARDIAC CATHETERIZATION

In the 1970s we studied the value of postoperative cardiac catherization [7] and found that if patients have clinical deterioration and are catheterized, the chances of finding a significant hemodynamic abnormality are higher than if they do not have clinical deterioration. In contrast, if a patient has a small embolus, the chance of finding an abnormality on a hemodynamic study is small. If patients are not doing well but are studied aggressively, the chances are good that some abnormality will be found that can, perhaps, be corrected if it is related to a valve substitute.

CONCLUSION

The recommendation for valvular heart surgery and replacement is made anticipating that the prognosis with surgery will be better than without surgery. In the majority of patients, improvement is achieved. However, on occasion an unsatisfactory result will occur. The causes of unsatisfactory results after valve replacement can be related to complications occurring during valve replacement, valve substitute dysfunction after surgery, another valve disease that was mild at operation and has worsened, associated coronary artery disease and other heart disease. Any and all of these can result in mortality after valvular surgery. With careful postoperative care these adverse outcomes can be anticipated and perhaps avoided.

REFERENCES

1. Ivert TSA, Dismukes WE, Cobbs CG, et al: Prosthesis valve endocarditis. Circulation 1984; 69:223–232.
2. Teply JF, Grunkemeier GL, Sutherland HD, et al: The ultimate prognosis after valve replacement: An assessment at twenty years. Ann Thorac Surg 1981;32(2):111–119.
3. Richardson JV, Karp RB, Kirklin JW, et al: Treatment of infective endocarditis: A 10-year comparative analysis. Circulation 1978;58:589.

4. Edmunds LH Jr: Thromboembolic complications of current cardiac valvular prostheses. Ann Thorac Surg 1982;34:96.
5. Karp RB, Cyrus RJ, Blackstone EH, et al: The Björk-Shiley valve: Intermediate term follow-up. J Thorac Cardiovasc Surg 1981;81:602–614.
6. Oyer PE, Miller DC, Stinson EB: Clinical durability of the Hancock porcine bioprosthetic valve. J Thorac Cardiovasc Surg 1980;80:824.
7. Morton MJ, McAnulty JH, Rahimtoola SH, et al: Risks and benefits of postoperative cardiac catherization in patients with ball-valve prosthesis. Am J Cardiol 1977;40:870–875.

2. THROMBOEMBOLISM AFTER CARDIAC VALVE REPLACEMENT

LAWRENCE H. COHN

The use of two entirely different types of cardiac valve substitutes centers primarily on the continuing debate on the risks of thromboembolism and anticoagulation morbidity associated with prosthetic valves and the long-term durability problems of bioprostheses. After the development of the STARR-EDWARDS® ball valve, which was hemodynamically quite sound, bioprosthetic valves were developed because these valves allegedly did not require anticoagulation, nor did they have a significant incidence of associated thromboembolism. This presentation will try to elucidate some of the mechanisms and causative factors of thromboembolism after valve replacement.

AORTIC VALVES
In figure 2-1 data by Tepley, et al, [1] summarize in actuarial form, the 20-year thromboembolism experience with the STARR-EDWARDS aortic ball valve. Data in the same paper show similar findings after mitral valve replacement. The probability of freedom from embolus in two different time periods, using the same valve by the same surgeons, is illustrated. In the implant years prior to 1973, the 5-year percentage of freedom from thromboembolism was $77 \pm 4\%$, while the percentage from 1973–81 was $89 \pm 3\%$, $p < .01$. In part, these data may reflect improvement in preoperative patient factors, so that operations in the later period were done on patients far less catastrophically ill than in the previous period. Figure 2-2 shows data from the same paper giving the event rates in terms of percent per patient-year of follow-up. Though the embolism rate falls, we note that the rate

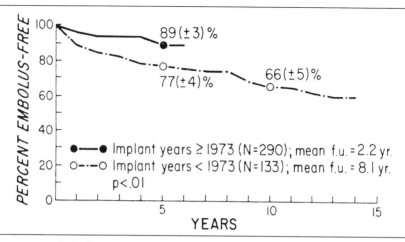

Figure 2-1. Embolus-free curve with the current silastic ball aortic valve according to time frame of implantation. (Reproduced with permission: Tepley et al: Ann Thorac Surg 1981; 32:116.)

Event	1960-72 (%/pt-yr)	1973-80 (%/pt-yr)	p value
Embolus	6.3	4.4	< 0.001
Prosthetic Thrombosis	0.7	0.7	NS
Hemorrhage	1.3	4.3	< 0.001
Ball Variance	0.9	...	< 0.001
Rereplacement	1.0	1.7	NS
Endocarditis	0.8	0.8	NS

[a]Aortic and mitral single caged-ball implants only.

NS = not statistically significant.

Figure 2-2. Differences in combined fatal and non-fatal events in two time eras. (Reproduced with permission: Tepley et al: Ann Thorac Surg 1981; 32:115.)

of hemorrhage associated with use of anticoagulation is increased. It is not possible to determine if this is a cause and effect relationship, but it tends to suggest that the decrease in the incidence of embolism is associated with an increase in anticoagulation morbidity.

Recently, we reviewed our personal experience over a 12-year period with aortic valve replacement using a bioprosthetic porcine valve or the BJÖRK-SHILEY® tilting disc valve [2]. In general, the low profile prosthetic valve has its best use in the small aortic root. The natural history of patients with aortic valve disease does not generally include chronic atrial fibrillation and associated thromboembolism. The primary postoperative rhythm of patients with aortic valve disease is normal sinus rhythm with minimal thromboembolic potential. So, prosthetic valve implantation in the aortic root has the potential of introducing a new natural history into a patient's life requiring anticoagulation and the possibility, however low it may be, of thromboembolism.

In our series we concurrently used the tilting disc valve in about one-third of our patients and bioprostheses in about two-thirds. The reasons patients received tilting disc valves were either anatomic, or, in the earlier years 1972–1975, based on the feeling that tilting disc valves had significantly better hemodynamics and might be more appropriately used in patients with compromised ventricular function. The data from our recent analysis of this large cohort of patients, numbering 912, indicated that the percent of embolism and thrombosis per patient year was about the same in both valve types (table 2-1). However, the probability of anticoagulant hemorrhage was much greater in patients with tilting disc valves who required long-term anticoagulation, than in the 10% of the patients with bioprostheses who required anticoagulation for chronic atrial fibrillation. The incidence of anticoagulant related hemorrhage and death was vastly different in the two groups. In addition to thromboembolism, there is the problem of total valve thrombosis. In the group of tilting disc valves, total valve thrombosis was 0.34% per patient-year [3]. This resulted from changing the patients' anticoagulant programs because of hemorrhagic complications. In two patients with bioprostheses, thrombosis occurred because of low cardiac output, one in the perioperative period and one 5 months postoperatively.

Selecting a valve substitute for a patient with aortic valve disease is based on clinical and anatomic criteria. In various clinical series around the world there is a wide variation in predilection for various valve types. The type of practice (private versus academic, congenital versus acquired) and age of patient group determine the type of valve that is implanted. In our clinic, predilection for a

Table 2-1. Incidence of thromboembolism after implantation of two types of aortic valve prostheses 1972 to 1982

	BPV	TDV
Emboli/Thrombosis	1.89 + 0.23*	2.02 + 0.42
Thrombosis	0.07 + 0.05	0.34 + 0.17
Anticoag Hemorrhage	0.15 + 0.07	1.82 + 0.40

BPV = bioprosthetic valve
TDV = tilting disc valve
* % per patient-year of follow-up + standard error of mean

bioprosthesis in two-thirds of the patients is determined primarily by the patient's age. In the 912 patients with aortic valve replacement the mean age was 61, and the median age was 63 years. Most patients in our clinic requiring aortic valve replacement are over 60 years of age. It is felt that older patients do much better without anticoagulation because they suffer from an increasing incidence of other medical and surgical conditions. With anticoagulation, all of these conditions can become more complicated to treat.

Even in the aortic area, chronic atrial fibrillation plays a role in thromboembolism, regardless of valve type. In patients with bioprostheses the incidence of emboli, though low, predominates in patients in chronic atrial fibrillation (figure 2-3). The difference is statistically significant.

MITRAL VALVES

Mitral valve replacement continues to be an enigma. Despite advances over the past 25 years, the incidence of thromboembolism following mitral valve replacement is still relatively high and considerably higher than that following aortic valve replacement. There are five factors that seem to have an effect on the incidence of thromboembolism: valve design, the presence or absence of anticoagulation, cardiac rhythm and atrial and patient factors.

Patient factors include the presence of chronic, low cardiac output, predisposing to stasis within the cardiac chambers and thromboembolism. For example, a patient who has a mitral valve replacement for severe long-standing mitral regurgitation

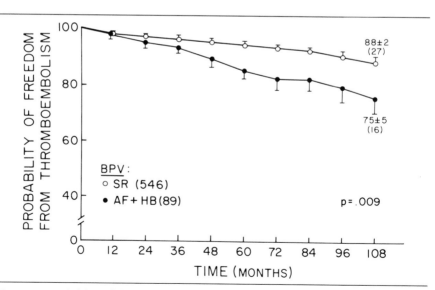

Figure 2-3. Probability of freedom from thromboembolism with bioprosthetic valves according to postoperative rhythm, atrial fibrillation and heart block versus sinus rhythm. (Reproduced with permission: Cohn et al: J Thorac Cardiovasc Surg, in press)

with a low cardiac output will have a tendency toward thromboemboli because of an enlarged heart, low cardiac output and enlarged left atrium.

Interestingly, there is not a great deal of recent data on the morbidity and mortality of patients undergoing long-term anticoagulation. The problem of morbidity following anticoagulation varies enormously. Anticoagulation in some areas is associated with a high morbidity due to lack of patient compliance, but in other areas, physicians and patients are meticulous about anticoagulation, and few problems occur. Still unknown is the actual level of anticoagulation at which a patient is protected from thromboembolism occuring in the presence of a prosthetic valve. We currently use a regimen of COUMADIN® for a patient with a ST. JUDE MEDICAL® or BJÖRK-SHILEY valve to bring the prothrombin time to approximately 18–20 seconds with a control value of about 12 seconds. This is considerably less than the 2 times control that is advocated with the STARR-EDWARDS ball valves. At this level the incidence of anticoagulant-related hemorrhage is low. What the ultimate long-term result will be in terms of prevention of thromboembolism is, as yet, unknown.

Table 2-2 shows data from major series of mitral valve replacements from centers with long-term follow up. [4] These include the STARR-EDWARDS, the BJÖRK-SHILEY, the ST. JUDE MEDICAL valve and the porcine and pericardial bioprostheses. As the hemodynamics of the various devices improve, the rate of freedom from embolism also improves. That is, with central flow, tilting-disc valves there is a lower thromboembolic incidence than with the STARR-EDWARDS valve, which has a more-or-less circumferential flow around the poppet. The pericardial valves have a lower incidence of thromboembolism than the porcine valves because of better overall hemodynamics.

Cardiac rhythm appears to be critical in determining thromboemboli in the mitral valve area because of the large numbers of patients with chronic atrial fibrillation. Atrial fibrillation *per se* is not as benign a rhythm as we once thought. In two large epidemiologic series, from the insurance industry [3] and the Framingham study [5], patients with chronic atrial fibrillation had a worse long-term survival rate than control patients who did not have atrial fibrillation.

Table 2-2. Incidence of thromboemboli after mitral valve replacement

Type of valve	% Per patient-year
Starr-Edwards	6.5
Björk-Shiley	4.0
St. Jude Medical	3.5
Porcine Valves	3.5
Ionescu-Shiley	1.5

From Edmunds LH: Ann Thorac Surg 1982; 34:96.

In the long-term study by Gajewski and Singer (figure 2-4), 3,500 patients with atrial fibrillation from many different conditions, including mitral stenosis, were evaluated against a standard expected curve of survival in patients who did not have atrial fibrillation. There were significant alterations in cumulative survival rate. Similarly, in the Framingham study (figure 2-5) on the long-term natural history of cardiovascular deaths, patients who had chronic atrial fibrillation had signifi-

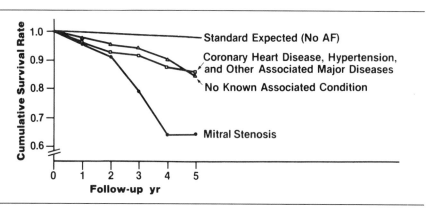

Figure 2-4. Cumulative survival rate of patient groups with atrial fibrillation compared to standard expected survival rate. (Reproduced with permission: Gajewski and Singer: JAMA 1981; 245:1543.)

MORTALITY	MEN			WOMEN		
	CASES	CONTROLS	RISK RATIO	CASES	CONTROLS	RISK RATIO
	per cent of group *			*per cent of group* *		
Total deaths	59.2 † (29)	34.3 (84)	1.7	44.9 † (22)	25.3 (62)	1.8
Deaths from cardiovascular causes	42.9 † (21)	21.2 (52)	2.0	40.8 † (20)	15.1 (37)	2.7
Average time to death	*5.9 yr* †	*7.7 yr*		*6.6 yr*	*6.7 yr*	

*Figures in parentheses denote number of subjects.

†Significant difference between values for cases and those for controls among all subjects 38 to 78 years old at death (P<0.05).

Figure 2-5. Comparison mortality rates in patients with and without chronic atrial fibrillation. (Reproduced with permission: Kannell el al: N Engl J Med 1982; 306:1021.)

cantly higher death rates from all causes and from cardiovascular deaths. Such an observation presents a challenge to cardiologists in that patients with other symptoms should be considered for cardiac surgical therapy before the onset of chronic atrial fibrillation, if possible. I think this will make an important, positive impact on long-term survival after cardiac surgery. Also, the earlier patients are referred for surgery, the higher the probability for mitral valve reconstruction rather than replacement.

In the Brigham experience with porcine valve replacement data on 459 patients, followed long-term, after mitral valve replacement, significant differences have been noted between patients in normal sinus rhythm and atrial fibrillation. The question is often asked: If a patient is in atrial fibrillation and has a successful valve reconstruction/replacement, what is the probability of return to sinus rhythm after surgery? If the patient has been in atrial fibrillation for less than one year prior to surgery, there is a reasonable probability of return to normal sinus rhythm [6].

Finally, if patients are in chronic atrial fibrillation and need a mitral valve replacement, they probably will require long-term anticoagulation regardless of the valve substitute chosen. Thus, if long-term anticoagulation is needed, a mechanical prosthetic valve should be considered in these patients. However, there are data which suggest that patients with a bioprosthesis who are in chronic arterial fibrillation do just as well in long-term freedom from thromboembolism on aspirin and PERSANTINE® as they do on COUMADIN [7]. Other intraoperative atrial factors, such as, the presence of intra-atrial clot, previous embolism or a large, dilated left atrium indicate the need for anticoagulation. The presence of one or more of these atrial factors place patients at a very high risk for embolism, regardless of the type of valve used, and anticoagulation must be prescribed.

Chronic atrial fibrillation may be less important when choosing a valve replacement for young women who are pregnant or in the childbearing age group. Management of pregnancy with anticoagulants is extremely difficult. Recent data from Salazar et al. [8] from Mexico City showed that neither aspirin and PERSANTINE nor subcutaneous heparin are effective in preventing thromboemboli or valve thrombosis in patients with prosthetic heart valves who are pregnant. COUMADIN, on the other hand, had a very high associated incidence of cerebral hemorrhage and abortion. However, patients with bioprostheses had virtually event-free pregnancies with normal deliveries, no abortions and no hemorrhage or emboli (table 2-3).

CONCLUSIONS

This brief review has touched on some of the factors responsible for thromboembolism after cardiac valve replacement. Aortic valves are considerably less prone to thromboembolic events, and because the vast majority of these patients are in normal sinus rhythm, bioprostheses are preferred, particularly in elderly patients. The causative factors of thromboembolism with mitral valves are considerably more complex, making valve selection difficult. Chronic atrial fibrillation is not a completely benign rhythm and leads to decreased long-term survival. A challenge

Table 2-3. Pregnancy, anticoagulation and prosthetic valves

Prosthetic valve groups	Valve thrombosis	Cerebral emboli	Hemorrhage	Abortion
Gp. I (68)—ASA/Pers.	4%	25%	1.5%	10%
Gp. II (128)—Coumadin	0	2.3%	7%	28%
Gp. III (12)—SubQ Heparin	0	8%	8%	0
Bioprosthetic Valve Group Gp. IV (15)—Zero	0	0	0	0

From Salazar, et al: Circulation 1983; 68 (III):III-318.

to surgeons and cardiologists is to refer patients for mitral valve surgery before the onset of chronic atrial fibrillation, which in turn may lead to more reconstructive rather than replacement operations.

REFERENCES

1. Tepley JF, Grunkemeier GL, Sutherland HD, et al: The ultimate prognosis after valve replacement: An assessment at twenty years. Ann Thorac Surg 1981; 32:111–119.
2. Cohn LH, Allred EN, DiSesa VJ, et al: Early and late risk of aortic valve replacement: A 12-year concomitant comparison of the porcine bioprosthetic and tilting disc prosthetic aortic valves. J. Thorac Cardiovasc Surg (in press).
3. Gajewski J, Singer RB: Mortality in an insured population with atrial fibrillation. JAMA 1981; 245:1540–1544.
4. Edmunds LH: Thromboembolic complications of current cardiac valvular prostheses. Ann Thorac Surg 1982; 34:96–106.
5. Kannel WB, Abbott RD, Savage DD, et al: Epidemiologic features of chronic atrial fibrillation. N Engl J Med 1982; 306:1018–1021.
6. Betriu A, Chaitman BR, Almazan A, et al: Preoperative determinants of return to sinus rhythm after valve replacement, in Cohn LH, Gallucci V (eds), Cardiac Bioprostheses, New York, Yorke Medical Books, 1982, pp 184–191.
7. Nunez L, Gil Aguada M, Celemin D, et al: Aspirin or Coumadin as the drug of choice for valve replacement with porcine bioprosthesis. Ann Thorac Surg 1982; 33:354–358.
8. Salazar E, Zajarias A, Gutierrez N, et al: The problem of cardiac valve prostheses, anticoagulants and pregnancy. Circulation 1983; 68 (III): III-318.

3. NONPROSTHETIC FACTORS PRODUCING THROMBOEMBOLISM IN PATIENTS WITH CARDIAC VALVE SUBSTITUTES: THEIR NATURE AND THE PROBLEMS OF ASSESSING THEIR ROLE

R. LEIGHTON FISK

Frequently the patient presents after a clinically obvious systemic embolic episode. . . . Studies in this situation usually show no evidence of thrombus on the prosthesis or abnormal function
—F. E. KLOSTER, M.D. [1]

A large number of factors contribute to thromboembolism in patients with cardiac valvular disease including: underlying primary disease, the prosthesis mechanism and function, the operation itself and alterations during the follow-up period [2]. This chapter concerns the factors that contribute to thromboembolism in patients with cardiac valvular disease regardless of which prosthesis is used.

PRIMARY DISEASE
Primary factors related to the underlying disease which contribute to endocardial thrombus formation are shown in the summary in figure 3-1. Rheumatic carditis can result in severe endocardial fibrosis and calcification that produce foci for superimposed thrombus formation. Clearly, areas within the heart where thrombus has been debrided leave roughened and disturbed endothelium which act as foci for postoperative thrombus formation. These areas include those around the pulmonary vein entry sites to the left atrium, chamber surface of the atrial appendage, free wall surfaces and, of course, the paravalvular anulus.

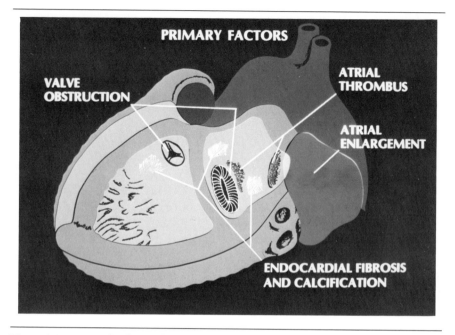

Figure 3-1. Factors related to underlying pathology and pathophysiologic phenomena that contribute to endocardial thrombus formation.

THE PROSTHESIS

Chronic stasis and flow disturbance created by valvular malfunction may lead to chamber enlargement, a well-recognized contributor to thrombus formation. This propensity is aggravated by coexistent supraventricular dysrhythmias of the fibrillation or flutter variety. The combination of enlarged atrium, dysrhythmia and less than adequate valve function produce marked stasis or *back waters* where the possibility of thrombus formation is increased.

SURGICAL DISTURBANCES

The clinician intuitively attributes thromboembolism after surgical replacement to the prosthesis, forgetting that the maneuvers and manipulations required for the valve implantation also contribute to thrombus formation. Some of these factors are shown in figure 3-2. Raw surfaces are left following debridement of thrombus, calcium and destroyed valve tissue.

Considerable injury to endocardium results from retraction and compression on the heart that occurs while exposing valves for these procedures. Other raw surfaces are left, such as on a divided papillary muscle, which can develop superimposed thrombus. Also, endocardial injury can be caused by jet flow, injury from catheters, or by underlying tissue ischemia resulting from these procedures.

Surgical interruption of the endocardium can result in irregular, roughened and

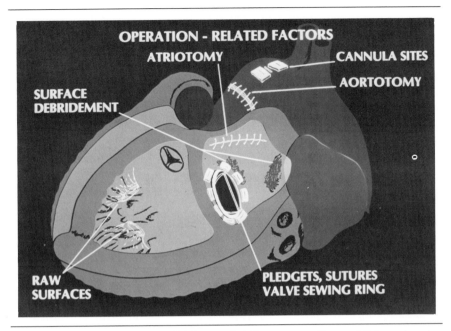

Figure 3-2. Surgical disturbances in left heart endothelium can contribute to left heart thrombus formation.

ridged tissue. These include the suture lines in the aorta from aortic valve replacement, the atriotomy from mitral valve replacement, and catheter sites in the ascending aorta which are also possible foci for thrombus formation. The anulus of the excised valve represents an irregular surface susceptible to thrombus formation. This focus can be further aggravated by inadequate debridement, by instability of the underlying abnormal tissue and by the passage of many sutures through the valve anulus.

Foreign material introduced at operation, other than the valve mechanism, is undoubtedly a contributor to thrombus formation. This includes pledgets, sutures and valve sewing ring material. Therefore, a number of factors, totally independent of the nature of the valve design, can contribute to the postoperative thromboembolism.

There are many obstacles to the objective assessment of the relative roles of the foregoing factors in the broad field of valve surgery. First, there is considerable variation in practice, experience and technique from center to center and even surgeon to surgeon within each center. Patient profiles vary with geographic locale and many contrasting subgroups of patients are treated. Even after successful operation, some valve patients have disturbances in hydration, metabolism and coagulation mechanisms that can contribute to a relative hypercoagulation state.

Surgical techniques vary widely. For example, whether or not the diseased posterior leaflet of the mitral valve is left or excised could well result in a variation between two series of patients with different mitral prostheses.

FOLLOW-UP

Variability of follow-up is a recognized problem. First, the protocols for the management of anticoagulants is tremendously variable. Although this is a recognized phenomenon, greater attention must be directed to this factor when comparing results of contrasting valve patient series. Second, the number of patients who are lost to follow-up differs among various series. How many of these patients died of thromboemboli and how many of them from other factors? Third, most centers tend to study valve patients consecutively rather than concurrently. As techniques improve, the most recent experience of a given research group would favor the valve currently in use.

Events that suggest valve-related thromboembolism may be totally unrelated to the central flow mechanism of the valve prosthesis and thereby be falsely represented as postoperative events.

For example, calcium embolization usually occurs in the perioperative period but it can occur as the disease progresses and prosthesis and anulus wear occur. Granulated tissue can embolize in patients who have a focal infectious process in the region of the valve sewing ring. This certainly does not seem to be a phenomenon more likely to occur in one valve type than another. Also, suture and pledget material can embolize on rare occasions.

It is important to document the cause of death in patients who experience primary cerebrovascular thrombosis and hemorrhage which can take place in anticoagulated patients. We recently lost a patient who developed a stroke as a result of hemorrhage into a previously undiagnosed cerebral tumor. Without an autopsy this event may have been attributed erroneously to a thromboembolism from the prosthesis.

Also, the cardiac valve patient is particularly susceptible to cardiac syncope from postural hypotension or cardiac dysrhythmia. And toxic neurologic syndrome that is temporary, might be mistaken for transient ischemic attack or recurrent cerebral embolism.

Sudden, unexpected death can be caused by cerebral or coronary thromboembolism or thrombosis of a prosthesis, certainly, but it might well be caused by a number of other factors that are more likely to occur in valve patients than in the general population. Myocardial infarction, cardiac dysrhythmia, massive pulmonary embolism and bleeding with cardiac tamponade have all occurred among patients in most large series. Again, cerebral thrombosis, hemorrhage and embolism are an ever-present threat and may be totally unrelated to the flow mechanism at the valve replacement site. Severe cerebral hemorrhage or gastrointestinal hemorrhage can be fatal and, of course, trauma can claim patients. Failure to accurately document the cause of the sudden, unexpected death from any of these events might result in erroneously attributing the death to a thrombotic event, thus adversely affecting the appraisal of the valve under study.

OTHER FACTORS

Bias alone can be introduced into patient assessment by a number of factors that influence our interpretation of results. Concurrent study is obviously helpful in minimizing these factors. We all desire to demonstrate that our currently preferred valve is superior to that previously abandoned. In the future, cost will be an increasingly important consideration, but it introduces the possibility of bias into our consideration of merit. There is a tendency to prefer new valves as they become available, since they are designed to eliminate problems. One of our greatest challenges is to retain objectivity and propriety when giving reasons why a therapy or device might be superior.

Aesthetics plays a role in determining preference. I believe heterograft prostheses have created a considerable interest because of their structural sophistication and biological components. The very compliant, yet bulky, sewing ring of the porcine xenograft prosthesis is a fine handling feature but introduces an unnecessary amount of foreign material into the circulation.

Certain valves are chosen for the small aortic anulus, the mitral position or the tricuspid position for subjective reasons, occasionally based on anecdotal accounts. The preferred location for various valves creates major difficulty in assessing the thromboembolic propensity of the various devices.

Error created by poor study design can be illustrated by citing an example. At one center that I am aware of, most of the very uncomplicated mitral valve patients were referred to one surgeon who used one valve for many years. Most of the reoperations, complex and very ill patients, and multiple valve patients were referred to other surgeons who used a variety of other prostheses, including new introductions to the marketplace. An internal review of the experience at that center, relating all postoperative events to the valve type alone, showed better early and late results in patients with the valve mechanism used by the one surgeon for uncomplicated patients. That report was inaccurate by omission of context and by suggesting the superiority of a valve that was used in a select, low-risk patient group.

TOPICS FOR STUDY

It must be accepted that factors other than the valve mechanism can strongly influence the incidence of postoperative thromboembolism. Ways in which we might assess some of these factors are available, but very challenging.

Nonprosthetic factors indirectly influencing the incidence of thromboembolism might be defined by examining certain subsets of the population rather than the valve prosthesis used. Thromboembolism occurring in the general population should be studied further. Patients with valve disease treated medically and those following valvotomy should also be evaluated in greater depth. For example, valvotomy relieves the hemodynamic compromise in patients with mitral valve disease without imposing the variables associated with a prosthesis or factors related to the operation.

Delayed thromboembolism has been observed in coronary bypass patients with left heart and aorta cannula sites which would suggest that thromboembolism may originate at the same sites in valve patients. Patients with ventricular aneurysm have a myocardial incision and thus, raw surface areas which are somewhat analogous to those of the mitral valve patient following papillary muscle division. Repair of atrial septal defect introduces suture lines in the right and left atria similar to those used for mitral valve replacement. Thromboembolism following adult atrial septal defect repair has certainly been observed and should be considered.

MINIMIZING THROMBOEMBOLISM

How can we minimize thromboembolism from nonprosthetic factors in our ongoing practice of valve surgery? We can attempt to reduce the amount of suture material and fabric within the heart by minimizing suture knots, tail lengths on sutures and the use of pledgets.

It would seem worthwhile to optimize the degree of debridement when removing offending material, while limiting the amount of raw surface conducive to thrombus formation. Excessively large prostheses with very large sewing rings introduce unnecessarily large amounts of foreign material into the circulation. Optimizing patient support through proper hydration and better control of anticoagulation should serve to further reduce morbidity and mortality from thromboembolism.

The gap is narrowing in the incidence of thromboembolism seen among groups of patients having various prostheses. In a 1981 collective review [3], Dr. Henry Edmunds summarized that in patients who had biological valves without COUMADIN® and patients who had mechanical valves with COUMADIN, there was a 2% per patient-year incidence of thromboembolism after aortic valve replacement. The incidence increased to 4% per patient-year for biological mitral valve recipients with or without COUMADIN and for mechanical valves on COUMADIN. It was also noted that the mortality of COUMADIN is 0.2% per patient-year and the morbidity incidence is 2.2% per patient year [3].

CONCLUSION

The close proximity of these statistics further suggests that a number of factors might be collectively responsible for the decreasing number of thromboembolic events observed as time passes. When accurate follow-up information is available in the future, it may become apparent that the flow control mechanism of various cardiac valve prostheses has less causal relationship to thromboembolism in valve recipients than previously supposed.

In summary, many *nonprosthetic* factors can contribute to thromboembolism in cardiac valve recipients. Further study of the incidence of systemic thromboembolism in various groups of patients who do not have valve prostheses may indirectly provide insight into the contribution these nonprosthetic factors make to thromboembolism. The components of the flow control mechanisms of prosthetic valves have probably been overemphasized with respect to their role in producing thromboembolism in cardiac valve recipients.

REFERENCES

1. Kloster, FE: Diagnosis and management of complications of prosthetic heart valves. Am J Cardiol 1975; 35:872.
2. Roberts WC, Fishbein MD, Golden A: Cardiac pathology after valve replacement by disc prosthesis. Am J Cardiol, 1975; 35:740.
3. Edmunds LH: Thromboembolism complications of current cardiac valve prostheses. Ann Thorac Surg, 1981; 34:96.

4. ANTICOAGULANT THERAPY AND CARDIAC VALVULAR SURGERY: COUMADIN® AND OTHER ALTERNATIVES

SHAHBUDIN RAHIMTOOLA

The thesis of this chapter is that anticoagulation therapy that is inadequate, inappropriate or discontinued contributes to thromboembolism. It must be remembered that thromboembolism is frequently related to the patient's disease or its effects.

RATES OF FATAL THROMBOEMBOLISM

A study from the Montreal Heart Institute [1] shows there is a significant difference in mortality among patients with mechanical valves who are anticoagulated and those who are not. The data clearly show that at the end of 3 years, 42% of patients not treated with anticoagulants either died or had thromboemboli.

Similar data from England [2] show that patients with BJÖRK-SHILEY® valves who were treated with warfarin sodium had an incidence of fatal and nonfatal thromboembolism of 7%. Those treated only with dipyridamole had an incidence three times higher, at 22%.

RATES ACCORDING TO THERAPY

Björk's 1975 data [3] show a 0.3% per patient-year incidence of thromboembolism for patients on COUMADIN® with BJÖRK-SHILEY valves. Patients given no anticoagulation therapy had a rate of 22% per patient-year as did patients treated with dipyridamole and aspirin. Patients given dicumarol after 6 months had an incidence of 10%. If dicumarol is discontinued and then readministered, the incidence is 5.5% per patient-year. These data show that for patients without

COUMADIN, or with aspirin and dipyridamole, or with dipyridamole alone, the thromboembolism rates will be unacceptable.

Other data from the Montreal Heart Institute [4] show the incidence of thromboemboli when patients are well-controlled on anticoagulant therapy is 3% and when they are not well-controlled the incidence is 19%. Similar data from the Mayo Clinic [5] show the incidence is much higher for patients with mitral prostheses who are inadequately controlled than with those who are adequately controlled. The difference between patients with aortic prostheses in this study was not statistically significant.

ADDITIONAL ANTICOAGULANTS

In an important study performed at the Brigham and Women's Hospital in 1971 [6], patients with mechanical prostheses were split into groups and given warfarin sodium, warfarin sodium with dipyridamole or warfarin sodium with a placebo. Success was defined as a patient alive, with no emboli and still on the drugs given; the results were 64% success in the group given warfarin sodium plus a placebo and 70% in the group given sodium warfarin and dipyridamole. The incidence of thromboemboli in those treated with warfarin sodium alone was roughly 10 times higher than those treated with warfarin sodium and dipyridamole. A similar study performed at the Mayo Clinic 10 years later [7] showed essentially the same data and no difference in the incidence of bleeding. These studies show that warfarin sodium plus dipyridamole appears, in certain patients, to reduce the incidence of thromboembolism with mechanical valves. There was a significant increase in bleeding when aspirin was used, suggesting that patients with mechanical valves should not be treated with aspirin and warfarin sodium.

Steele, et al. [8] in 1979 showed there is a select group of patients who have reduced platelet survival who would particularly benefit by an addition of an antiplatelet agent to their COUMADIN therapy.

HEMORRHAGE

Major bleeding is the price patients must pay for anticoagulant therapy. Starr [9] quotes the incidence of fatal bleeding at 1.3% per patient-year for 1960–1972 and 4.3% per patient-year for 1973–1980.

SUGGESTED REGIMEN

The anticoagulation regimen I use for all patients with mechanical valves is COUMADIN. I consider dipyridamole (and/or aspirin and/or sulfinpyrazone) if thromboemboli occur in spite of COUMADIN therapy. The first choice for an additional drug is dipyridamole since aspirin may cause a much higher bleeding rate.

Anticoagulation therapy should be given to all patients with bioprostheses until the second to sixth postoperative months. We give it long-term to patients who have atrial fibrillation, who have had a thromboembolic episode or who have a large left atrium, particularly when a thrombus is present.

CONCLUSION

When a patient must be withdrawn from anticoagulant therapy, we must remember that it is the patient who is taking the risk. Nearly every study indicates that 80% or more patients who have thromboemboli will have it in the cerebral circulation, so the risk must be recognized.

REFERENCES

1. Limet L, Lepage E, Grondin CM: Thromboembolic complications with the cloth-covered Starr-Edwards aortic prosthesis in patients not receiving anticoagulants. Ann Thorac Surg 1977;23:529.
2. St. John Sutton MG, Miller GAH, Oldershaw PJ, et al: Anticoagulants and the Bjork-Shiley prosthesis: Experience of 390 patients. Br Heart J 1978;40:558.
3. Björk VO, Henze A: Management of thromboembolism after aortic valve replacement with the Björk-Shiley tilting disc valve. Scand J Thorac Cardiovasc Surg 1975;9:183–191.
4. Friedli B, Aevichide N, Grondin P, Campeau L: Thromboembolic complications of heart valve prostheses. Am Heart J 1981;81:702.
5. Barnhorst DA, Oxman HA, Connolly DC, et al: Long-term follow-up of isolated replacement of the aortic or mitral valve with the Starr-Edwards prosthesis. Amer J Cardiol 1975; 35:228–233.
6. Sullivan JM, Harken DE, Gorlin R: Pharmacological control of thromboembolic complications of cardiac valve replacement. N Engl J Med 1971;284:1391.
7. Chesebro JH, Fuster V, Elveback LR, et al: Trial of combined warfarin plus dipyridamole or aspirin therapy in prosthetic heart valve replacement: Danger of aspirin compared with dipyridamole. Am J Cardiol 1983;51:1537.
8. Steele P, Rainwater J, Vogel R: Platelet suppressant therapy in patients with prosthetic cardiac valves. Circulation 1979;60:910.
9. Teply JF, Grunkemeier GL, Sutherland HD, et al: The ultimate prognosis after vavle replacement: An assessment at twenty years. Ann Thorac Surg 1981;32(2):111–119.

5. REOPERATION AFTER CARDIAC VALVE SURGERY: ELECTIVE, URGENT AND EMERGENT

JAMES R. PLUTH

During the 1970s there was a trend toward the use of tissue or heterograft valves in order to avoid the high rate of thromboembolism and anticoagulant related complications associated with mechanical prostheses. Use of bioprostheses appears to have reduced thromboembolic complications, but unfortunately, bioprosthesis must still be considered a temporary valve substitute. Due to its limited durability, one must consider the risks of future reoperation for valve replacement when weighing the potential benefits of a bioprosthesis. This chapter assesses the risks of valve reoperation and its effect on subsequent longevity.

PATIENT POPULATION

The records of all patients undergoing valve reoperation at the Mayo Clinic between January 1961 and December 1980 were reviewed. There were 551 patients with 617 valve reoperations. Patients with congenital heart defects and valve conduits were excluded. Previous commissurotomies, previous valvotomies and coronary revascularization procedures were not considered first operations. Only patients who had a second operation for a previously replaced valve were included.

Patients were grouped by indication for the first valve reoperation: 117 (22%) Braunwald–Cutter replacement; 37 infectious endocarditis; 13 repeated episodes of thromboembolism; 197 thrombosed disc valves or catastrophic tears of the heterograft valves; 151 paravalvular regurgitations; and 15 miscellaneous.

Patients were also divided by degree of urgency of reoperation. *Elective* procedures were those that could be scheduled. *Urgent* operations could be scheduled

29

in the next available operative slot, usually within 24 to 48 hours. *Emergent* operations were performed within a few hours of evaluation. The majority of aortic replacements were elective, undoubtedly reflecting experience with the BRAUNWALD-CUTTER series. In mitral patients, the majority of reoperations were urgent or emergent.

Cases were subdivided by preoperative New York Heart Association Classification (NYHA) at reoperation. Of the 392 aortic valve patients, 50% were Class I and II. The opposite was true of the mitral valve patients in which 80% were Class III and IV.

RISK OF MORTALITY

The influence on early mortality of age, sex, year of operation, NYHA Class, urgency of operation, indications for surgery and concomitant surgical procedures was evaluated. In the aortic position only urgency of operation and concomitant revascularization significantly affected mortality. With mitral valve replacement significant variables were NYHA Classification, urgency of operation and year of surgery.

In the first 7 years of this study the risk of reoperation was 15%. In the second 7 years the risk dropped to 7%. In the most current 7-year period (1979 to 1983), the risk was 5.7%. For those patients who had second reoperations, the risk was 14%, while for those with a third operation, the risk was 7%. There was no mortality in the 4 patients having their fourth reoperation. For elective reoperation in the aortic position the risk was less than 1.5%, for urgent reoperation the risk was 8% and for emergent conditions the risk was 37%. In the mitral valve series, only 22 patients had elective procedures and there was no mortality. In contrast, the mortality for emergent replacement of mitral valves was 54%.

Risk of mortality for aortic patients in NYHA Classes I and II was 2% and for Class IV it was 20%. Similarly, in the mitral position, the risk was 4% for Class II patients and 41% for Class IV patients.

We found no statistical difference between valve models when we correlated type of valve with mortality. Differences were related to the percentage of Class IV patients with certain valve designs. Patients requiring emergent reoperations (30%) and the number of patients with heterografts or disc valves was similar. Regurgitation was the leading reason for early tissue valve failure.

The highest risk of mortality during reoperation was for patients with infectious endocarditis (24.3%). This difference was not statistically significant from other indications for reoperation since the mortality appeared to be related to the high percentage of Class IV patients with infectious endocarditis.

In this series, concomitant procedures (most being coronary revascularization) appeared to have a significant influence on mortality. Risk of mortality was 11.5% when revascularization was performed before or at initial valve implant with reoperation following. Risk remained about the same (14%) if coronary revascularization occurred between the first surgery and the second surgery. However, risk increased to 21% if coronary revascularization was performed at valve replacement reoperation.

In the mitral position, concomitant revascularization did not reach statistical significance when compared with mortality. However, aortic valve reoperation carried a 5% risk factor. As a result, we recommend caution when choosing to perform revascularization at the time of reoperation of aortic valves.

COMPLICATIONS

Postoperative complications following reoperation were similar to those of the first operation. Postoperative bleeding in the first 24 hours after reoperation was 793 ml versus 754 ml at the initial operation. Reoperation for excessive postoperative bleeding was 3% after reoperation versus 4% after the initial procedure. Tamponade developed in 2% of the patients and prosthetic valve endocarditis occurred in 1%. Paravalvular regurgitation and the need for intra-aortic balloon assist occurred in less than 1% of patients. Low cardiac output following surgery occurred in 4% of aortic valve patients and in 10% of mitral valve patients.

SURVIVAL

Actuarial survival at 5 years following reoperation was 73% and at 7 years 70%. These figures are somewhat lower than what we anticipate following initial valve replacement. A similar group of patients undergoing first valve operations who were followed from 1973 to 1978 had an actuarial survival of 84%.

Although reoperation may have a negative effect on survival, the lower survival rates appear to be related to preoperative NYHA Classification. For Class I and Class II mitral patients, survival at 7 years following reoperation was 94% and for aortic patients of the same Classes the survival was 80%. Survival following reoperation for patients in Classes I and II actually matched or exceeded that of initial valve replacement. Only in Classes III and IV did patient survival differ markedly from that achieved after initial operation.

NYHA CLASSIFICATION IMPROVEMENT

Improvement in NYHA Classification occurred in virtually all categories of patients. Over 90% of Class III and Class IV patients improved by at least one or two Classes postoperatively.

CONCLUSION

On the basis of this study we conclude that the risks of elective reoperation for Class I or Class II patients is no higher than for initial valve replacement. Since the mortality of reoperation appears to be relatively low, qualified support for the use of valves of limited durability seems appropriate. However, reoperation should be elective and done only when the patient is in Class I or Class II.

I do not wish to minimize the risks of reoperation, but within this review, Class I and Class II patients could have a reoperative mortality of less than 1.5%. We must, therefore, look at the alternatives when selecting a mechanical prosthesis.

Generally, most mechanical prostheses in the mitral position have an incidence of thromboembolism of 4.5% to 6.5% per patient-year. One must then add the risk of thrombosis at 0.7% per patient-year. In this series the risk of anticoagulant related complications, including death or hemorrhage severe enough to require hospitalization and transfusions, is 3.5% per patient-year. Thus, it is conceivable that after 10 years there would be an 80% to 90% chance of either valve thrombosis, thromboembolism or a major anticoagulant related complication. Although the majority of thromboemboli are probably not recognized, 90% of those that are affect the cerebral circulation. Likewise, a high percent of anticoagulant related complications are cerebral.

When one compares the risk of strokes with the relatively small mortality associated with reoperation in an elective situation, I would choose reoperation rather than incapacitation by thromboembolism or anticoagulant-related hemorrhage.

PART I. DISCUSSION

LAWRENCE H. COHN, MODERATOR

ANTICOAGULATION

LORENZO GONZALEZ-LAVIN: Dr. Cohn, I am the first to strongly endorse your belief of operating on patients with mitral valve disease before they establish thromboembolic risk factors. I think once patients establish these factors, the outlook is much worse.

I would like to share with you some of our findings in assessing the incidence of thromboembolism and hemorrhagic complications in patients on anticoagulant therapy in a series of 206 porcine valves implanted in the mitral position. Patients were divided into two groups. Group I was patients with a high number of thromboembolic risk factors. Group II patients had fewer thromboembolic risk factors.

Oral anticoagulation, which was used in both groups was not effective in preventing thromboembolsm in the patients in Group I. Patients having TE were considered well anticoagulated in 18 of 21 incidents. Anticoagulant related hemorrhage occurred in both groups. In Group II hemorrhagic events outnumbered the thromboembolic events.

Based on this experience, we suggest that patients, requiring mitral valve replacement with a bioprosthesis, who are without thromboembolic risk factors and in regular sinus rhythm, should not be anticoagulated. They should be placed on antiplatelet drugs. In high risk patients (Group I) perhaps some combination of heparin and warfarin sodium therapy is indicated.

LAWRENCE H. COHN: I want to direct a question to our presenters. We have alluded to this question, but I believe it is deserving of further discussion. We assume that everyone who has a prosthetic valve requires anticoagulation. I want to know from each of you, if I could, when you have a patient with a prosthetic mitral valve, what is the desirable level of prothrombin time to be achieved when compared to a control value of 12 seconds?

SHABUDIN RAHIMTOOLA: Let me refer to a control of 10 seconds. We would try to achieve a prothrombin time between 16 and 19 seconds. In other words, 1.6 to 1.9 times control. The reason for this is that once you go above 2 times control, the incidence of bleeding is greatly increased and there are virtually no data to show that the incidence of thrombo-embolism is reduced by going above 2 times control. By focusing the prothombin time between 1.6 and 1.9, you allow for occasional lapses when the prothrombin will go to 2 times control.

R. LEIGHTON FISK: Our preference is exactly the same as Dr. Rahimtoola's.

JAMES PLUTH: We use 1.5 to 2 times the control and tend towards 1.5 when we combine dipyridamole with COUMADIN® therapy.

LAWRENCE H. COHN: How often do you combine COUMADIN and dipyridamole therapy?

JAMES PLUTH: 100% now.

LAWRENCE H. COHN: Thus, every patient with a prosthetic valve, say a ST. JUDE MEDICAL® valve, is placed on COUMADIN and dipyridamole.

Can I have a show of hands in the audience as to how many use the ST. JUDE MEDICAL valve? A high percentage, apparently. How many use anticoagulation at the 1.5 to 1.8 times control level for long-term anticoagulation? How many use a minimum of 2 times the control value of the prothrombin time? While more appear to favor the 1.5 to 1.8 level, there are still a fair number that prefer 2 times the control value.

How many use dipyridamole in conjunction with warfarin derivatives? Only 6 positive responses. Dr. Rahimtoola would you like to comment on that? You raised the question, "Should we be using dipyridamole with COUMADIN in every patient?"

SHABUDIN RAHIMTOOLA: I am not convinced one needs to use dypridamole with COUMA-DIN in the aortic position in all patients. However, the incidence of thromboembolism is much higher in the mitral position. If we can get an additional study which compliments the Mayo Clinic data, I believe we would then be in a situation for determining whether dipyridamole should be combined with COUMADIN. What dose of dipyridamole is being used?

JAMES PLUTH: We are using 75 mg, three times a day.

II. CARDIAC VALVE SUBSTITUTES: CURRENT STATUS

6. CLINICAL EXPERIENCE WITH THE CAGED-BALL STARR-EDWARDS® PROSTHESIS

JAMES R. PLUTH

The STARR-EDWARDS® valve is associated with the birth of prosthetic valve surgery. Although it was not the first successful valve to be implanted in the anatomical position, it was the first prosthetic valve to gain universal acceptance.

The original design had inherent problems, such as high rates of thromboembolism and swelling of the SILASTIC® poppet, which were noted a few years after implantation. By the fall of 1965, engineering changes and changes in the cure of the SILASTIC poppet produced the valve design that remains with us to this date. With over 23 years of experience with the caged-ball concept and with 19 years of experience with the current model, the STARR-EDWARDS valve remains the standard of durability among valvular prostheses.

Harken [1] established a set of criteria in the mid-1960s for valve comparison. This list is now partially outdated because all prosthetic valves are easily available, have similar ease of insertion and have reliable function. However, longevity, durability, thromboembolics rate and hemodynamic function remain a basis for valve comparison.

DURABILITY

The durability of the STARR-EDWARDS is without parallel. Following 19 years of implantation, valve failures are virtually unknown. The poppet on explantation may be more opaque or slightly discolored, but valve function is unimpaired. Numerous other valve models have been introduced and heralded as durable only to be no longer available. It is important to note that in the test of a valve's durability, *in vitro* data often do not correlate with *in vivo* performance.

SURVIVAL

Generally, poor valve designs demonstrate flaws within a few years of implantation. Those that survive that initial period will probably have similar actuarial survival rates, because valve-related deaths are uncommon and most valve-related factors, i.e., infection or dehiscence, are common to all valves. In Starr's 20-year follow-up of the STARR-EDWARDS valve [2], survival at 10 years was 60% and at 15 years it was 45%. Our results at Mayo Clinic are identical to those of Starr.

HEMODYNAMICS

In contrast, hemodynamic differences among valves do exist. Pressure gradients can be shown *in vitro*. However, *in vivo* performance is usually worse than that obtained in a laboratory. Pressure gradients for the small-sized STARR-EDWARDS valves are worse than any other mechanical valve, but as size increases, the differences become fewer and are indistinguishable in the largest valve sizes, except when physiological flow rates are exceeded. Generally, a STARR-EDWARDS valve of less than 9A or 3M is inadequate for women and a 10A or 4M should be considered minimal for most males. With these limitations in mind, excellent relief of symptoms correlating with good performance can be obtained with a STARR-EDWARDS valve.

It is impressive that the small prosthetic valve can provide excellent symptomatic palliation. Schaff [3] reviewed a group of 50 children with STARR-EDWARDS valves. The majority (40) of these children had an adult-sized prosthesis, but 10 could only be implanted with a small size. Four of these 10 came to reoperation after 10 years when body surface area had nearly doubled. A larger STARR-EDWARDS valve was implanted in 2 and a larger disc valve was placed in the other 2.

The average age of the entire group of 50 children was 10 years, ranging from 6 months to 18 years. Follow-up averaged 8 years with a maximum of 17 years. Overall survival at 5 years was 86%; at 10 years aortic survival was 90% and mitral survival was 76%. Seven patients had a major thromboembolic event; and 5 experienced transient neurological symptoms suggestive of thromboembolism. At 10 years embolus-free survival for aortic patients was 60% and for mitral patients it was 90%. The overall incidence of thromboembolism was 5% per patient-year for the aortic position and 2% per patient-year for the mitral or systemic atrioventricular valve. Half of the thromboembolic complications occurred in children who had stopped anticoagulant therapy.

THROMBOEMBOLISM

The major concern with mechanical valves is thromboembolism. In 1972 at The Society of Thoracic Surgeons meeting in Toronto, a consensus developed advocating anticoagulant therapy for all mechanical valves. Despite changes in valve design and materials, this recommendation still seems valid. In contrast to tilting disc valves, valve thrombosis with the STARR-EDWARDS valve is rare. Nevertheless, thromboembolism is a major concern. The incidence of thromboembolism with the STARR-EDWARDS valve varies by implant site. Previous reviews from our institution [4] and from other series [5–17] show the risk of thromboembolism to be about 2% per patient-year in the aortic and 5% per patient-year in the mitral. During the last 4 years we have used antiplatelet adhesive agents with standard anticoagulation to reduce the risk of thromboembolic events. A preliminary study [18] indicates that dypridamole with warfarin sodium can reduce thromboembolic events by 70%. In contrast, aspirin had little effect on the incidence of emboli and, in fact, compounded bleeding problems.

CONCLUSION

In summary, the STARR-EDWARDS valve remains the standard for valve durability by virtue of 20 years of follow-up after implantation. The valve may not be the ideal prosthesis from a hemodynamic or thromboembolic aspect, but with the use of antiplatelet adhesive agents and proper size selection, the valve remains an excellent mechanical valve substitute.

REFERENCES

1. Harken DE: Prosthetic heart valves: Perfection may be the enemy of good. Med Instrum 1977;11:70–71.
2. Tepley JF, Grunkemeier GL, Sutherland HD, et al: The ultimate prognosis after valve replacement: An assessment at twenty years. Ann Thorac Surg 1981;32(2):111–119.
3. Schaff HV, Danielson GK, DiDonato RM, et al: Late results after Starr-Edwards valve replacement in children. J Thorac Cardiovasc Surg 1984;88:583–589.
4. McGoon MD, Fuster V, McGoon DC, et al: Aortic and mitral valve incompetence: Long-term follow-up (10 to 19 years) of patients treated with the Starr-Edwards prosthesis. J Amer Coll Cardiol 1984;3:930–938.
5. Miller DC, Oyer PE, Mitchell RS, et al: Performance characteristics of the Starr-Edwards Model 1260 aortic valve prosthesis beyond ten years. J Thorac Cardiovasc Surg 1984;88(2):193–207.
6. Pellegrini A, Peronace B, Marcazzan E, et al: Results of valve replacement surgery with mechanical prostheses. Int J Artif Organs 1982;5(1):27–32.
7. Mikaeloff P, Van Haecke P, Frieh JP, et al: Prognosis following mitral valve replacement with the Starr-Edwards 6120 prosthesis. Arch Mal Coeur 1981; 74(7):799–807.
8. Dale J, Myhre E: Can acetylsalicylic acid alone prevent arterial thromboembolism? A pilot study in patients with aortic ball valve prostheses. Acta Med Scand 1981:645(Suppl):73–78.
9. Peronace B, Cornelli U, Marcazzan E, et al: Aortic valve replacement with Starr-Edwards and Björk-Shiley prosthesis: Long-term results and statistical analysis of some risk factors. G Ital Cardiol 1980;10(8):1024–1030.
10. Macmanus Q, Grunkemeier G, Houseman L, et al: Early results with composite strut caged ball prostheses. Am J Cardiol 1980;46(4):566–569.
11. Schoevaerdts JC, Jaumin P, Ponlot R, et al: Twelve year results with a caged-ball mitral prosthesis. Thorac Cardiovasc Surg 1979;27(1):45–47.
12. Sakashita I, Ohtani S, Nakamura C, et al: Clinical evaluation of a new anticoagulant therapy in prosthetic valve replacement. Jpn Heart J 1978;19(3):324–331.
13. Moggio RA, Hammond GL, Stansel HC Jr, et al: Incidence of emboli with cloth-covered Starr-Edwards valve without anticoagulation and with varying forms of anticoagulation: Analysis of 183 patients followed for 3½ years. J Thorac Cardiovasc Surg 1978;75(2):296–299.

14. Starr A, Grunkemeier GL, Lambert LE, et al: Aortic valve replacement: A ten-year follow-up of non-cloth-covered vs cloth-covered caged-ball prostheses. Circulation 1977;56(3 pt 2 suppl): III33–III39.
15. Dale J: Arterial thromboembolic complications in patients with Björk-Shiley and Lillehei-Kaster aortic disc valve prostheses. Am Heart J 1977;93(6):715–722.
16. Cachera JP, Laurent F, Poulain H, et al: Mitral replacement using a ball-valve prosthesis under hypothermic protection of the myocardium: 230 cases. Nouv Presse Med 1977;6(5):341–344.
17. Dale J: Arterial thromboembolic complications in patients with Starr-Edwards aortic ball valve prostheses. Am Heart J 91(5):653–659.
18. Chesebro JH, Fuster V, Elveback LR, et al: Trial of combined warfarin plus dipyridamole or aspirin therapy in prosthetic heart valve replacement: Danger of aspirin compared with dipyridamole. Am J Cardiol 1983;51:1537.

7. OVERVIEW OF EXPERIENCE WITH THE BJÖRK-SHILEY® VALVE

DONALD B. DOTY

The BJÖRK-SHILEY® cardiac valve prosthesis was produced in 1969. The original design was unique and revolutionary in the manufacture of cardiac valve substitutes. The tilting disc mechanism was a considerable departure from the types of prosthetic devices in use at that time. The low profile and improved hemodynamic properties made the device especially attractive so that it rapidly became very popular and widely utilized for cardiac valve replacement. The original disc was made of DELRIN® and opened to 50°.

The DELRIN disc was replaced by the conical pyrolytic carbon disc in 1971 because of the improved durability of this material. The original DELRIN disc functions very well for periods in excess of 10 years but the pyrolytic carbon device should have further prolonged the functional durability of the prosthesis. The BJÖRK-SHILEY Spherical disc valve opened to 60° and was generally a very reliable device with very rare structural problems (mechanical failure 0.001% per patient-year). The pyrolytic carbon discs apparently rotated freely and no static wear patterns or surface indentations were found in late follow-up of explanted valves. The wear of the surface of the disc was so little as to be negligible. A few fractures of the inlet valve strut which retain the disc were reported.

Thromboembolic events reported by Lindbloom [1] in isolated aortic valve replacement was 1.2% per patient-year and for mitral valve replacement the rate was 4.2% per patient-year (table 7-1). Thrombotic obstruction of the prosthesis was an especially alarming complication because it was often fatal. Actual incidence

Table 7-1. Thrombosis and embolism with the Björk-Shiley prosthesis [1]

	% Per patient-year	
	Clotted valve	Embolism
Aortic Delrin	0.2	1.6
Standard	0.8	0.4
C-C	0.2	1.0
Mitral Delrin	1.1	3.8
Standard	1.7	2.4
C-C	0	2.1

of this complication is not known, but in known cases the rate appears to be about 1–2% clotted prostheses per patient-year in anticoagulated patients and as high as 8% clotted valves per patient-year in nonanticoagulated patients. A radiopaque, ring-shaped marker was added in 1975 to aid in the diagnosis of this complication.

The Convexo-Concave disc and other modifications of the prosthesis were first tested clinically in 1975 and introduced into the United States market in 1979. The Convexo-Concave disc was developed to diminish the incidence of thromboembolic complications. The shape of the disc and its method of retention created clearance, allowing movement of the disc away from the valve flange. The flow distribution through the minor orifice was increased by 30%. These changes should have created a *washing* effect that would lower the incidence of thromboembolism.

The thromboembolic rate did decrease to 2.1% per patient-year for mitral valve replacement and the incidence of clotted valves decreased to less than 1% per patient-year. The rates of thromboembolism in collected series [2–7] are shown in table 7-2 and are quite low.

Structural problems may have increased slightly in this new design as a result of greater stress on the retaining struts and also on the disc due to the fact that the disc closes 15% faster. The inlet strut became an integral part of the flange mechanism eliminating two welds, but the outlet or minor strut remained subject

Table 7-2. Thromboembolism with the Björk-Shiley Convexo-Concave prothesis reported from collected series [2–7]

	% Per patient-year		
	Aortic	Mitral	Double
Björk	1.0	2.3	0
Shipara	1.4	2.8	2.2
Shipara	1.5	3.8	1.6
Doty	3.4	5.5	3.6
Stalpaert	0.9	1.5	1.5
Edmunds	2.4	2.3	

to great forces which produced disruption in some cases. This event is often fatal when the disc escapes from the device.

Data on strut fractures are difficult to accurately determine, but estimates are summarized in table 7-3. The incidence is about 0.04% per patient-year for all sizes. The risk is higher in the mitral position and in larger sizes because it appears to be primarily a closure problem in which the outlet strut is pulled off by closure contact with the disc. There were 21 known deaths due to this complication in 1983. The manufacturer reportedly took steps to better control the strut-to-disc clearance, to reduce the residual stress in the strut after disc insertion and to improve welding techniques and inspection.

The most recent design modification of the BJÖRK-SHILEY prosthesis is clearly the result of increased concern for strengthening the outlet strut, which was attempted by utilizing an integral monstrut to retain the Convexo-Concave disc. The disc occluder opening angle has been further increased to 70° by moving the inlet strut approximately 0.2 mm toward the center of the valve. There is a single cantilevered outlet strut of thicker metal replacing the wire retention strut of the former design. The entire metal configuration of the valve is formed by electro-chemical machining to selectively remove metal from a single disc of Haynes 25 (STELLITE®), a cobalt-based super alloy. There are no weld points in the prosthesis so that durability should be markedly improved. Hemodynamics of the device should be improved by the greater opening angle of the occluder. Many devices have been implanted in Europe and throughout the world. Clinical trials in the United States have not started because of FDA restrictions.

Overall, clinical experience with the various designs of the BJÖRK-SHILEY valve prostheses have been good. It is apparent that the device is generally durable and reliable. Thrombotic events are rare and seem to be well controlled with anticoagulants. It is generally agreed that anticoagulants are required when using this device and the complications related to medication are significant.

Table 7-3. Summary of strut fracture experience with the Björk-Shiley Convexo-Concave prosthesis

Incidence All Sizes = < 0.04
              29 mm* =   0.35 (recall group)
              29 mm* =   0.12 (present)

Mortality—1983 = 21 patients (known)

Cause = A closure problem, hence more frequent in mitral.
        Outlet strut is pulled off by disc contact.
        Weld or negative residual stress in strut.

Prevention = 1. Control strut to disc clearance
              2. Residual stress testing
              3. Weld inspection

*Includes all sizes 29 mm and larger

REFERENCES

1. Lindbloom D. Thromboembolic complications following valve replacement with the Convexo-Concave Björk-Shiley prosthesis. *Cardiac Prosthesis Symposium,* Shiley Inc. 1982, pp 157–195.
2. Björk V: Comments. J Thorac Cardiovasc Surg 1981; 82:674.
3. Shipara N, Salazar C, Patel J, et al: Early and late results with the Björk-Shiley Convaco-Convex prosthesis in relation to etiology. Abstr 49th Assembly Amer Coll Chest Phys, Chicago, Oct 1983.
4. Shipara N, Salazar C, Patel J, et al: Björk-Shiley Convexo-Concave valve prosthesis. Abstr 16th World Congress of the Int Soc for Cardiovasc Surg, Rio de Janeiro, Sept 1983.
5. Doty D, Elliott D, Hiratzka L: Thrombosis of the Björk-Shiley prosthesis. *Cardiac Prosthesis Symposium,* Shiley Inc. 1982, pp 143–148.
6. Stalpaert G, Vandermast M, DeKeyser L, et al: Experience with standard and Convexo-Concave Björk-Shiley valvular replacement. *Cardiac Prosthesis Symposium,* Shiley Inc. 1982, pp 149–152.
7. Edmunds LH: Thromboembolic complications of current cardiac valvular prostheses. Ann Thor Surg 1982; 34:96–106.

8. EXPERIENCE WITH STANDARD AND SUPRA-ANNULAR CARPENTIER-EDWARDS® PORCINE BIOPROSTHESES

W. R. ERIC JAMIESON, MICHAEL T. JANUSZ, G. FRANK O. TYERS, ALFRED N. GEREIN, DONALD R. RICCI, LAWRENCE H. BURR, ROBERT T. MIYAGISHIMA

Since 1975 porcine bioprostheses have been the valve substitute of choice for cardiac valvular replacement at Vancouver General Hospital and St. Paul's Hospital in Vancouver, Canada. From 1975 to May 1984 porcine bioprostheses were implanted in 2066 patients (99%) and mechanical prostheses, in 23 patients (1.0%), the majority being ST. JUDE MEDICAL® (SJM) valves.

Evaluation of a greater than 5 years experience with the HANCOCK® prosthesis showed that primary tissue degeneration was affecting long-term durability. This chapter will evaluate our greater-than-5-year experience with first generation CARPENTIER-EDWARDS® (CE) standard valves (high-pressure fixed with glutaraldehyde) and our early experience with the newer generation CARPENTIER-EDWARDS supra-annular valve (low-pressure fixed with glutaraldehyde). The supra-annular model was developed to improve hemodynamic performance and durability.

PATIENTS AND METHODS

By May 1984 the CARPENTIER-EDWARDS valve had been implanted in 2066 patients: 1167 standard and 726 supra-annular. A 5-year evaluation was available on 235 patients with the standard model by May 1983; early experience with 255 patients with supra-annular prostheses concluded in February 1983.

Operative techniques were similar in both series. Since late 1976, hypothermic, asanguinous potassium cardioplegia has been used for myocardial protection.

Long-term anticoagulation was prescribed for patients with chronic atrial fibrillation, intracardiac thrombus or dilated left atrium. The majority of mitral valve replacements (MVR) and multiple valve replacements (MR) received early postoperative anticoagulation; the majority of patients undergoing aortic valve replacements (AVR) did not receive anticoagulation.

DEFINITIONS

This chapter evaluates valve-related complications with both the standard and supra-annular models. Valve-related complications included: thromboembolism, anticoagulant-related hemorrhage, prosthetic valve endocarditis, paravalvular leak and prosthetic failure. Reoperation or death resulting from these complications were considered valve related.

Thromboembolism was defined as all new, focal neurological deficits, either transient or permanent, or peripheral emboli diagnosed at embolectomy. Cerebrovascular accidents occurring intraoperatively were not considered valve-related thromboembolism. Anticoagulant-related hemorrhage included internal or external bleeding necessitating hospital care, transfusion or extensive outpatient care.

Prosthetic valve endocarditis was defined as any documented infection of the prosthesis. Operative management of prosthetic valve endocarditis was determined by the presence of progressive and severe congestive heart failure, systemic emboli and/or persistent sepsis.

All episodes of paravalvular leak were documented by cardiac catheterization, reoperation or autopsy. Paravalvular leak caused by infective endocarditis was listed as prosthetic valve endocarditis.

Prosthetic failure was documented by cardiac catheterization, reoperation or autopsy and defined as any structural failure of the prosthesis causing stenosis or insufficiency, including leaflet disruption, calcification, stent failure or thrombosis. Valve failures resulting from infective endocarditis or paravalvular leak were excluded and listed separately.

Reoperation was defined as re-replacement for any cause. Reoperation for repair or replacement of another native valve or other cardiac pathology unrelated to the prosthesis, e.g., coronary artery disease, was not included.

The multiple decrement analysis method of Bodnar and colleagues [1] was used for assessment of these valve series. This assessment allows for separation of valve survival from patient survival. Freedom from all valve-related complications is the actuarial proportion of patients remaining free from any valve-related complications, including those causing death or reoperation. Freedom from mortality due to valve-related complications denotes the actuarial proportion of patients alive or who have died from a nonvalve related cause. Freedom from valve-related mortality or reoperation denotes the actuarial proportion of patients remaining free from valve-related death or from reoperation for a valve-related cause.

CARPENTIER-EDWARDS STANDARD PATIENT POPULATION

The CARPENTIER-EDWARDS standard porcine bioprosthesis was implanted in 235 patients, utilizing 252 prostheses: AVR = 106; MVR = 107; tricuspid valve replacement (TVR) = 5; MR = 17. Previous cardiac surgery had been performed in 31 patients (13.2%). Concomitant procedures were performed in 34 patients (14.5%), of whom 24 had coronary artery bypass.

Follow-up information for clinical evaluation was obtained by direct contact with patients and/or attending physicians during a four-month period. Cumulative follow-up for all patients was 900 patient-years (AVR = 419 patient-years; MVR = 423 patient-years; TVR = 12 patient-years and MR = 46 patient-years). Patient follow-up was 99% complete.

Results

Early mortality and complications
Operative mortality (< 30 days) was 6.8% (16): AVR = 2.8% (3); MVR = 8.4% (9); TVR = 20% (1); and MR = 17.6% (3). Low output syndrome was identified in and contributed to 37.5% of operative mortality.

Late mortality and complications
In this series of patients there were 35 (14.9%) late deaths. Overall late mortality, expressed as a linearized occurrence rate, was 3.9% per patient-year: AVR = 3.6% per patient-year (15); MVR = 3.1% per patient-year (13); MR = 10.9% per patient-year (5); and TVR = 16.7% per patient-year (2). Valve-related causes of late mortality were thromboembolism (4), prosthetic valve endocarditis (2) and paravalvular leak (1). Two patients died at reoperation, one from prosthetic valve endocarditis and one from paravalvular leak.

Overall patient survival, including operative deaths, is expressed by the life table method and is shown in figure 8-1. At 2 years the overall rate was 85.6 ± 3.4% and at 6 years it was 75.4 ± 5.7%. At 6 years AVR = 82.5 ± 7.4%; MVR = 76.4 ± 10.4%; and MR = 53.8 ± 18.2%.

Valve-related complications
As stated above, significant valve-related complications were thromboemboli, prosthetic valve endocarditis, primary tissue failure, paravalvular leak and anticoagulant related hemorrhage. The linearized occurrence rate for valve-related complications was 2.9% per patient-year (26) and the fatality rate was 0.7% per patient year (7). Freedom from valve-related complications at 2 years was 93.1 ± 3.5% and at 6 years was 87.5 ± 4.7% (figure 8-2).

Linearized occurrence rates and number of events for all valve related complications are shown in table 8-1. The overall linearized occurrence rate for thromboembolism is 1.6% per patient-year (14): AVR = 1.0% per patient-year (4); MVR = 1.65% per patient-year (7); and MR = 6.5% per patient-year (3). There were three fatalities from thromboembolism following MVR and one following MR. The linearized occurrence rate for prosthetic valve endocarditis overall was 0.6% per patient-year (5): AVR = 0.5%; MVR = 0.24%; and MR = 4.3%. There were two fatalities due to prosthetic valve endocarditis, one following AVR and

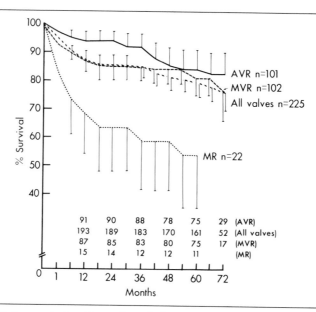

Figure 8-1. Patient survival to 72 months with the Carpentier-Edwards standard model.

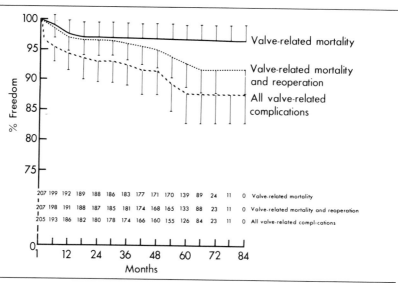

Figure 8-2. Freedom from valve-related mortality and complications to 84 months with the Carpentier-Edwards standard model.

Table 8-1. Linearized morbidity and mortality rates and events for the Carpentier-Edwards *standard* prosthesis.

Morbidity mortality	% Per patient-year (no. patients or events)		
	AVR	MVR	MR
Thromboembolism			
overall	1.0 (4)	1.7 (7)	6.5 (3)
fatal	0	0.7 (3)	2.2 (1)
Prosthetic valve endocarditis			
overall	0.5 (2)	0.24 (1)	4.3 (2)
fatal	0.24 (1)	0	2.2 (1)
Primary tissue failure			
overall	0	0.7 (3)	4.3 (2)
fatal	0	0	0
Paravalvular leak			
overall	0	0.24 (1)	0
fatal	0	0.24 (1)	0
Anticoagulation-related hemorrhage			
overall	0	0.24 (1)	0
fatal	0	0	0

one following MR. For primary tissue failure, the linearized occurrence rate was 0.6% per patient-year (5): AVR = 0; MVR = 0.7%; and MR = 4.3%. No fatalities were attributed to primary tissue failure. One serious episode of anticoagulant-related hemorrhage occurred following MVR (0.24% per patient-year). Paravalvular leak occurred in one MVR patient (0.24% per patient-year) who died at reoperation. The other death at reoperation occurred from prosthetic valve endocarditis.

Reoperation for valve-related complications occurred in 9 patients: AVR = 1; MVR = 5; and MR = 3. Reoperation was performed in 5 patients for primary tissue failure, in 3 patients for prosthetic valve endocarditis and in 1 patient for paravalvular leak. Two fatalities from reoperation were due to valve-related complications and are noted above.

Freedom from valve-related complications
Freedom from valve-related complications and death is shown in figure 8-3. Freedom from all valve-related complications at 2 years was 93.1 ± 3.5% and at 6 years was 87.5 ± 4.7%. Freedom from valve-related mortality at 2 years was 97.0 ± 2.4% and at 6 years was 96.4 ± 2.6%. Freedom from valve-related mortality and reoperation at 2 years was 96.5 ± 2.5% and at 6 years was 91.8 ± 4.0%.

CARPENTIER-EDWARDS SUPRA-ANNULAR PATIENT POPULATION

The CARPENTIER-EDWARDS supra-annular porcine bioprosthesis was implanted in 255 patients (271 prostheses: AVR = 121; MVR = 130; and MR = 20). Previous cardiac surgery had been performed in 20 patients (7.8%). Concomitant procedures were performed in 82 patients (32.2%). Cumulative follow-up for all patients was 229 patient-years: AVR = 108 patient-years; MVR = 109 patient-years; and MR = 12 patient-years. Follow-up was 99% complete.

Results

Early mortality and complications

Overall operative mortality (< 30 days) was 6.7% (17): AVR = 3.3% (4); MVR = 10.0% (13). There was no mortality for multiple valve replacements.

Late mortality and complications

There were 10 late deaths in the series (3.9%). Overall late mortality, expressed as linearized occurrence rate, was 4.4% per patient-year: AVR = 4.1% per patient-year (5); MVR = 3.1% per patient-year (4); and MR = 5.0% per patient-year (1). There were no valve-related causes of late mortality or deaths from reoperation.

Survival

Overall patient survival at 2 years, including operative deaths expressed by the life table method is 89.4 ± 2.4%: AVR = 92.4 ± 3.6%; MVR = 85.8 ± 3.2%; and MR = 93.3 ± 12.6% (figure 8-3).

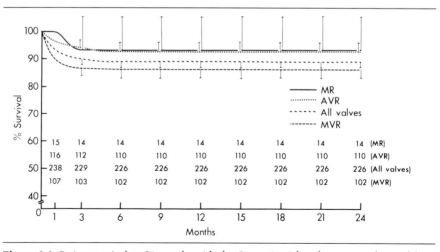

Figure 8-3. Patient survival to 24 months with the Carpentier-Edwards supra-annular model.

Valve-related complications

The linearized occurrence rate for valve-related complications was 4.3% per patient-year (11). There were no fatalities. Freedom from all valve-related complications at 2 years was 95.1 ± 2.8% (figure 8-4).

All valve-related complications by linearized occurrence rates and number of events are show in table 8-2. The overall linearized occurrence rate for thromboembolism was 1.7% per patient-year (4): AVR = 0.9% per patient-year (1); and MVR = 2.8% per patient-year (3). There were no cases of thromboembolism in MR patients or any fatalities from thromboembolism. The overall linearized occurrence rate for prosthetic valve endocarditis was 1.3% per patient-year (3): AVR = 0; MVR = 1.8% and MR 8.3%. There were no cases of primary tissue failure in this series. One case of anticoagulant-related hemorrhage followed MVR (0.9% per patient-year). Paravalvular leak occurred in 3 MVR patients (2.8% per patient-year).

Reoperation for valve-related complications occurred in 2 patients without fatality: AVR = 1 (paravalvular leak); MVR = 1 (prosthetic valve endocarditis).

Freedom from valve-related complications

Freedom from valve-related complications and death is shown in figures 8-4 and 8-5. Freedom from all valve-related complications at 2 years was 95.1 ± 2.8%. Freedom from valve-related mortality was 100%. Freedom from valve-related mortality and reoperation at 2 years was 99.1 ± 1.2%. Freedom from each complication was: thromboembolism = 98.2 ± 1.7%; anticoagulant-related hemorrhage = 99.6 ± 0.86%; prosthetic valve endocarditis = 98.7 ± 1.5%; and paravalvular leak = 98.7 ± 1.5%. There were no cases of primary tissue failure in this series.

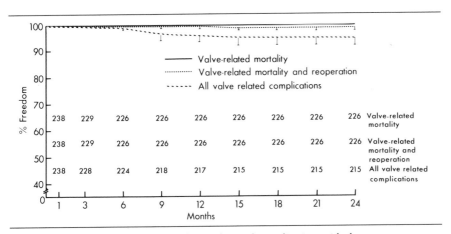

Figure 8-4. Freedom from valve-related mortality and complications with the Carpentier-Edwards supra-annular model.

Table 8-2. Linearized morbidity and mortality rates and events for the Carpentier-Edwards *supra-annular* prosthesis.

Morbidity mortality	% Per patient-year (no. patients or events)		
	AVR	MVR	MR
Thromboembolism			
overall	0.9 (1)	2.8 (3)	0
fatal	0	0	0
Prosthetic valve endocarditis			
overall	0	1.8 (2)	8.3 (1)
fatal	0	0	0
Primary tissue failure			
overall	0	0	0
fatal	0	0	0
Paravalvular leak			
overall	0	2.8 (3)	0
fatal	0	0	0
Anticoagulation-related hemorrhage			
overall	0	0.9 (1)	0
fatal	0	0	0

Hemodynamic assessment

Hemodynamic evaluation of the CARPENTIER-EDWARDS supra-annular prosthesis has begun. In 6 patients with 21 mm and 23 mm prostheses in the aortic position, the average resting mean pressure gradient across the valve was 10 mm

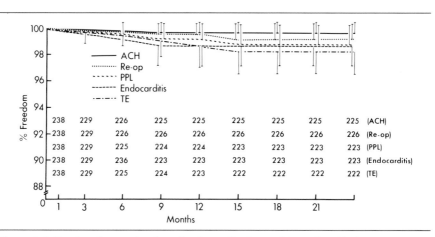

Figure 8-5. Freedom from each valve-related complication to 24 months with the Carpentier-Edwards supra-annular model.

Hg and the calculated aortic valve area was 2.3 cm² (range of 2.0-2.8 cm²). In 4 patients with 27 mm and 29 mm prostheses in the mitral position, the average resting mean diastolic gradient across the valve was 7 mm Hg and the calculated valve area was 1.7 cm² (range of 1.15-2.43 cm²).

DISCUSSION

Tissue prostheses, both porcine and pericardial, have provided a very satisfactory quality of life for patients requiring valvular replacement. [2–12] The bioprostheses have afforded a low incidence of valve-related complications, especially thromboembolism. In our experience, incidence of thromboembolism has been consistently less than 2.0% per patient-year. [2–6]

Edmunds [13] has provided extensive documentation on thromboembolism with tissue and mechanical prostheses. His study shows the incidence of thromboembolism in the aortic position is less than 2% per patient-year with biological valves and no anticoagulation and with mechanical valves and anticoagulation. With MVR, the incidence of thromboembolism was approximately 4% per patient-year for biological valves with or without anticoagulation and for mechanical valves with anticoagulation.

Concern about durability of bioprostheses remains, even though glutaraldehyde-preserved bioprostheses have reduced thromboembolism and anticoagulant-related hemorrhage (which are well documented with mechanical prostheses) [6, 8, 10, 11]. The two prime concerns are leaflet failure and calcification. Ishihara et al. [14] have documented four types of primary leaflet failure: 1) cusp tear near the commissures and in the right coronary cusp; 2) linear perforations forming arc perforations parallel to the sewing ring; 3) large, round or oval perforations in the central region; and 4) pinhole perforations in the central region and left and right noncoronary cusps. These leaflet failures are due to the structural failure of the connective tissue components, primarily collagen degeneration. Fatigue failures may be due to mechanical forces or calcium [15].

To reduce or eliminate the leaflet failures and calcification, extensive research has been conducted on structural support design and tissue preservation [16]. Broom et al. [17] reported that pressure fixation of porcine tissue below 1 mm Hg will preserve tissue compliance closer to that of fresh tissue and provide less constraint with better coaptive margins. Broom also showed that the circumferential collagen of the fibrosa and ventricularis take the bulk of the stress.

Carpentier [16] incorporated low-pressure fixation of the porcine tissue in the present investigational CARPENTIER-EDWARDS supra-annular bioprosthesis. The supra-annular design may reduce turbulence, and improved preservation should reduce calcification. Low pressure fixation may prevent the collagen bundle from splitting and prevent the loss of the elastic fiber crimp currently seen in high-pressure fixed valves.

Our data in this study show initial tissue failure in our standard high-pressure fixed valves and no evidence of tissue failure with the low-pressure fixed valve within a short evaluation interval. In our series the failure mode of the CARPEN-

TIER-EDWARDS valve has been primarily tears and perforations which have not been catastrophic and have allowed re-replacement surgery to be performed electively [10]. The re-replacement prostheses has been either the low-pressure fixed CARPENTIER-EDWARDS supra-annular valve or the ST. JUDE MEDICAL valve, selected at the discretion of the surgeon, cardiologist and patient.

To allow comparison with other prostheses, this study has used indicators of valve performance given in recent publications by the University of British Columbia and Stanford University [10, 18, 19]. Miller et al. [18, 19] use the broad term valve failure to denote any mortality or reoperation related to a valve-related complication. This corresponds to our term of valve-related mortality and reoperation. Their term valve-related late deaths corresponds to our terminology of valve-related mortality; and their terms overall valve-related morbidity and mortality or occurrence of valve failure plus complications not leading to reoperation or causing death correspond to our encompassing term of overall valve-related complications. Using the same definitions allows a composite assessment (table 8-3) of all valve-related complications showing effect on performance and structural durability.

A reoperation rate of 80% at 10 years has been shown for porcine bioprostheses and the STARR-EDWARDS and BJÖRK-SHILEY® valves [11, 19, 22]. At the 10-year interval overall valve-related complications and mortality due to these complications are not distinguishable between mechanical prostheses and bioprostheses. The 15-year evaluation may distinguish superiority for one type of prosthesis. However, these evaluations are for old generation prostheses. The new generation mechanical valves, such as the monostrut disc of BJÖRK-SHILEY, the bileaflet of ST. JUDE MEDICAL and Duromedics, and the low-pressure fixation porcine and pericardial valves, will need long-term evaluation.

Intraoperative hemodynamic evaluation of the CARPENTIER-EDWARDS supra-annular porcine bioprosthesis have shown encouraging data. [23] Chaitman and colleagues [24] have conducted an evaluation of the CARPENTIER-EDWARDS standard bioprosthesis. Our data show the supra-annular prosthesis in the aortic position is superior to the standard prosthesis: a resting gradient of 10 mm Hg compared to 21 mm Hg and a valve area of 2.3 cm^2 compared to 1.2 cm^2. In the mitral position, our data for the supra-annular prosthesis are very similar to Chaitman's results of the standard CARPENTIER-EDWARDS mitral prosthesis.

CONCLUSION

The performance of the CARPENTIER-EDWARDS standard and supra-annular porcine bioprostheses has afforded our patients a low incidence of valve-related complications and mortality. The porcine bioprosthesis remains a satisfactory substitute for valvular performance. Long-term assessment will determine the influence of low-pressure glutaraldehyde prostheses on durability and performance.

ACKNOWLEDGEMENT

The authors extend appreciation to Ms. Joan MacNab and Ms. Florence Chan, research assistants, for their efforts in patient follow-up and data formulation. The

Table 8-3. Freedom from valve-related morbidity and complications.

Prosthesis	Valve-related complications	Valve-related mortality	Valve-related mortality and reoperation
Hancock (Stanford) [18]	AVR 74 ± 5% @ 8 yrs. MVR 60 ± 3% @ 9 yrs.	AVR 97 ± 1% @ 6 yrs. MVR 90 ± 4% @ 9 yrs.	AVR 82 ± 5% @ 8 yrs. MVR 71 ± 4% @ 10 yrs.
Hancock (UBC) [20]	Overall 66.2 ± 9.3% @ 8 yrs.	Overall 95.0 ± 3.9% @ 8 yrs.	Overall 84.7 ± 7.1% @ 8 yrs.
Carpentier-Edwards (UBC-MHI) [10,21]	AVR 89.4 ± 5.5% @ 6 yrs. MVR 81.8 ± 8.2% @ 6 yrs.	AVR 99.3 ± 1.4% @ 6 yrs. MVR 96.8 ± 3.1% @ 6 yrs.	AVR 95.6 ± 3.9% @ 6 yrs. MVR 89.7 ± 6.2% @ 6 yrs.
Starr-Edwards (Stanford) [19]	AVR 51 ± 3% @ 10 yrs.	AVR 88 ± 2% @ 10 yrs.	AVR 82 ± 2% @ 10 yrs.

authors also acknowledge the support of Drs. A. I. Munro, P. Allen, H. Tutassaura and H. Ling for inclusion of their patients in the study.

REFERENCES

1. Bodnar E, Wain WH, Haberman S: Assessment and comparison of the performance of cardiac valves. Ann Thorac Surg 1982;34:146–156.
2. Jamieson WRE, Janusz MT, Miyagishima RT, et al: Embolic complication of porcine hetero-graft cardiac valves. J Thorac Cardiovasc Surg 1981;81:626–631.
3. Janusz MT, Jamieson WRE, Allen P, et al: Experience with the Carpentier-Edwards porcine valve prosthesis in 700 patients. Ann Thorac Surg 1982;34:625–633.
4. Janusz MT, Jamieson WRE, Allen P, et al: Long-term follow-up of patients with procine cardiac valve prostheses. Can J Surg 1983;26:160–162.
5. Jamieson WRE, Janusz MT, Tyers GFO, et al: Early durability of the Carpentier-Edwards porcine bioprosthesis, in Kaplitt MJ, Borman JB (eds): *Concepts and Controversies in Cardiovascular Surgery*. New York, Appleton-Century-Crofts, 1983, pp 111–133.
6. Minale C, Bardos P, Bourg NP et al: Early and late results of porcine bioprostheses versus mechanical prostheses in aortic and mitral positions, in Cohn LH, Gallucci V (eds): *Cardiac Bioprostheses: Proceedings of the Second International Symposium*. New York, Yorke Medical Books, 1982, pp 143–153.
7. Schonbeck M, Egloff L, Kugelmeier J, et al: Porcine bioprostheses versus mechanical valvular substitutes: A retrospective comparative analysis, in Cohn LH, Gallucci V (eds): *Cardiac Bioprostheses: Proceedings of the Second International Symposium*. New York, Yorke Medical Books, 1982, pp 192–204.
8. Oyer PE, Stinson EB, Miller DC, et al: Clinical analysis of the Hancock porcine bioproshtesis, in Cohn LH, Gallucci V (eds): *Cardiac Bioprostheses: Proceedings of the Second International Symposium*. New York, Yorke Medical Books, 1982, pp 539–551.
9. Marshall WG Jr, Kouchoukos NT, Karp RB, et al: Late results after mitral valve replacement with the Björk-Shiley and porcine prostheses. J Thorac Cardiovasc Surg 1983;85:902–910.
10. Jamieson WRE, Pelletier LC, Janusz MT, et al: Five year evaluation of the Carpentier-Edwards porcine bioprosthesis. J Thorac Cardiovasc Surg 1984;88:324–333.
11. Magilligan DJ, Lewis JW, Lilley B: The porcine bioprosthetic valve: Twelve years later. J Thorac Cardiovasc Surg (in press).
12. Ionescu MI, Smith DR, Hasan SS, et al: Clinical durability of the pericardial xenograft valve: Ten years' experience with mitral replacement. Ann Thorac Surg 1982;34:265–277.
13. Edmunds LH Jr: Thromboembolic complications of current cardiac valvular prostheses. Ann Thorac Surg 1982;34:96–105.
14. Ishihara T, Ferrans VJ, Boyce SW, et al: Structure and classification of cuspal tears and perforations in porcine bioprosthetic cardiac valves implanted in patients. Circulation 1981;48:665–678.
15. Broom ND: Fatigue induced damage in glutaraldehyde-preserved heart valve tissue. J Thorac Cardiovasc Surg 1978;76:202–211.
16. Carpentier A, Dubost C, Lane E, et al: Continuing improvements in valvular bioprostheses. J Thorac Cardiovasc Surg 1982;83:27–42.
17. Broom ND, Christie GW: Effect of fixation pressure on the function of porcine valvular xenografts, in Cohn LH, Gallucci V (eds): *Cardiac Bioprostheses: Proceedings of the Second International Symposium*. New York, Yorke Medical Books, 1982.
18. Miller DC: Late results with bioprosthetic valves. American College of Surgeons Postgraduate Course, 1983.
19. Miller DC, Oyer PE, Mitchell RS, et al: Performance characteristics of the Starr-Edwards model 1260 aortic valve prosthesis beyond 10 years. J Thorac Cardiovasc Surg 1984;88:193–207.
20. Jamieson WRE: Personal communication, University of British Columbia.
21. Jamieson WRE, Pelletier LC: Personal communication, University of British Columbia and Montreal Heart Institute.
22. Karp RB, Cyrus RJ, Blackstone EH, et al: The Björk-Shiley valve: Intermediate long-term follow-up. J Thorac Cardiovasc Surg 1981:81;602–614.
23. Cosgrove DM, Lytle BW, Gill CC, et al: In vivo hemodynamic comparison of porcine and pericardial valves. J Thorac Cardiovasc Surg 1985; 89(3):358–368.
24. Chaitman BR, Bonan R, Lepage G, et al: Hemodynamic evaluation of the Carpentier-Edwards porcine xenograft. Circulation 1979;60:1170–1182.

9. AORTIC VALVE REPLACEMENT WITH THE IONESCU-SHILEY® BOVINE PERICARDIAL VALVE: AN 81 MONTH EXPERIENCE

LORENZO GONZALEZ-LAVIN, SEONG CHI, T. CALVIN BLAIR, J.Y. JUNG, A.G. FABAZ, BETTY LEWIS, GEORGE DAUGHTERS

Abstract. The type of tissue and design of the IONESCU-SHILEY® valve coupled with its excellent hemodynamics and low incidence of thromboembolism motivated us to initiate the routine use of this valve in the aortic position shortly after it became commercially available. Between February 1977 and December 1983, 240 patients underwent aortic valve replacement with an IONESCU-SHILEY valve. Concomitant procedures were performed in 110 patients (45.8%). Hospital mortality was 6.7%. Among patients with isolated aortic valve replacement (IAVR), hospital mortality was 4.6%. None of the hospital deaths was valve related. All 224 hospital survivors have been followed for up to 81 months (100% follow-up) for a 621.6 patient year follow-up and a mean of 33.6 months. Only three instances of intrinsic valve failure have occurred for an incidence of 0.5% per patient-year. Actuarial freedom from intrinsic tissue failure is 95 ± 2.9%. Thromboembolism (all nonfatal) occurred in 5 patients or 0.83% per patient-year (2 of these had concurrent mitral valve disease). Patients with IAVR were not anticoagulated. Actuarial freedom from thromboembolism is 96.4 ± 1.6%. Of the 194 surviving patients, only 2 remained in Class IV and all others were in NYHA Class I or II. Overall patient survival is 78.5 ± 5.2%; it is 85.2 ± 5.3% for those with IAVR. The low thrombogenicity and excellent clinical results obtained in these patients, even those with a small aortic anulus (17–21 mm), are believed to be due to the excellent hydraulic characteristics of the IONESCU-SHILEY valve. Durability, so far, surpasses that of other xenobioprostheses in clinical use; this is believed to be due to the collagen content of bovine pericardium as well as to the preservation of collagen fiber waviness and multidirectional arrangement after fixation.

INTRODUCTION

Availability and reliability have established the xenobioprosthesis as the most commonly used tissue valve in the last decade. It has been learned that the most important factors dictating the overall performance of these hybrid valves (bovine pericardial and porcine tissue valves) are: valve design, type of tissue and preparation method. Valve design dictates the hydraulic and hemodynamic function and, to a degree, determines the thrombogenicity of a given valve. The tissue employed to fabricate the valve and the pressure it is subjected to during fabrication, as well as the methods of sterilization and stabilization, dictate the durability of each device.

The design of the bovine pericardial valve allows for superb hydraulic function and excellent performance [1–4]. The high collagen fiber content of bovine pericardium, the waviness that is preserved during stabilization and sterilization, and the fact that the valve is fabricated without being subjected to pressure, are very desirable characteristics of this xenobioprosthesis. These features motivated us to initiate the routine use of the IONESCU-SHILEY bovine pericardial valve (ISBPV) in the aortic position.

MATERIALS AND METHODS

In the 81 months between February 1977 and December 1983, 240 patients underwent aortic valve replacement with an ISBPV. One hundred forty-seven patients were male and 82 were female, a 1.6 to 1 ratio. Ages ranged from 17 to 86 years, with a mean of 62.5 years. Isolated aortic valve replacement (IAVR) was performed in 130 patients (54.2%). The other 110 patients underwent a concomitant procedure (45.8%). Among the concomitant procedures, 67 operations were for coronary revascularization (27.9%). Multivalvular procedures, some including coronary revascularization, were performed in 33 patients (13.7%). The other 10 patients had either resection of ascending aortic or ventricular aneurysms, or left ventricular myomectomies (4.2%). Valve lesions were aortic stenosis in 155 patients (64.6%); pure aortic regurgitation in 40 patients (16.7%); and mixed aortic valvular disease in 45 patients (18.7%).

Classified according to the criteria set forth by the New York Heart Association (NYHA), 3 patients (1.3%) were in Class I; 76 (31.6%) were in Class II; 126 (52.5%) were in Class III; and 35 (14.6%) were in Class IV. Therefore, 67.1% of the patients had been or were in congestive heart failure at the time of operation. Most of the patients in Classes I and II had concurrent coronary artery disease or other complicating lesions (i.e., ascending aortic aneurysm).

Cardiopulmonary bypass was employed using moderate flows, a bubble oxygenator, hemodilution and moderate systemic hypothermia to 28° C. Crystalloid potassium cardioplegia and topical hypothermia were used for myocardial protection. The aortic xenobioprosthesis was inserted with multiple everting interrupted mattress sutures of 3-0 DACRON® reinforced with TEFLON® pledgets. Valve sizes used ranged from 17 to 31 mm: 17 mm = 10 patients; 19 mm = 45 patients; 21 mm = 82 patients; 23 mm = 58 patients; 25 mm = 31 patients; 27 mm = 9 patients; 29 mm = 4 patients; and 31 mm = 1 patient. One hundred thirty-seven patients (57.1%) received a 17, 19 or 21 mm valve. Patients undergoing IAVR were not placed on anticoagulant or antiplatelet drugs. Patients undergoing multivalve replacement received oral warfarin sodium; those in chronic atrial fibrillation, or those with atrial clots found at operation, were maintained on long-term oral anticoagulant therapy.

RESULTS

Hospital mortality

Sixteen patients died in the hospital for a 6.7% hospital mortality. None of these deaths was valve related. Among the cohort of 130 patients undergoing IAVR, there were 6 hospital deaths (4.6%) (table 9-1).

Follow-up and actuarial analysis

The fate of all 224 hospital survivors was ascertained, for a 100% follow-up. A computerized questionnaire was completed following examination of the patient by the cardiologist or cardiac surgeon and also after telephone interview with the referring physician and/or the patient. The cumulative duration of follow-up is 621.6 patient-years, with a mean follow-up of 33.6 months. Ninety-six patients (42.9% of the series) have been followed for at least 3 years. Actuarial curves were constructed according to the method of Kaplan and Meier [5] to compensate for censored observations. Censoring of data was by date of analysis. There were no patients lost to follow-up so patient status could not change mortality figures or other variables studied. Statistical comparison of actuarial data was made using the method of Gehan [6]. One of the authors (GD) made the statistical analysis.

Parameters analyzed

Valve durability, infective endocarditis, thromboembolic complications, clinical performance of the survivors and overall patient survival were analyzed.

Table 9-1. Hospital mortality

Cause of death	Isolated aortic valve replacement (N = 130)	With concomitant procedures (N = 110)	All patients (N = 240)
Low cardiac output		5	5
Myocardial infarction	3	1	4
Arrhythmia		2	2
Renal failure		2	2
Pulmonary embolism	1		1
Rupture right ventricle	1		1
Septic shock	1		1
Totals	6 (4.6%)	10 (9.1%)	16 (6.7%)

Late mortality

There were 26 late deaths (11.6%) or 4.2% per patient-year (table 9-2). Fourteen of these were cardiac related (6.3%), 5 with valve dysfunction due to endocarditis (2.2% mortality).

Valve durability

To clarify the concept of intrinsic tissue failure the definition of Borkon et al. [7] was adopted:

Bioprosthetic failure resulting from structural deterioration without preceding infection which required reoperation or resulted in death was considered intrinsic tissue failure. Infection of the valve was not considered as intrinsic tissue failure as the mechanism of infective endocarditis is more closely related to the host or environment than to the valve substitute, *per se* [8].

Intrinsic tissue failure occurred in three instances and was due to calcification of all three leaflets. One had a tear and rupture of one of the calcific leaflets. These

Table 9-2. Late mortality

Cause of death		Number of patients
Cardiac related:		
Infective endocarditis:		7
with valve involvement	5	
without valve involvement	2	
Arrhythmia		3
Myocardial infarction		2
Left ventricular failure		2
		14(6.3%)
Other:		
Subarachnoid hemorrhage		2
Carcinoma of the lung		2
Cirrhosis of the liver		1
Ruptured abdominal aortic aneurysm		1
Agranulocytosis		1
Hepatitis		1
Mesenteric thrombosis		1
Histocystic lymphoma		1
General demise		1
Adverse drug reaction		1
		12
Total		26*

*11.6% of 224 hospital survivors

failures occurred at 38, 45 and 60 months after implantation. All occurred in males, one 47 years old and two 50 years old. The linearized incidence of intrinsic tissue failure is 0.5% per patient-year. The actuarial freedom from intrinsic tissue failure is 95 ± 2.9% at 6 years (figure 9-1).

Infective endocarditis
Fourteen patients acquired infective endocarditis, for a linearized rate of 2.2% per patient-year. Seven patients survive (50%), six with the original bovine pericardial valve and one after replacement of the infected valve with another ISBPV.

Thromboembolism
Thromboembolism, defined as all new focal neurological deficits (either transient or permanent) as well as clinically detectable noncerebral arterial emboli, occurred in 6 patients for a linearized rate of 1.0% per patient-year. Three patients, however, had concurrent mitral valve disease, 1 with significant mitral stenosis. The other 2 patients had undergone prior mitral valve replacement with a HANCOCK® porcine valve. Interestingly, 1 of these porcine valves was replaced at 77 months because of calcification and thrombosis; at the time of reoperation the ISBPV in the aortic position was found to be without evidence of degenerative changes or thrombus formation. Three thrombotic events occurred among the cohort of the 130 patients undergoing IAVR who were not placed on anticoagulant or antiplatelet drugs. All were nonfatal. The linearized rate in this cohort is 0.83% per patient-year. The actuarial freedom from thromboembolic events (including patients with concomitant procedures) is 96.4 ± 1.6% (figure 9-2).

Clinical performance
Clinical performance based on NYHA functional classification was assessed postoperatively in all 194 survivors. Only 2 patients remain in Class IV; both were found to

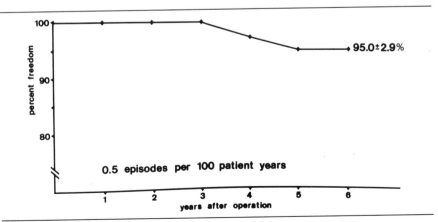

Figure 9-1. Actuarial curve depicting freedom from intrinsic valve failure.

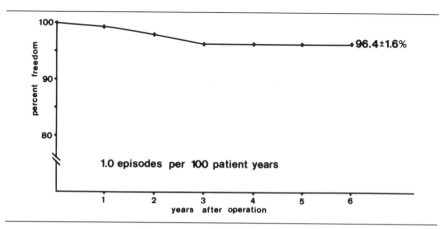

Figure 9-2. Actuarial curve depicting freedom from thromboembolic events.

have a significant cardiomyopathic element at the time of valve replacement. All other patients are in Class I or II (figure 9-3). Of particular interest is that all the 111 surviving patients with a 17, 19 or 21 mm valve are in Class I or II (figure 9-4).

Patient survival

Of the 224 patients leaving the hospital, 78.5 $\pm$ 5.2% are alive and retain their original prosthesis at 6 years. In the cohort undergoing IAVR, of the 124 hospital

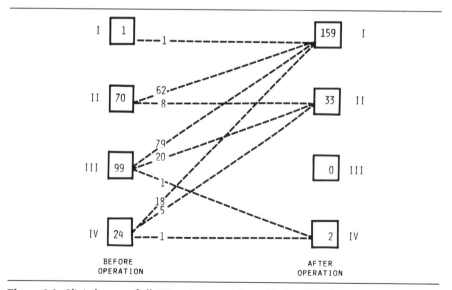

Figure 9-3. Clinical status of all 194 patients surviving with the original ISBPV as compared to their preoperative NYHA Classification.

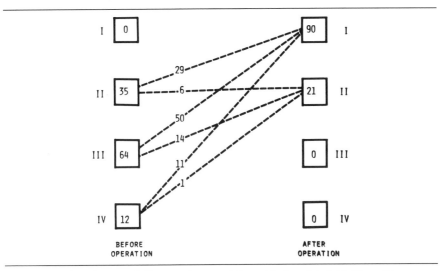

Figure 9-4. Clinical status of all 111 patients surviving with the original 17, 19, or 21 mm ISBPV as compared to their preoperative NYHA Classification.

survivors 85.2 $\pm$ 5.3% are alive and retain their original xenobioprosthesis. Actuarial patient survival curves are depicted in figure 9-5. The 6 year survival of patients after IAVR is significantly better than those with concomitant procedures (p = 0.01).

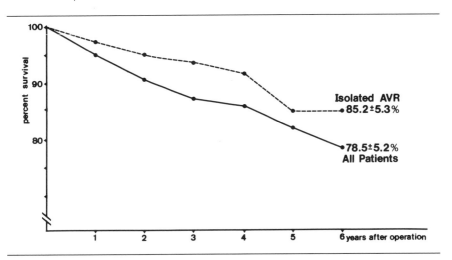

Figure 9-5. Actuarial curves depicting patient survival (with the original ISBPV) for all 224 patients leaving the hospital and for the 124 patients with isolated aortic valve replacement.

DISCUSSION

This retrospective analysis based on a 100% follow-up and multivariate determinants of valve-related complications of the IONESCU-SHILEY bovine pericardial valve in the aortic position during an 81-month experience, allows for a thorough evaluation of the clinical performance characteristics of this xenobioprosthesis. The findings of this study also corroborate well-established facts about patients undergoing aortic valve replacement.

Although valve durability is an important factor in overall patient survival, the degree of myocardial reserve as measured by NHYA functional classification, and the presence of associated lesions requiring concomitant procedures, affect overall patient survival. There has been no valve-related death in the absence of infective endocarditis. Among the 79 patients in preoperative NYHA Classes I and II there was no hospital mortality and 7.8% late mortality at 81 months, for a 92.2% survivorship. The group of 126 patients in NYHA Class III had an 8.7% hospital and 13% late mortality with a survivorship of 79.4%. The 35 patients in NHYA Class IV had the highest hospital and late mortality: 14.3% and 16.7% respectively, with a 71.4% survivorship. The difference between each group is statistically significant (p = 0.02). The survival of patients with IAVR is significantly better than those with concomitant procedures (p = 0.01).

Evaluating the ISBPV itself, the inherent valve design with its large, effective central orifice due to the simultaneous and symmetrical opening of the three leaflets provides excellent hemodynamics even in those patients with a small aortic anulus. This is particularly indicated for the elderly patient with calcific aortic stenosis in whom aortic valve replacement can be carried out without aortic anular enlargement, simplifying the procedure and lowering the surgical risk in this cohort of patients in whom operative and hospital mortality tend to be higher than in younger patients. The fact that 137 patients (57.1%) received a valve size 17 to 21 mm in diameter also reflects our confidence in the hydraulic features and hemodynamic performance of ISBPV. The low thrombogenicity in this series without the use of anticoagulant therapy is also believed to be related to the hydraulic and hemodynamic function of this device.

Important features in the durability of this bovine pericardial xenobioprosthesis are its high collagen content, multidirectional orientation of the collagen fibers, the preservation of collagen waviness after stabilization, and sterilization and valve fabrication without the use of pressure [9]. The fact that it does calcify, although to a lesser extent in comparison to other tissue valves, is worrisome [10–12]. Perhaps the introduction of surfactants during valve preparation to avoid calcium phosphate impregnation of the tissue will further decrease the incidence of calcification.

Nevertheless, at present we believe that the ISBPV is one of the valve substitutes of choice for aortic valve replacement because of its reliability and excellent hemodynamic performance in up to 81 months follow-up. In addition, it permits aortic valve replacement without the need for anticoagulation, thus avoiding the associated risk of anticoagulant-related hemorrhage.

REFERENCES

1. Walker DK, Scotten LN, Modi VJ, et al: In vitro assessment of mitral valve prostheses. J Thorac Cardiovasc Surg 1980; 79:680.
2. Wright JTM: Hydrodynamic evaluation of tissue valves, in Ionescu MI (ed): *Tissue Heart Valves*. London, Butterworth, 1979, pp 29–88.
3. Rainer WG, Christopher RA, Sadler TR Jr, et al: Dynamic behavior of prosthetic aortic tissue valves as viewed by high-speed cinematography. Ann Thorac Surg 1979; 28:274.
4. Tandon AP, Smith DR, Mary DAS, et al: Sequential hemodynamic studies in patients having aortic valve replacement with the Ionescu-Shiley pericardial valve. Ann Thorac Surg 1977; 24:149.
5. Kaplan EL, Meier P: Non-parametric estimation from incomplete observations. J Am Stat Assoc 1958; 53:457.
6. Gehan EA: A generalized Wilcoxon test for comparing arbitrarily singly-censored samples. Biometrika 1965; 52:203.
7. Borkon AM, McIntosh CL, Von Rueden TJ, et al: Mitral valve replacement with the Hancock bioprosthesis: Five- to ten-year follow-up. Ann Thorac Surg 1981; 32:127.
8. Tandon AP, Whitaker W, Ionescu M: Multiple valve replacement with pericardial xenograft: Clinical haemodynamic study. Br Heart J 1980; 44:534.
9. Broom ND, Thomson FJ: Influence of fixation conditions on the performance of glutaraldehyde-treated porcine aortic valves: Towards a more scientific basis. Thorax 1979; 34:166.
10. Gonzalez-Lavin L, Al-Janabi N, Ross DN: Long term results after aortic valve replacement with preserved aortic homografts. Ann Thorac Surg 1972; 13:594.
11. Oyer PE, Miller DC, Stinson EB, et al: Clinical durability of the Hancock porcine bioprosthetic valve. Ann Thorac Surg 1978; 26:303.
12. Lakier JB, Khaja F, Magilligan DJ Jr, et al: Porcine xenograft valves. Long-term (60–89 month) follow-up. Circulation 1980; 62:313.

PART II. DISCUSSION

DIETER HORSTKOTTE, MODERATOR

HEMODYNAMIC MEASUREMENTS

BRUCE MINDICH: I have a question for Dr. Gonzalez-Lavin. I was quite surprised by your stunning results in the 17, 19 and 21 mm valve sizes. I routinely measure pressure gradients at the time of surgery and in valves of these sizes, the gradients in the tissue prostheses have always been excessively high. Do you indeed measure gradients at that time or at another time postoperatively?

LORENZO GONZALEZ-LAVIN: We did measure gradients immediately after coming off bypass, but I think that is a bad time to assess them. However, the highest gradient we observed in patients with a small aortic anulus was less than 20 mm. I think we were satisfied.

BRUCE MINDICH: Did you measure cardiac output at the time you were measuring gradients?

LORENZO GONZALEZ-LAVIN: Yes.

STRUT FRACTURES

DIETER HORSTKOTTE: Dr. Doty, the strut failures in the BJÖRK-SHILEY valve group, if I remember right, was cited as 23. In Europe, we already have more than 20 strut fractures; and the FDA recently reported 11 or 12 instances in the month of September. So, I would think 23 is rather low.

DONALD B. DOTY: I do not think the number of strut fractures is truly known, any more than the number of clotted valves. It is very difficult to determine a number because patients who die suddenly may have such a complication without its being identified or reported. What we do know is what gets talked about—like the numbers that you have just cited.

I think these mechanical failures are so dramatic, that most of the time they get reported primarily by word of mouth rather quickly to the manufacturers. You know, everybody likes to bring a failure to the manufacturer's attention. While we say it is a known number, you certainly have to multiply that by some factor; but I do not think it is a factor of 10 or anything like that.

VALVE SUBSTITUTE SELECTION

DIETER HORSTKOTTE: I have a question for all the speakers. What valve do you use and what are your indications for using either a bioprosthesis or a mechanical prosthesis?

JAMES PLUTH: The mechanical valve that we are currently using is the ST. JUDE MEDICAL® valve, unless the patient is on a valve research protocol. For our tissue valve, the preference is still the IONESCU-SHILEY®. We follow these guidelines: the patient who is old or very elderly would be more likely to receive a tissue valve than a ST. JUDE MEDICAL valve so as to avoid the risks of anticoagulation.

DONALD B. DOTY: I do not know how to answer that because we use the IONESCU-SHILEY, the CARPENTIER-EDWARDS®, the STARR-EDWARDS®, the MED-TRONIC HALL™ and the ST. JUDE MEDICAL valves. The decision varies according to soft criteria. If a patient has a small aortic root, we often use a ST. JUDE MEDICAL or MEDTRONIC HALL valve. If there is a very generous mitral anulus and the patient does not wish to consider a reoperation, we will often select the STARR-EDWARDS valve. Tissue valves, obviously, are for patients who cannot tolerate anticoagulation. In that situation, we would use the IONESCU-SHILEY in the aortic position and the CARPEN-TIER-EDWARDS in the mitral position because of the way the valve is constructed.

W.R. ERIC JAMIESON: In Vancouver at both the St. Paul and Vancouver General Hospitals we have 10 surgeons presently doing valve replacements and in 98% of the replacements the CARPENTIER-EDWARDS tissue valve is used. We are evaluating the supra-annular model and this is the only tissue valve that we are using at the present time. In the other 2%, we are using ST. JUDE MEDICAL valves when replacing a tissue valve in adolescents or in some adults with a very small tissue anulus.

LORENZO GONZALEZ-LAVIN: I have been using bioprostheses most of my life. Currently, I am using the IONESCU-SHILEY in the aortic and mitral positions, except when the patient is younger than 17 years of age.

JACK MATLOFF: I hesitate to comment two sessions in a row, but there is something that is bothering me. We have been talking about the issues of valve durability, hemodynamic function and thromboembolism as complications of valvular replacement. What no one has said, but certainly has been implied, is that we have to have a clear time reference for each model. For instance, when we talk about, the BJÖRK-SHILEY valve, the frame of reference that most of us have is not that of the Convexo-Concave models; it is that of the original DELRIN® disk and the initial pyrolytic carbon disk. The Convexo-Concave BJÖRK-SHILEY valve is a new valve. It is even *younger* than the ST. JUDE MEDICAL valve. Bringing out a new valve has always been difficult because of the relative lack of a significant temporal clinical experience. Now, every time a change is made in valve design, presumably to make it better, a new FDA review is in order. I think Dr. Pluth really nailed this down today when he talked about the various models of the STARR-EDWARDS valve: a design change is made in a valve to achieve an improvement, usually to lessen the thromboembolism rate, and almost always this change has resulted in new complications that may take us a while to discover. I think that as we talk about these valves, we have to keep this model change very much in mind, because despite all of the good things we can say about improved hemodynamic function, the fact of the matter is, the reference point is durability over time. We have to understand that although the same name adorns the valve, the model number is a critical issue, which Dr. Rahimtoola mentioned in his first presentation (Chapter 1). We have to constantly keep that in front of us. My comment in not meant to have negative implications for one valve or another; but in the generic sense I want to bring this issue into focus.

One other thing that bothers me is the method of analysis that excludes operative or one-month mortalities and begins with survivors only, or that refers to any end point that excludes mortality. No matter what kind of analysis we carry out, no matter how we define the criteria for that analysis, the one single end point that none of us can argue with is whether the patient lives or dies. I think it is a mistake to totally give that up too quickly in our attempts to better assess survival.

III. CARDIAC VALVE REPLACEMENT IN SPECIAL CIRCUMSTANCES

10. ANNULOAORTIC ECTASIA: SURGICAL REPAIR USING A COMPOSITE ST. JUDE MEDICAL® VALVE AND DACRON® TUBE GRAFT

DENTON A. COOLEY

Annuloaortic ectasia, a term that we coined in 1962 [1], is a disease that includes fusiform aneurysmal dilitation of the aortic sinuses of Valsalva and ascending aorta with aortic regurgitation. The disease has proven to be much more prevalent than previously thought. The enlarged anulus on angiography has the appearance of a Florence flask (as used in the chemistry laboratory). In some instances, the annulo-aortic ectasia is confined to the proximal aortic anulus.

In the classic case, aortic incompetence is produced by stretching of the aortic valve leaflets and displacement of the commissures. The coronary orifices are also displaced upward, making standard valve replacement unsatisfactory. At times, the disease extends into the ascending aorta and transverse arch. Progressive dilation and degeneration of this region of the aorta may result in death from aortic rupture or left ventricular decompensation.

The fundamental defect in the aortic medial lamina is cystic medionecrosis, first described histologically by Erdheim [2]. Necrosis and disappearance of muscle cells occur in the elastic laminae, and there are often cystic spaces filled with a mucoid material. The resulting aneurysm is fusiform, nearly equally affecting all areas of the circumference. Dissection and separation of layers of the aorta are common. Perhaps as a result of the dissection, pericarditis is often seen, particularly adjacent to the aneurysm. Annuloaortic ectasia is frequently present in patients who manifest the clinical symptoms of Marfan's syndrome, but may occur without these findings. The cause of cystic medionecrosis is, as yet, unknown.

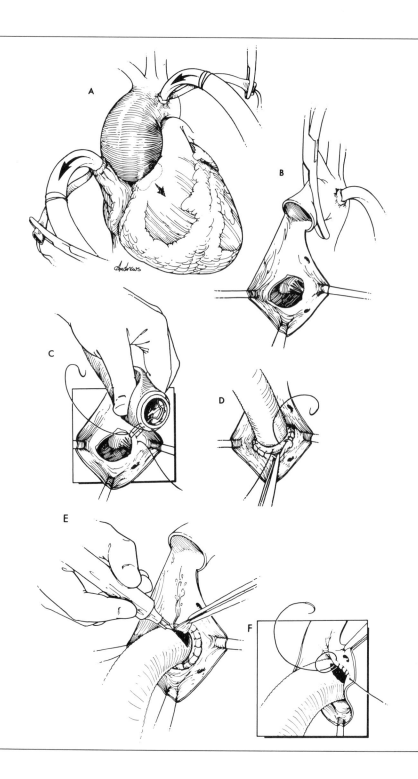

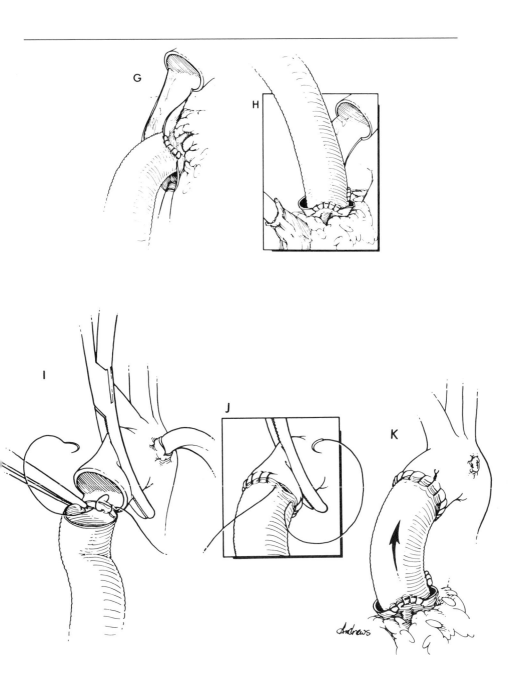

Figure 10-1. Operative technique used for surgical repair of annuloaortic ectasia using a Dacron tube graft and St. Jude Medical valve.

DIAGNOSIS

Diagnosis of ascending aortic aneurysms can be made by many techniques, including echocardiography [3] and computerized axial tomography (CAT) scan [4], but the definitive diagnosis is made by aortography in preparation for surgery. Widened pulse pressure, bounding pulses and an aortic diastolic murmur are usually present. Chest roentgenogram often shows enlargement of the ascending aorta and left ventricle. Most of the aneurysms associated with annuloaortic ectasia are found at examination for patients with symptoms of aortic regurgitation, the most frequent indication for operation. Acute or chronic dissection or rupture of the aneurysm are other indications for surgical therapy and all patients diagnosed should be considered for operation to prevent subsequent rupture.

OPERATIVE TECHNIQUE

Surgical management of annuloaortic ectasia should include total replacement of the aortic sinuses and ascending aorta with a low porosity, woven fabric graft. Replacement of the incompetent aortic valve is necessary, and the coronary ostia must also be reimplanted to maintain myocardial circulation. The conventional method of repair employs a supracoronary graft to replace the aneurysm and a standard valve replacement [5,6]. Since patients with annuloaortic ectasia, however, demonstrate a degenerative process in their aortic wall, operative techniques using supra-aortic anastomosis have been hampered because a residual tongue of possibly abnormal proximal wall is left behind, which has the potential for later aneurysm formation [7–14], dissection [15] or paravalvular leakage [16,17]. In 1968, Bentall and De Bono [18] described a technique that overcame this limitation by employing a conduit composed of a TEFLON® graft and a STARR-EDWARDS® valve. This technique is commonly used today.

Cannulation of the right atrium is done with a large bore tube to provide venous outflow (figure 10-1A). If the patient had a previous operation, drainage is via the pulmonary artery through the right ventricle. Arterial return is made distal to the aneurysm and often in the transverse aortic arch. If a dissection of the arch is encountered, the arterial catheter must be placed in a common femoral or external iliac artery. After cold cardioplegic arrest is obtained, the aneurysm is opened longitudinally on the anterior surface and resected, leaving the posterior portion intact (figure 10-1B). The coronary orifices are identified and are displaced cephalad. The Bentall technique is applicable if the coronary ostia are 2.0 cm or more above the aortic anulus; otherwise, the repair of the aneurysm is made above the ostia using a separate fabric graft and prosthetic valve.

A composite, low-porosity woven DACRON® graft is then preclotted and autoclaved in autologous plasma [19] (figure 10-2). Although other materials such as human albumin and whole blood can be used, we have found that homologous plasma is most impervious and until the FDA approves use of beef collagen (currently under investigation), we will continue to preclot using this material. The graft contains a presewn prosthetic valve that is secured within by a continuous suture of 2-0 or 0 monofilament polypropylene (figures 10-1C and 10-1D). We

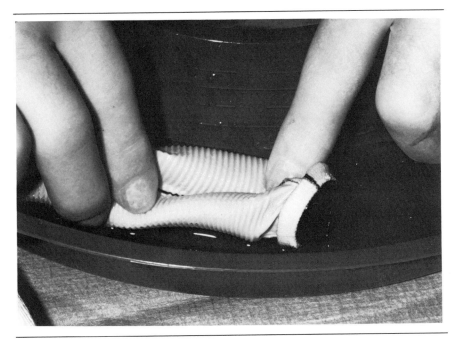

Figure 10-2. Preclotting of composite conduit with homologous plasma prior to autoclaving.

currently use a composite conduit graft prepared by St. Jude Medical (figures 10-3 and 10-4) which is being modified to make the proximal sewing ring impervious by inserting nonporous material prior to covering with velour. The proximal anastomosis of the tube graft and valve is made to the aortic anulus with a running polypropylene suture (figures 10-1C and 10-1D). Disposable, hot cautery is used to make openings in the graft adjacent to the left coronary ostium (figure 10-1E). Wide berth is allowed for the coronary ostium so that no suture would impinge on the coronary lumen. The direct anastomosis is performed with a running 4-0 polypropylene suture with through-and-through bites taken in the aortic wall. A similar anastomosis is performed between the graft and right coronary orifice (figure 10-1F to 10-1H). Following completion of these anastomoses, the graft is trimmed with an appropriate bevel. The distal anastomosis is completed using a 3-0 polypropylene suture, which may be reinforced externally with a wrap of Dacron velour tube graft (figures 10-1I to 10-1J). After air is aspirated from the graft and cardiac action resumes, the cannulae are removed from the right atrium and aortic arch (figure 10-1K).

RESULTS

In a recently reported series from our institution [15], 140 patients underwent repair of ascending aortic aneurysms with concomitant aortic valve replacement from June 1979 to December 1982. Annuloaortic ectasia was the most common

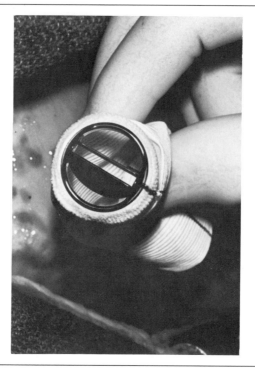

Figure 10-3. Conduit composed of a Dacron tube graft and St. Jude Medical valve after autoclaving.

indication for this operation, occurring in 50.7% (71 out of 140) patients, followed by acute and chronic dissection, which occurred in 33.6% (47 out of 140) patients. Patients undergoing composite replacement with coronary reimplantation were 63.6% (89); and 36.4% (51) had separate graft/valve repair or primary repair of the aneurysm. Hospital mortality for the entire series was 7.9%, with 5.6% of patients having conduit replacements and 13.7% of patients having separate graft/valve repair. Mortality correlated with separate graft/valve repair in patients with annuloaortic ectasia. No patient has required reoperation for conduit malfunction. Of the 89 cases using a valved conduit, there were five hospital deaths, one from stroke, one from arrhythmia, one from multisystem failure and sepsis, one from distal dissection, and one suicide on the third day of his hospitalization.

Because of our satisfactory experience with the ST. JUDE MEDICAL® prosthesis for aortic valve replacement, we requested that a composite graft be designed containing the ST. JUDE MEDICAL valve and a low-porosity, woven MEADOX-COOLEY® graft (figure 10-3). When these prostheses became available recently, we implanted three in patients with annuloaortic ectasia. The functional result was good, as expected. Because of some increased porosity in the standard velour-knitted DACRON sewing ring on the valve prosthesis, some troublesome

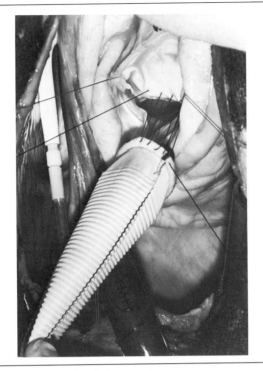

Figure 10-4. Conduit being secured with 2-0 monofilament suture.

bleeding occurred from the proximal suture line. The prosthesis had been treated by autoclaving in autologous plasma, but this was not sufficient to reduce the bleeding from needle holes. Accordingly, new prostheses are being fabricated for our use, in which an additional layer of fabric will be placed in the sewing ring. We anticipate that this modification will make the composite graft containing a ST. JUDE MEDICAL valve a superior product.

In 1983, we replaced the ascending aorta in 40 patients, and in 17 of these we used composite grafts. There was one death from myocardial failure.

CONCLUSION

In degenerative diseases, such as annuloaortic ectasia, conduit repair is usually most effective, because it eliminates the abnormal tissue between the aortic anulus and the distal extent of the aneurysm. The operation can be performed in this subgroup with a very acceptable mortality; morbidity and early results have been very encouraging. Patients experience symptomatic improvement with over 90% of patients asymptomatic or mildly symptomatic (NYHA Functional Class I or II) [9,20]. The separate graft/valve repair, incorporating a separate supracoronary graft, does not eliminate enough diseased aorta and can lead to recurrences below the proximal suture line in patients with cystic medial degenerative changes [15]. The reoperative mortality for these recurrences may be high, generally at 5 to 7 years after operation [12]. Using a composite conduit in this group of patients also eliminates significant bleeding from the anastomotic suture lines. Operative time has been reduced, and adequate cardiac function has been maintained postoperatively.

SUMMARY

Based on our experience, aneurysms should be excised completely in patients with annuloaortic ectasia when it extends into the sinuses of Valsalva. Reimplantation of the coronary arteries should not increase the incidence of postoperative hemorrhage. I do not believe, however, that it is necessary to reimplant the coronary ostia in patients with a normal anulus. When the coronary ostia are not elevated cephalad, a supracoronary anastomosis can be done. Thus, unless the coronary orifices are at least 2 cm above the anulus, we do not reimplant them.

REFERENCES

1. Ellis PR Jr, Cooley DA, DeBakey ME: Clinical considerations and surgical treatment of annuloaortic ectasia. J Thorac Cardiovasc Surg 1961; 42:363–370.
2. Erdheim J: Medionecrosis aortae idiopathica. Virchows Arch Pathol Anat 1959; 273:454–479.
3. DeMaria AN, Bommer W, Neumann A, et al: Identification and localization of aneurysms of the ascending aorta by cross-sectional echocardiography. Circulation 1979; 59:755–761.
4. Sanders JH, Molove S, Nieman HL, et al: Thoracic aortic imaging without angiography. Arch Surg 1979; 114:1326–1329.
5. Groves LK, Effler DB, Hawk WA, et al: Aortic insufficiency secondary to aneurysmal changes in the ascending aorta. Surgical management. J Thorac Cardiovasc Surg 1964; 48:362–379.
6. Wheat MW, Wilson JR, Bartley TD: Successful replacement of the entire ascending aorta and aortic valve. JAMA 1964; 188:717–719.
7. Cabrol C, Pavie A, Gandjbakhch I, et al: Complete replacement of the ascending aorta with reimplantation of the coronary arteries. New surgical approach. J Thorac Cardiovasc Surg 1981; 81:309–315.
8. Mayer JE, Lindsay WG, Wang T, et al: Composite replacement of the aortic valve and ascending aorta. J Thorac Cardiovasc Surg 1978; 76:816–823.
9. Kouchoukos NT, Karp RB, Blackstone EH, et al: Replacement of the ascending aorta and aortic valve with a composite graft. Results in eighty-six patients. Ann Surg 1980; 192:403–413.
10. Symbas PN, Baldwin BJ, Silverman ME, et al: Marfan's syndrome with aneurysm of ascending aorta and aortic regurgitation: Surgical treatment and new histochemical observations. Am J Cardiol 1970; 25:483–489.
11. Symbas PN, Raizner AE, Tyras DH, et al: Aneurysms of all sinuses of Valsalva in patients with Marfan's syndrome: An unusual late complication following replacement of aortic valve and ascending aorta for aortic regurgitation and fusiform aneurysm of ascending aorta. Ann Surg 1971; 174:902–907.
12. McCready RA, Pluth JR: Surgical treatment of aortic aneurysms associated with aortic insufficiency. Ann Thorac Surg 1979; 28:307–317.
13. Egloff L, Rothlin M, Kugelmeier J, et al: The ascending aortic aneurysm. Replacement or repair? Ann Thorac Surg 1982; 34:117–124.
14. Borst HG: Replacing the ascending aorta and aortic valve. Ann Thorac Surg 1981; 32:613–614.
15. Grey DP, Ott DA, Cooley DA: Surgical treatment of aneurysm of the ascending aorta with aortic insufficiency. J Thorac Cardiovasc Surg 1983; 86:864–877.
16. Miller DC, Stinson EB, Oyer PE, et al: Concomitant resection of ascending aortic aneurysm and replacement of the aortic valve. J Thorac Cardiovasc Surg 1980; 79:388–401.

17. Davis Z, Pluth JR, Giuliani ER: The Marfan syndrome and cardiac surgery. J Thorac Cardiovasc Surg 1978; 75:505–509.
18. Bentall H, De Bono A: A technique for complete replacement of the ascending aorta. Thorax 1968; 23:338–339.
19. Cooley DA, Romagnoli A, Milam JD: A method of preparing woven Dacron grafts to prevent interstitial hemorrhage. Cardiovasc Dis Bull Tex Heart Inst 1981; 8:48–52.
20. Helseth HK, Haglin JJ, Monson BK, et al: Results of composite graft replacement for aortic root aneurysms. J Thorac Cardiovasc Surg 1980; 80:754–759.

11. VALVE REPLACEMENT IN THE GERIATRIC PATIENT USING THE ST. JUDE MEDICAL® PROSTHESIS

DEMETRE M. NICOLOFF, WILLIAM G. LINDSAY, KIT V. AROM, WILLIAM F. NORTHRUP, III, THOMAS E. KERSTEN

Abstract. The results of valve replacement with the ST. JUDE MEDICAL® prosthesis in three age groups are compared. Six hundred and eighty patients underwent 735 valve replacements. Operative mortality for the entire group of patients was 6.6%. Patients were divided into three groups: Group I = < 60 years of age, Group II = 60 to 69 years and Group III = 70+ years. Operative mortality for each group was: Group I = 5%, Group II = 5% and Group III = 11.5%. Late mortality for the entire group was 7.7%. Late mortality for each group was: Group I = 5%, Group II = 7% and Group III = 12.5%. The incidence of thromboembolism and permanent major sequelae was not higher in Group III following aortic valve replacement (AVR), but was higher following mitral valve replacement (MVR). Survival at 6 years for the entire group was 86%. Six year survival for each group was: Group I = 90.5%, Group II = 88% and Group III = 77%. Operative and late mortality was markedly higher in Group III patients following these procedures: AVR + miscellaneous, MVR + coronary artery bypass (CAB) and MVR + miscellaneous. The ST. JUDE MEDICAL prosthesis is associated with satisfactory short-term and long-term results in the geriatric age group.

INTRODUCTION

Use of prosthetic valves to replace severely diseased cardiac valves has been an accepted mode of therapy for over 20 years. Considerable change in valve design and construction has occurred over this time period. During the last 10 years, several mechanical and bioprosthetic valve designs have become available. Many papers have been written on the pros and cons of each type of valve substitute, with a variety of recommendations on the appropriate choice for a given patient.

Age of the patient is often used as a major factor in deciding which valve substitute to select. Important information to have when selecting a valve for the geriatric age group would be whether or not there is a higher operative and late mortality in this age group and whether valve-related complications dictate the need for anticoagulation.

The purpose of this study is to compare the results of valve replacement with the ST. JUDE MEDICAL prosthesis in three age groups: Group I = < 60 years; Group II = 60 to 69 years; Group III = 70+ years (geriatric). Operative and late mortality and incidence of thromboembolic and hemorrhagic complications are compared.

PATIENT MATERIAL

From October 3, 1977 to October 3, 1983, 680 patients had 735 cardiac valves replaced with ST. JUDE MEDICAL prostheses. Ages ranged from 6 months to 87 years. The surgical technique was similar in all patients and utilized interrupted 2-0 DACRON® everting mattress sutures for implantation. TEFLON® felt pledgets were used if indicated by anatomic findings at surgery. Postoperatively, all patients were advised to maintain their prothrombin time at 1.5 to 2 times the control value with COUMADIN®. Follow-up was for a minimum of 6 months and a maximum of 6 years. All but 33 patients were contacted by questionnaire or phone interview resulting in a 95% follow-up.

The number of patients by group are: Group I = 254 (37.3%); Group II = 246 (36.2%); Group III = 180 (26.5%). Distribution of patients by sex and type of procedure is shown in table 11-1. Note there are more males than females in Group I and in Groups II and III the number is equal. Isolated AVR was performed more frequently in males in Group I and in Groups II and III, the distribution for that procedure was equal. When CAB was performed with AVR, the male

Table 11-1. Number of patients by group, procedure and sex (male/female)

	Group I	Group II	Group III	Total
AVR	69/22	38/29	31/29	218
AVR and CAB	16/1	39/13	42/18	129
AVR and misc	6/1	1/3	1/2	14
MVR	32/60	16/49	7/14	178
MVR and CAB	11/5	21/17	8/9	71
MVR and misc	3/6	0/3	0/3	15
DVR	5/15	4/6	3/7	40
DVR and CAB	0/0	3/4	3/2	12
DVR and misc	0/2	0/0	0/1	3
Total	142/112	122/124	95/85	680

predominance remained in all three age groups. Isolated MVR was more commonly done in females in all three age groups. MVR + CAB was performed more frequently in males in Group I but was performed in males and females equally in Groups II and III.

Isolated AVR was performed more frequently in Group I and equally in Groups II and III. When CAB was combined with AVR, most procedures were done in Groups II and III, with Group III being the largest group. Isolated MVR was performed most frequently in Group I with Group III being the smallest group. MVR + CAB was done most frequently in Group II with Groups I and III being equal in size. Double valve replacement (DVR) was most frequent in Group I with Groups II and III being equal. DVR + CAB was performed only in Groups II and III.

The number of coronary artery bypass grafts done in each age group with AVR, MVR and DVR is shown in table 11-2. Coronary artery bypass was performed in 36% (129) of patients with AVR. In Groups II and III, approximately 50% of patients had concomitant CAB procedures done, but in Group I this was only 14%. The number of patients with multiple grafts was the same in Groups II and III. Coronary artery bypass was performed in 27% (71) of patients having MVR. Groups I and III were equal in number of patients having MVR + CAB, with Group II having twice as many. CAB was performed in 45% of Group III patients and 36% of Group II patients. Multiple graft procedures were performed more frequently in Group II. CAB + DVR was performed in 12 patients in Groups II and III.

RESULTS

Operative mortality

Overall operative mortality for the entire group was 6.6%. Operative mortality for each group is shown in figure 11-1. In Groups I and II it was 5%; and for Group III it was 11.5%. The risk of valve replacement is slightly more than two times greater in patients over 70 years of age; being 60 to 69 years of age does not carry a higher risk than being < 60 years of age.

However, significant differences in operative mortality among the age groups occurs, depending on the operative procedure performed. Operative mortality for isolated AVR is 10% for Group III and 1.2% for Groups I and II. There is no

Table 11-2. Number of patients undergoing coronary artery bypass surgery (CAB) with valve replacement by group

	Group I	Group II	Group III	Total
AVR and CAB	17	52	60	129
MVR and CAB	16	38	17	71
DVR and CAB	0	7	5	12

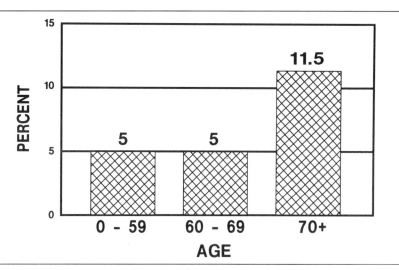

Figure 11-1. Overall operative mortality for each age group.

difference in the three groups when AVR is combined with CAB. When AVR and MVR are combined with miscellaneous procedures (closure of ventricular septal defect, resection of left ventricular aneurysm, replacement of ascending aorta) operative mortality increases two to threefold in Group III patients. MVR + CAB carries a sixfold increase in operative mortality in Group III patients. The only operative mortality in DVR patients occurred in Group III patients.

Predominant causes of operative mortality are given in figure 11-2. The majority

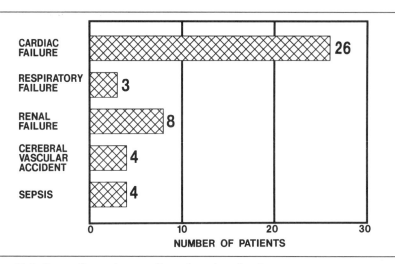

Figure 11-2. Causes of operative mortality and number of patients per cause.

of deaths were due to cardiac failure or low cardiac output (26 patients). Respiratory failure (13), renal failure (8), cerebrovascular accident (4) and sepsis (4) accounted for the other deaths. Approximately one-half of operative deaths occurred in Group III patients. The remainder of deaths occurred equally in Groups I and II. None of the deaths were due to valve malfunction.

Late mortality

Overall late mortality for the entire group was 7.7%. Overall late mortality of the three groups is given in figure 11-3: Group I = 5%, Group II = 7% and Group III = 12.5%. Late mortality for Group III is approximately twice that of the other two groups. AVR + miscellaneous procedures, which had a high operative mortality rate in Group III patients, also had a very high late mortality. Late mortality of isolated MVR in Group III patients was 5 times that of Groups I and II. There was no late mortality for MVR + CAB in Group III patients, but the operative mortality for this same group was quite high. Late mortality for MVR + miscellaneous and DVR for Group II was 3 to 4 times that of the other two groups.

Thromboembolism

A large number of patients had anticoagulation discontinued because of major trauma or subsequent surgical procedures. The incidence of thromboembolism per patient-year for all AVR and MVR patients with or without CAB, is given in figure 11-4. The incidence of thromboembolism in Group III (1.1%) following AVR is slightly less than for Groups I (1.3%) and II (1.7%). Following MVR the incidence of thromboembolism is 3 times higher in Group III (4%) than in

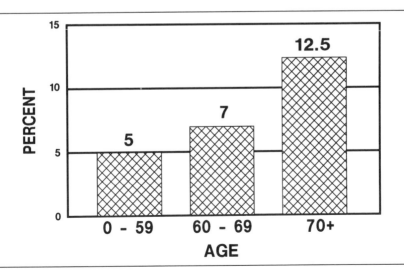

Figure 11-3. Overall late mortality for each age group.

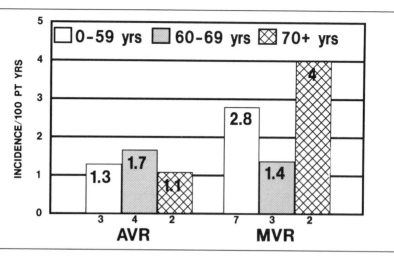

Figure 11-4. Incidence of thromboemboli for each age group following valve replacement. Number below bar is the number of patients.

Group II (1.4%) and 1.5 times higher than in Group I (2.8%). The incidence of permanent major sequelae following embolization for the three groups is given in figure 11-5. For Group III patients, it was 0.5% per patient-year (AVR) and 2.0% per patient-year (MVR). The incidence of thromboembolism in MVR patients is highest in Group III.

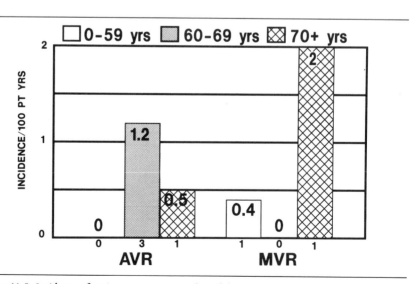

Figure 11-5. Incidence of major permanent sequelae of thromboemboli in each age group. Number below bar is the number of patients.

HEMORRHAGIC COMPLICATIONS

A major complication of anticoagulation is excessive bleeding or hemorrhage. All instances of easy bruising, melena, hemoptysis, hematemesis, hematuria and cerebrovascular hemorrhage were considered a complication of anticoagulation. The incidence of bleeding for each group by valve procedure is given in figure 11-6. The incidence in Group III following AVR (0.2%) is less than in Groups I (4.3%) and II (5%). Following MVR, Group III patients have a higher incidence of bleeding (4%) with Groups I and II being nearly equal (1.7%, 1.9% respectively). No significant bleeding problems occurred in Groups II and III following DVR.

SURVIVAL RATE

The survival rate at 6 years for the entire group was 86%: Group I = 90.5%; Group II = 88% and Group III = 77%. However, there is a significant difference between the groups, by procedure (figure 11-7). For all procedures, Group III patients do not survive as well as patients in Groups I and II. This decreased survival rate is more marked following MVR, MVR + CAB, MVR + miscellaneous and AVR + miscellaneous.

DISCUSSION

Overall operative and late mortality in the geriatric age group (Group III) is 2 to 3 times greater than that of the other age groups. There was little difference between Groups I and II. Group III had a higher incidence of CAB procedures combined with valve replacement and also had a large number of complex procedures, such as closure of ventricular septal defect, resection of left ventricular

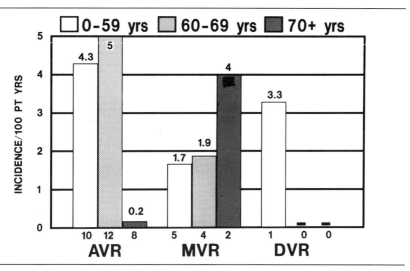

Figure 11-6. Incidence of bleeding complications in each age group. Number below bar is number of patients.

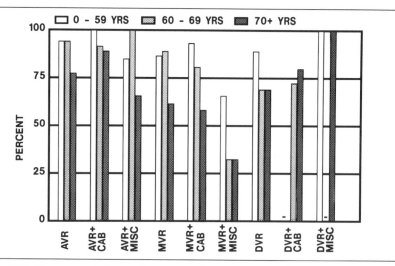

Figure 11-7. Six-year survival for each age group by operative procedure.

aneurysm and/or resection of ascending aortic aneurysm. Isolated AVR in Group III was evenly divided between females and males, but in Group I the patients were predominantly male. In Group III approximately 50% had AVR + CAB and 40% had MVR + CAB, both male and female.

For Group III patients, operative (11.5%) and late (12.5%) mortality was not prohibitive. However, because mortality can be quite high for some procedures, the recommendation for certain procedures in the geriatric group may be questioned.

Following AVR, the incidence of bleeding complications, thromboembolism and permanent major sequelae was not higher in Group III patients. Following MVR, there was a higher incidence of thromboembolism and permanent major sequelae in Group III patients. For an unknown reason, the incidence of bleeding complications was also higher in this group; but it was not in the AVR group. Whether this was due to a higher level of anticoagulation is not clear.

Even though there was a higher incidence of thromboembolism and hemorrhagic complications in this group of geriatric patients, when compared to the other 2 groups, it should not prohibit the use of the ST. JUDE MEDICAL prosthesis. Continued follow-up, however, will be necessary to determine whether the ST. JUDE MEDICAL valve should be used in patients over 70 years of age who require mitral valve replacement. Patients requiring AVR or DVR in the geriatric age group do as well with the ST. JUDE MEDICAL prosthesis as do patients less than 70 years old.

12. TRICUSPID VALVE REPLACEMENT—A COMPARATIVE EXPERIENCE WITH DIFFERENT VALVE SUBSTITUTES

FRANCIS WELLENS, JEAN-LOUIS LECLERC, F. DEUVAERT, G. VAN NOOTEN, J. GOLDSTEIN, G. PRIMO

INTRODUCTION

The need for tricuspid valve surgery remains a difficult problem for the cardiac surgeon. Conservative repair is always preferable in the treatment of tricuspid valve disease, but tricuspid valve replacement (TVR) is a necessity in some cases.

The choice of a valve substitute is difficult, mainly because of the high rate of prosthetic valve dysfunction and thrombotic occlusions of ball and disc valves in the tricuspid position [1–3].

In order to evaluate whether or not these adverse consequences could be moderated by use of the ST. JUDE MEDICAL® valve in the tricuspid position, we updated our experience with TVR, using several valve substitutes.

PATIENTS AND METHODS

Between January 1967 and December 1981, 93 patients underwent tricuspid annuloplasty (TA) and 143 patients had TVR. During this period, 1442 patients had a single or combined mitral valve replacement (MVR) and 289 had a mitral commissurotomy (MC). From 1967 until 1975 Kay-Shiley (KS), BJÖRK-SHILEY® (BS) and Smeloff-Cutter (SC) prostheses were implanted. HANCOCK® (H) and CARPENTIER-EDWARDS® (CE) porcine heterografts were used from 1975 until 1980 and the ST. JUDE MEDICAL prosthesis (SJM) was used from January 1979 to December 1981 (table 12-1).

Minimum follow-up was 2 years. Follow-up data were provided by clinical

Table 12-1. Number and types of prostheses implanted in the tricuspid position from 1967 to 1981

Period	Group I (mechanical)	Group II (bioprosthesis)	Group III (mechanical)
1967–1975	Kay-Shiley, 25 Björk-Shiley, 24 Smeloff-Cutter, 27		
1975–1980		Hancock, 29 Carpentier-Edwards, 34	
1979–1981			St. Jude Medical, 16
Reoperation	Smeloff-Cutter, 4 St. Jude Medical, 2	Carpentier-Edwards, 1	

examination at regular intervals in the outpatient clinic or by the referring cardiologist or family physician. Two patients were lost to follow-up.

RESULTS

Of the patients admitted for TVR, 98% were New York Heart Association (NYHA) Class III or IV. Previous valve surgery had been performed in 40% of the patients. Organic lesions accounted for 59% and functional lesions, for 41%. Early mortality was 15% for single TVR, 20% for double valve replacement (DVR) and 14% for triple valve replacement.

Follow-up data on patients by type of prosthesis implanted are summarized in table 12-2. Extensive data on patients KS, BS, SC, H and CE valves have been published previously [4].

St. Jude Medical valve experience

The 16 patients with tricuspid SJM implants all presented with severe valvular heart disease: 5 were Class III and 11 were Class IV. Eight patients had previous cardiac surgery: 1 patient underwent pericardiectomy for chronic constrictive pericarditis, 4 patients had 1 of 2 prior mitral commissurotomies and 3 others had DVR (2 MVR + TVR, 1 MVR + AVR). Seven patients had organic tricuspid lesions, 8 had functional lesions and 1 patient presented with prosthetic dysfunction (SC).

In the early postoperative period, 2 patients (13%) died due to low cardiac output. Both presented with preoperative end stage mitral valve disease and severe pulmonary hypertension. All patients received COUMADIN® 48 to 72 hours postoperatively. Total follow-up of the survivors was 517 months (mean 37 months). There were 3 late deaths at 8, 24 and 36 months postoperatively. One patient died after fulminant prosthetic endocarditis. Another patient died from an acute tricuspid valve thrombosis while on IV heparin, after COUMADIN therapy had been discontinued prior to elective cholecystectomy. The third patient died

Table 12-2. Data on patients with tricuspid valve replacement by type of prosthesis implanted

Type of prosthesis	Patient number	Early death	Late death	Survivors	Patient months follow-up	Lost to follow-up	Number of prostheses implanted	Valve months of follow-up
Group I								
Kay-Shiley	15	2	12	1	1039		15	885
Björk-Shiley	24	4	7	12	1966		24	1798
Smeloff-Cutter	27	7	13	8	1481		31	1624
Group II								
Hancock	29	6	6	17	1557	1	29	1557
Carpentier-Edwards	34	3	6	25	1580	1	35	1580
Group III								
St. Jude Medical	14	2	3	11	511		16	511

Table 12-3. Causes of late death

Cause	KS	BS	SJM	SC	H	CE
Myocardial failure	4	1	1	6	3	4
Arrhythmia	1			3		
Cerebral embolism	1	1		1	2	
Tricuspid valve thrombosis	3	3	1	3		
Hemorrhage (AC)		1				1
Prosthetic endocarditis	1		1			
Noncardiac					1	1
Not documented	2	1				
Total	12	7	3	13	6	6

(KS = Kay-Shiley; BS = Björk-Shiley; SJM = St. Jude Medical; SC = Smeloff-Cutter; H = Hancock; CE = Carpentier-Edwards; AC = Anticoagulants)

from low cardiac output; tricuspid valve thrombosis was suspected, but autopsy data were not available. There were no left-sided thromboembolic complications and only 3 minor hemorrhagic events occurred during the follow-up period.

Causes of late death and the incidence of late tricuspid valve thrombosis, related to the type of prosthesis used in the tricuspid position, for the whole series are summarized in table 12-3. Thrombosis was confirmed by autopsy, reoperation or angiography (1 patient). The annual incidence of valvular thrombosis per patient-year was: KS = 4.0%; BS = 2.7%; SC = 6.7%; CE = 0%; and H = 0.8%. In the most recent series with SJM prostheses, the thrombosis rate was 2.3% per patient-year. Actuarial survival and actuarial probability of freedom from tricuspid valve thrombosis for each type of valve substitute implanted are plotted in Figures 12-1 and 12-2.

DISCUSSION

From our previous study [4] we drew the conclusion that the behavior of a bioprosthesis in the tricuspid position was much better up to 7 years than for the KS, BS and SC prostheses. Being aware of the possibility of tissue valve degeneration even in the tricuspid position and in view of our excellent results with the SJM valve in the mitral position [5], 16 SJM prostheses were used in the tricuspid position and reviewed after a minimum follow-up of 2 years.

Early mortality in the SJM group did not differ from the other valve groups and is completely independent of the year of implantation, in spite of improvements in techniques of myocardial protection and perioperative and postoperative care. This experience reflects the very advanced functional status of the patient population undergoing tricuspid valve surgery and underscores how the preoperative functional class dramatically influences perioperative mortality. Such a conclusion was also reached by Stiles and Kirklin [6].

However, in contrast to early mortality, late survival was clearly influenced by the valve substitute implanted (figure 12-1). The 5-year survival for the SJM group

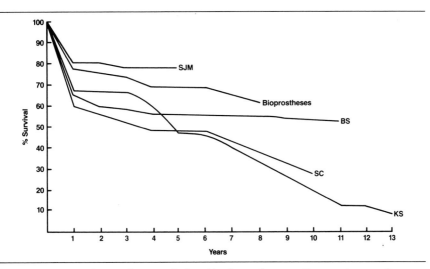

Figure 12-1. Actuarial survival curve of tricuspid valve replacement for several types of prostheses. (KS = Kay-Shiley; BS = Björk-Shiley; SC = Smeloff-Cutter; CE = Carpentier-Edwards; H = Hancock; SJM = St. Jude Medical)

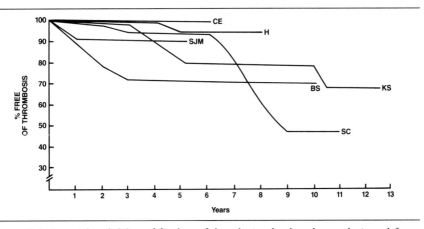

Figure 12-2. Actuarial probability of freedom of thrombosis related to the prosthesis used for tricuspid valve replacement.

was nearly 80%, although the confidence limits are large, and was comparable to the late survival of the bioprostheses group. Five-year survival of the KS, BS and SC valve groups was much lower (47%, 57% and 48%, respectively). This long-term survival is influenced by the high incidence of valve thrombosis (table 12-4), which was often fatal.

With the BS prosthesis, thrombosis occurred relatively early and was most often acute. The SC prosthesis was more often subject to late thrombosis and formation

Table 12-4. Incidence of late tricuspid valve thrombosis by type of prosthesis implanted

Valve type	No. valves at risk	Thrombosis		Mortality	Reoperation	Incidence of thrombosis (% per years of follow-up)
		Acute	Pannus			
Group I						
KS	13	1	2	2	1	4.0%
BS	20	4	0	2	2	2.7%
SC	23	1	8	5	3	6.7%
Group II						
H	24	1	0	0	1	0.8%
CE	28	0	0	0	0	0.0%
Total Group II	54	1	0	0	1	0.4%
Group III						
SJM	14	1	0	1	0	2.3%

of obstructing pannus. In contrast, the bioprosthesis group remains relatively free from valve thrombosis, with only one documented event up to 8 years. The recently implanted SJM valve did not remain free of this complication, in spite of its theoretical advantages of low profile, small size and low thrombogenicity due to central, laminar flow and very low transvalvular gradients [7]. One documented thrombotic event nevertheless occurred when COUMADIN therapy was switched to intravenous heparin for elective abdominal surgery.

Fluoroscopy is an effective noninvasive technique for the evaluation of SJM valve function. In view of the difficulty of assessing adequate tricuspid prosthetic function, fluoroscopy and echocardiography are routinely advocated for the SJM prosthesis at 6-month intervals and after periods of uncertain anticoagulant therapy.

CONCLUSION

Early experience with the SJM valve for tricuspid valve replacement is very encouraging in comparison with other mechanical prostheses used in that position. Five-year survival is very acceptable for the small number of patients at that interval, and this favorable trend will have to be confirmed by a longer follow-up period.

The behavior of the CARPENTIER-EDWARDS and HANCOCK bioprostheses, in terms of survival and incidence of valve thrombosis up to 8 years remains excellent.

Although the SJM valve is the valve of choice in our department (1400 SJM prostheses from October 1977 to December 1983) for mitral and aortic implantation, we currently continue to use a bioprosthesis whenever a tricuspid valve replacement is necessary.

REFERENCES

1. Bourdillon PDV, Sharratt GP: Malfunction of Björk-Shiley valve prosthesis in tricuspid position. Br Heart J 1976; 38:1149.
2. Peterfy A, Henze A, Savidfe GF, et al: Late thrombotic malfunction of the Björk-Shiley tilting disc valve in the tricuspid position: Principles for recognition and management. Scand J Thorac Cardiovasc Surg 1980; 14:33.
3. Jugdutt BI, Fraser RS, Lee SJK, et al: Long term survival after tricuspid valve replacement: Results with seven different prostheses. J Thorac Cardiovasc Surg 1977; 74:20.
4. Wellens F, Van Dale P, Deuvaert F, et al: The role of porcine heterografts in a 14 year experience with tricuspid valve replacement, in Cohn LH, Callucci V (eds): *Cardiac Bioprostheses,* New York, Yorke Medical Books, 1982, pp 502–515.
5. LeClerc JL, Wellens F, Deuvaert F, et al: Long term results with the St. Jude Medical valve, in DeBakey ME (ed): *Advances in Cardiac Valves: Clinical Perspectives,* New York, Yorke Medical Books, 1983, pp 33–40.
6. Stiles GE, Kirklin JW: Myocardial preservation symposium. J Thorac Cardiovasc Surg 1981; 82:870–877.
7. Bowen TE, Tri TB, Wortham DC: Thrombosis of a St. Jude Medical tricuspid prosthesis: Case report. J Thorac Cardiovasc Surg 1981; 82:257.

13. DOUBLE VALVE REPLACEMENT

RICHARD J. GRAY, LAWRENCE S. C. CZER, AURELIO CHAUX, TIMOTHY M. BATEMEN, MICHELE DEROBERTIS, JACK M. MATLOFF

Compared to single valve replacement, combined aortic and mitral replacement represents a major technical challenge, as it theoretically increases the possibility of early and late valve-related complications and is usually performed in the setting of the myocardial dysfunction of chronic multivalvular heart disease. The entire experience with 121 patients undergoing double valve replacement (DVR) at Cedars-Sinai Medical Center between 1969 and 1982 forms the basis of this report.

PATIENT POPULATION
The average age of the patients was 58 ± 13 years (mean $\pm$ standard deviation, range 22 to 81); 42% of whom were male. Preoperatively, 96% were either NYHA Class III or IV. Rheumatic heart disease was the most common etiology (86%), with myxomatous degeneration in 6% of patients; the remaining 8% had endocarditis, prosthetic valve dysfunction or ischemic mitral valve disease. The physiologic abnormality of the mitral valve was predominantly mitral stenosis in 16%, mitral regurgitation in 30%, and mixed stenosis and regurgitation in 54%; that of the aortic valve was stenosis in 11%, regurgitation in 39% and mixed in 50%.

Additional cardiac surgical procedures were performed on 35 patients (29%). Ten underwent tricuspid annuloplasty; 1 patient had left ventricular aneurysmectomy; and another had repair of a localized aortic root dissection. Coronary disease, as defined by the presence of $\geq 50\%$ diameter reduction in one or more vessels, was present in 26 patients. Single vessel disease was present in 10; double vessel in 6; triple vessel in 7; and left main disease in 3. Concomitant coronary artery bypass grafting was performed in 23 patients (19% of the entire cohort). Of these, coronary bypass grafting was incidental in 11 (9%) but was performed in response to severe angina pectoris or a strongly positive exercise treadmill test in 12 (10%).

Several types of *mitral* valve prostheses were employed, including the HANCOCK® standard orifice porcine valve (38%), the ST. JUDE MEDICAL® bileaflet prosthesis (31%), the Harken caged disc valve (24%) and the CARPENTIER-EDWARDS® porcine valve (6%). The choice of *aortic* prostheses included the ST. JUDE MEDICAL valve in 32%, the BJÖRK-SHILEY® spherical in 27%, the HANCOCK bioprosthesis in 20%, the Cutter-Smeloff in 13%, the CARPENTIER-EDWARDS bioprosthesis in 6% and the Harken caged-ball valve in 2%.

DATA COLLECTION AND FOLLOW-UP PROCEDURES

Preoperative variables studied include age, sex, NYHA classification, cardiac rhythm, type of valve lesion (stenosis, regurgitation or mixed), presence of coronary artery disease, stroke volume index, use of intra-aortic balloon pump, left ventricular ejection fraction and left ventricular end-diastolic volume index. Technically adequate left ventriculograms were available in 118 of 121 patients. Preoperative left ventricular ejection fraction was $62 \pm 16\%$, and left ventricular end-diastolic volume index was $120 \pm 53 \ cc/m^2$.

Operative variables examined were the use of cardioplegia and/or hypothermia, the type of aortic and mitral prosthesis employed, the performance of coronary bypass surgery, the intraoperative need for intra-aortic balloon counterpulsation, the concomitant performance of other cardiac surgical procedures and the year in which surgery was performed.

Follow-up ranged from 1 to 11 years with an average of 33 months. Follow-up data were available on 97% of the cohort. We found that 65% of the patients were alive, and 30% had died. Three patients had subsequently undergone reoperation and because of that fact were not entered in this analysis. Follow-up was conducted by means of yearly questionnaires supplemented by telephone interviews and in many cases, by personal office visit and physical examination.

RESULTS

Mortality

Early ($\leq$ 30 days) mortality was 9.1% overall and late mortality was 21%. Figure 13-1 shows the long-term survival for DVR compared to all single aortic (dotted line) and single mitral (solid line) valve recipients at this institution during the same time period. Although there is no significant difference between the actuarial curves of these three groups, the trend suggests that the outcome of DVR and mitral valve replacement (MVR) is similar and both are poorer than for the single aortic valve patients. DVR survival at 7 years is 53%.

The causes of the 34 deaths in our patients were classified as cardiac, nonvalve related in 23 (69%). This designation included congestive heart failure, cardiac

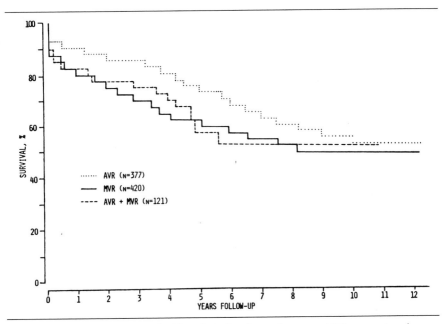

Figure 13-1. Survival following double and single valve replacement. AVR = aortic valve replacement; MVR = mitral valve replacement; AVR & MVR = double valve replacement.

pump failure, myocardial infarction and sudden cardiac death thought to be due to arrhythmia. Cardiac, valve-related deaths occurred in 7 patients (20%) and included cerebral vascular accident (CVA), COUMADIN®-induced hemorrhage, bacterial endocarditis and prosthetic dysfunction. Noncardiac deaths occurred in 3 (8%) and included trauma, cancer and combined respiratory and renal failure. The cause of death was classified as unknown in 1 patient (3%).

Preoperative variables were examined for their ability to predict a poor outcome. Age, sex, the physiological type of valve lesion and coexistence of coronary atherosclerosis (symptomatic in only 10% of patients) were not important factors. In descending order of importance, we found that the results were adversely affected by: the year surgery was performed (before or after 1978); the performance of tricuspid annuloplasty; preoperative NYHA Class IV (figure 13-2); preoperative atrial fibrillation (figure 13-3) and the preoperative use of intra-aortic balloon counterpulsation. Although the numbers were small, the performance of complex procedures, i.e., beyond DVR, also adversely affected outcome (figure 13-4). While the difference between the two curves in figure 13-3 is statistically significant, the biologic and/or clinical difference is greatest during the early postoperative period (≤ 30 days). In this series of patients, 53% were in atrial fibrillation preoperatively compared to 39% at late follow-up. Parenthetically, 6% of patients required a permanent pacemaker implantation after surgery.

As might be suspected, left ventricular function also played a prominent role

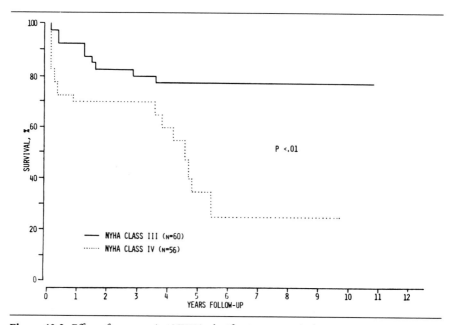

Figure 13-2. Effect of preoperative NYHA classification on survival.

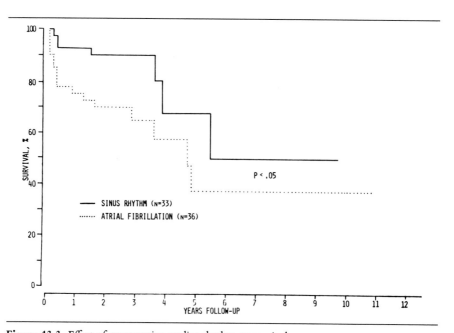

Figure 13-3. Effect of preoperative cardiac rhythm on survival.

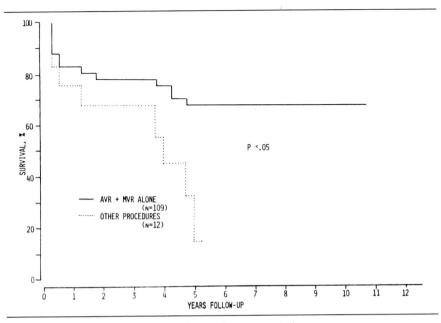

Figure 13-4. Effect of additional surgical procedures on survival.

in predicting long-term outcome (figure 13-5). Figure 13-5A shows the actuarial status of patients with varying ventricular function as determined by ejection fraction. There is both an immediate and long-term effect on survival in patients whose ejection fraction is below 45% compared to those above that level. In figure 13-5B patients are subgrouped with ejection fraction above 55%, between 35% and 55%, and below 35%. From this distribution it can be seen that the adverse effect on survival is noted predominantly in patients whose ejection fraction is below 35%. The impact on survival of an enlarged left ventricular end–diastolic volume is shown in figure 13-6. Here it can be seen that the outcome in those patients whose end–diastolic left ventricular volume index is larger than 150 cc/m² is worse than in those patients with smaller left ventricular volumes.

Several intraoperative variables potentially affecting survival were also examined. The year surgery was performed affected 30-day survivorship; early mortality in the 70 patients operated between 1969 and 1978 is 14% in contrast to 2% for the 51 patients operated since 1978. While this difference could be due to a number of factors, two potentially important explanations emerge. First, in 1978 we began to use moderate hypothermia and potassium cardioplegia, whereas prior to that time, intermittent cross-clamping with ischemic arrest and mild to moderate hypothermia had been used. Second, the type of prosthesis used in the majority of cases changed. In March 1978 we began to use the ST. JUDE MEDICAL prosthesis, and its use grew rapidly throughout the latter part of 1978 and 1979.

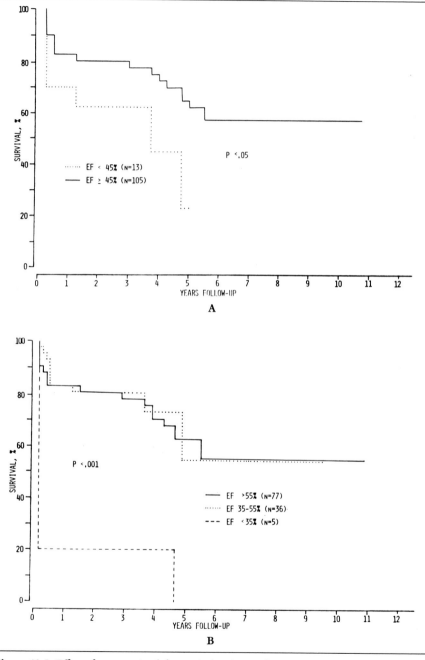

Figure 13-5. Effect of preoperative left ventricular ejection fraction on survival. EF = ejection fraction.

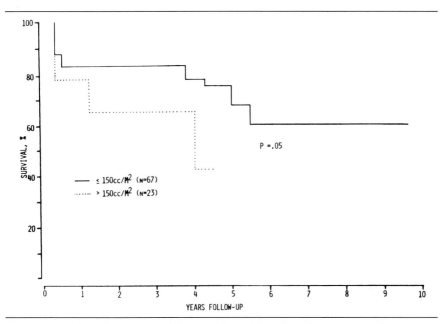

Figure 13-6. Effect of preoperative left ventricular end-diastolic volume on survival.

Figure 13-7 shows the actuarial data on patients depending on what type of aortic prosthesis (panel A) and what type of mitral prosthesis (panel B) was implanted. It appears that in the case of both aortic and mitral prostheses, use of the ST. JUDE MEDICAL valve was associated with a statistically better survival than that of patients receiving either the HANCOCK or CARPENTIER-EDWARDS bioprosthesis or the BJÖRK-SHILEY valve. No difference in outcome between the recipients of aortic bioprostheses or BJÖRK-SHILEY valves is discernible. In panel B however, it is apparent that patients receiving mitral bioprostheses had better long-term survival than patients receiving the mitral Harken valve. It should be pointed out however, that the use of the Harken valve was limited predominantly to the earlier era of surgery and was discontinued by 1975.

Intraoperative use of the intra-aortic balloon pump had a markedly adverse prognosis as all 5 such patients succumbed within 3 years of surgery. Of the 115 patients not requiring an intra-aortic balloon, 80% are alive at 3 years.

Postoperative functional classification

The postoperative functional classification in the 78 long-term survivors was compared to the preoperative functional status in the same patients. Of these 78 patients, preoperatively 74 were in functional Class III or IV. Postoperatively only 13 patients were in functional Class III or IV, 24 were in Class II and 42 were in Class I. Overall, the majority of patients had an improvement of one or more

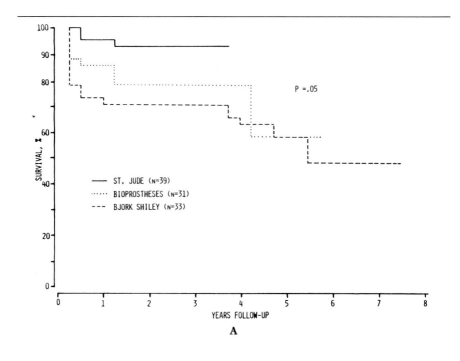

A

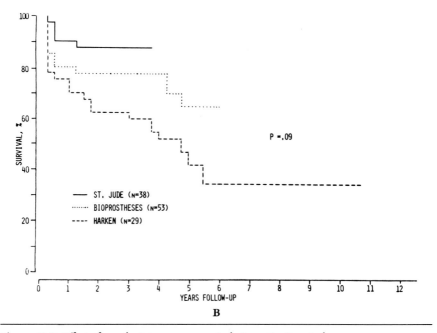

B

Figure 13-7. Effect of prosthesis type upon survival. A. aortic; B. mitral.

functional classifications after surgery; however, in 7 patients no change occurred, and 2 patients preoperatively in Class III are now in Class IV.

Thromboembolism

Preoperatively, 4.5% of our patients had experienced at least one thromboembolic episode. Thromboembolism after surgery was considered to be present with the occurrence of either a permanent or transient localized neurologic defect, transient visual aberration or recurrent unexplained dizziness and sudden occurrence of abdominal or peripheral pain and ischemia. Warfarin anticoagulation is recommended in all of our patients regardless of prosthesis type: 79% of patients were on warfarin; 4% were on an antiplatelet regimen, typically dipyridamole and aspirin; and 14% were on no antithrombotic medication.

The incidence of postoperative thromboembolism was 4.2% per patient-year. The incidence of CVA postoperatively was 3.1% per patient-year. The incidence of thromboembolism according to the status of anticoagulant therapy was analyzed: 22% of patients on no antithrombotic regimen had one or more occurrences of thromboembolism, whereas only 10% of patients on any antithrombotic regimen (consisting of warfarin, antiplatelet drugs or both) experienced thromboembolism.

DISCUSSION

Similar results with DVR over a comparable period of time have been reported by Björk [1] (figure 13-8) and Tepley [2] (figure 13-9). However, in these latter experiences single valves were used throughout. A significant difference occurred in our experience beginning in 1978 with institution of methods of specific myo-

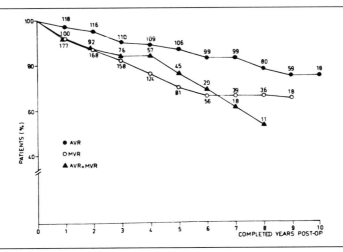

Figure 13-8. Actuarial survival with Björk-Shiley prosthesis [1]. From Björk VO, Henze A: Ten years' experience with the Björk-Shiley tilting disc valve. J Thorac Cardiovasc Surg 1979;78:331.

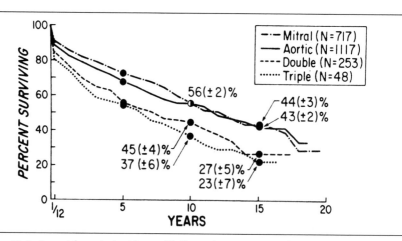

Figure 13-9. Actuarial survival with caged-ball prosthesis. From: Tepley JF, Grunkelmeier GF, Sutherland HD, et al: The ultimate prognosis after valve replacement: An assessment at twenty years. Ann Thorac Surg 1981; 32(2); 111–119.

cardial preservation and the use of St. Jude Medical valves. Thus, our overall experience is a summary of two very different experiences in operative mortality. However, it is not possible at this time to assign responsibility for the improvements noted to one or the other of these changes.

With respect to both early and late mortality, it appears that this particular group of *double valve recipients* behave in much the same manner as our patients receiving *single mitral prostheses.* The incidence of thromboembolism however, is similar to the additive incidence of thromboembolism in single mitral and single aortic recipients. Thus, the presence of two valve prostheses imparts an added incidence of thromboembolism over and above that expected to occur in patients with either mitral or single aortic implantation.

Another important message is that with the exception of the year in which surgery was performed and possibly the type of prosthesis employed, the most important predictors of outcome relate to the patient's preoperative status and more specifically, to the status of left ventricular function. Ejection fraction, left ventricular and end–diastolic volume, the need for additional surgical procedures (usually tricuspid annuloplasty) and requirements of intra-aortic balloon counterpulsation all point toward cardiac function as a major predictor of both early and late surgical outcome.

Physical activity and general daily life depend on the function of the heart as a pump. When cardiac pump efficiency is seriously impaired due to valvular heart disease, the impairment is very often irreversible in spite of correcting the mechanical valve defect. This concept is supported by the fact that the majority of late deaths are cardiac, nonvalve related and due to congestive heart failure. As the results of surgery continue to improve, it is reasonable to expect that patients will be referred for surgical therapy earlier, resulting in an even more optimistic long-term outcome, primarily based on preservation of myocardial function.

CONCLUSION

The patient with double valve disease, especially when there is coexisting disease requiring surgical correction, presents a formidable challenge. Interestingly, the early and late outcome of DVR is similar to that obtained after MVR.

Of the preoperative and perioperative variables that aid in predicting outcome, the most significant relate to the status of myocardial function at the time of surgery. Thus, the recommendation can be made that surgical therapy in such patients should be undertaken earlier, rather than later, in an attempt to preserve myocardial function.

Such a recommendation for earlier surgical therapy can be supported by the significantly reduced operative mortality that has been achieved in the past 6 years. Two intraoperative factors have been associated with this improvement: myocardial protection with hypothermic, hyperkalemic cardioplegic solutions and the use of ST. JUDE MEDICAL valves for both aortic and mitral valve replacement. Both can be regarded as improving cardiac function: the first by preserving myocardial integrity and the second by optimizing valvular function for a given level of myocardial function.

Long-term problems, other than cardiac, nonvalvular ones, also must be addressed. The primary ones relate to the incidence of thromboembolism and valve substitute durability. Whether better management of anticoagulation and improved design and fabrication of the valve substitute will have a beneficial effect will only be determined with further long-term follow-up of such patients.

REFERENCES

1. Björk VO, Henze A: Ten years' experience with the Björk-Shiley tilting disc valve. J Thorac Cardiovasc Surg 1979; 78:331.
2. Tepley JF, Grunkelmeier GF, Sutherland HD, et al: The ultimate prognosis after valve replacement: An assessment at twenty years. Ann Thorac Surg 1981; 32(2):111–119.
3. Chaux A, Czer LSC, Matloff JM, et al: The St. Jude Medical bileaflet valve prosthesis: A 5 year experience. J Thorac Cardiovasc Surg 1984;88:706–717.

14. CARDIAC VALVE REPLACEMENT IN THE PRESENCE OF CORONARY ATHEROSCLEROSIS

JACK M. MATLOFF, LAWRENCE S.C. CZER

This chapter will address the question: Does the presence of coronary atherosclerosis (CAD) affect the outcome of valvular replacement surgery, and if so, how and why?

Over the last 5 years, techniques of mitral valve surgery, particularly annuloplasty for mitral regurgitation, have affected the results of mitral valve surgery, especially with etiologically related coronary artery disease. Thus, the results of such surgical therapy may be clearly biased against valve replacement in these circumstances. For the purposes of this presentation our analyses have been confined to those pathologic conditions in which mitral, aortic and double valve replacement were carried out by necessity, without and with concomitant coronary artery bypass (CAB).

PATIENTS AND METHODS

From 1969 to 1977, single valve replacement at Cedars-Sinai Medical Center (figure 14-1) carried a one month mortality of 7.5% and a follow-up mortality to 8 years (mean = 3.5 years) of 12.5%. Furthermore, the operative mortality figures did not vary significantly from year to year, such that the mortality in 1977 was not significantly different from that in 1970 [1], or any of the intervening years.

Aortic and mitral valve surgery also carried the same risk, whether or not concomitant CAB was performed (figures 14-2 and 14-3). By examining the 85 early and late mortalities that occurred in these 423 cases [2], we found that our

111

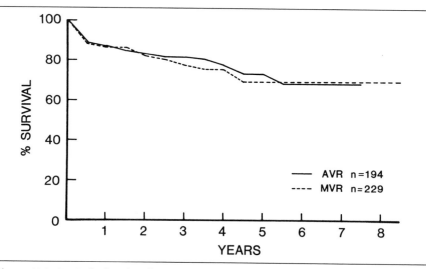

Figure 14-1. Survival of single valve replacement from 1969 to 1977.

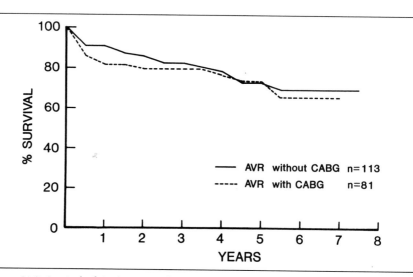

Figure 14-2. Survival of single aortic valve replacement (AVR) with and without coronary artery bypass (CABG) from 1969 to 1977.

highest mortality, especially early, was occurring in patients with what we considered primarily to be hemodynamic problems. Anatomically, these patients had combinations of limited left ventricular inflow or outflow and significant degrees of left ventricular dysfunction, especially when this was the result of coexisting coronary artery disease. In these circumstances, it was apparent that improved

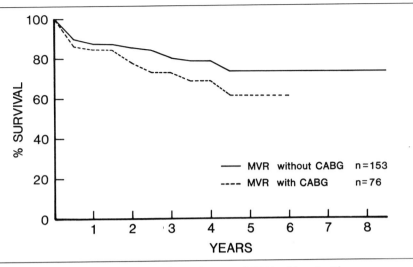

Figure 14-3. Survival of single mitral valve replacement (MVR) with and without coronary artery bypass (CABG) from 1969 to 1977.

results might be achieved by using a prosthesis with better hydraulic characteristics and by instituting the use of specific methods of myocardial preservation at surgery [3].

Because of these consideration, in April 1978 we began to use hypothermia to 25°C with hyperkalemic cardioplegia [4], and we began a limited trial of the ST. JUDE MEDICAL® prosthesis in what this earlier experience had indicated was our high risk patient subsets. We then analyzed our results for all valve replacement surgery performed between 1978 and 1980 to determine whether these changes, either alone or in combination had had an effect on outcome after surgery.

CARDIAC VALVE REPLACEMENT (1978–1980)

Overall, 9 operative deaths occurred in 261 patients for a 3.4% mortality (table 14-1). In single valve replacements, as compared to the earlier experience (1969–1977), operative mortality was reduced by two-thirds and mortality for all valve surgery was reduced by 50%. In the high-risk subset of patients who received ST. JUDE MEDICAL valves, our previous mortality of 7.5% was reduced to 2.3%. As a control group for the effect of cardioplegia, 173 patients received 212 porcine mitral and aortic valves or BJÖRK-SHILEY® aortic valves. The operative mortality of 4% for this control group was also lower than our previous mortality for single valve replacement.

In aortic valve replacement (AVR) patients, whether without or with CAD, mortality was reduced from 7.5% to 1% (1 mortality out of 102 cases). For double valve replacement patients (DVR), primarily without coronary artery disease, the decrease was from 14% to 4.7% (2 out of 42 cases). The overall mortality for

114   III. Cardiac valve replacement in special circumstances

Table 14-1. Cardiac valve replacement from March 1978 to April 1980.

		St. Jude		Other valves		Totals		
		N	Deaths	N	Deaths	Valves	Pts	Deaths
MVR	Isolated	24		28 P		52	52	
	CABG	14	2	43 P	3	57	57	5
AVR	Isolated	11		41 (P+B-S)	1	52	52	1
	CABG	16		34 (P+B-S)		50	50	
DVR	Isolated	11 M 12 A		38 P 7 B-S	2	68	34	2
	CABG	4 M 4 A		7 P 1 B-S		16	8	
Other	Isolated	3 M 1 A		7 P 1 B-S		12	5	
	CABG			5 P	1	5	3	1
	Valves	100		212		312		
	Patients	88	2	173	7		261	9
	Mortality	2.3%		4%			3.4%	

CABG = coronary artery bypass grafts; MVR = mitral valve replacement; AVR = aortic valve replacement; DVR = double valve replacement; Other = triple valve replacement, mitral and tricuspid valve replacement; mitral valve replacement, and repair post-infarction ventricular septal defect. P = porcine bioprosthesis; B-S = Björk-Shiley spherical prosthesis.

mitral valve replacement (MVR) was 4.5% (5 out of 109). No mortalities occurred among the 52 isolated mitral valve replacements and 5 mortalities occurred in the CAB group of 57 cases (9%).

In this prospective series of 261 patients, the early mortality for MVR and CAB was 9%. The mortality for all other valve replacements, including additional procedures was only 2% (4 out of 204). Statistically this is a significant difference when analyzed by Fisher's exact test.

MITRAL VALVE REPLACEMENT (1976–1982)

In order to determine what factors might account for this increased mortality in patients undergoing MVR and CAB, we increased our sample size by extending our analysis by two years in either direction to obtain a 6-year experience, extending from 1976–1982 [5]. From the resulting 380 MVR cases we excluded 131 with multiple procedures other than MVR and CAB. This left a cohort of 249, with roughly equal numbers of isolated MVR and MVR + CAB. With a logistic regression model, a multivariate analysis was performed of 25 variables, including preoperative, operative and postoperative factors [5].

Sex was not a significant factor, but age was significant for patients less than 60 or over 60 years of age (p = .01). The age of patients having coronary artery disease was higher than for those without coronary artery disease (64 vs. 58) which was statistically significant.

Coronary artery disease

The impact of coronary artery disease was significant overall (p < .05) [5] (figure 14-4). Results for patients with bypassed single and double vessel disease were identical to those of patients without coronary artery disease; 80% were 6-year survivors. These results were completely different from the larger number of patients (figure 14-5) who had triple vessel disease and left main artery disease which was bypassed and in whom there was 38% 6-year survival (p < .05). The detrimental effect of associated coronary artery disease was partially, but not completely, overcome by the performance of CAB surgery [6].

Ejection fraction

The effect of the preoperative left ventricular ejection fraction (LVEF) was also statistically significant. When patients are stratified by LVEF (figure 14-6) problems were evident in the group with an ejection fraction less than 0.35, who had

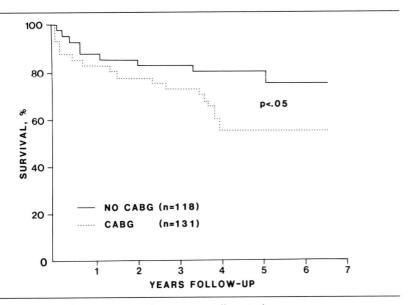

Figure 14-4. Impact of coronary artery disease on overall survival.

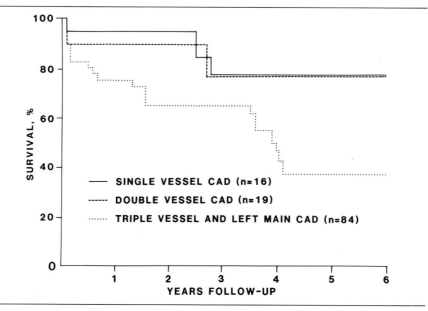

Figure 14-5. After 5 years, survival rates for patients with bypassed single and double vessel disease were identical to those of patients without coronary artery disease (figure 14-4).

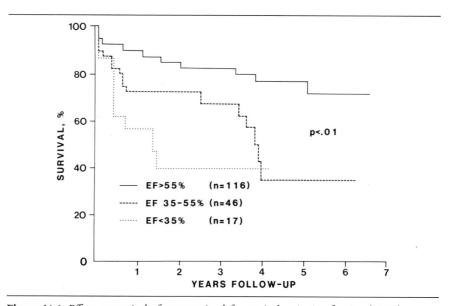

Figure 14-6. Effect on survival of preoperative left ventricular ejection fraction (LVEF).

a 40% 6-year survival. The intermediate group with LVEF from 0.35 to 0.55 did well for the first 3 years but at 4 years they dropped precipitously, so that at 4 to 6 years, their survival was no different than the group with a preoperative LVEF less than 0.35 (40% 6-year survival). Many of these patients had ischemic ventricles and ischemic mitral regurgitation. In contrast, 6-year survival with an ejection fraction over 0.55 was 78% (p < .05).

The difference between preoperative LVEF, with and without coronary disease (figure 14-7) was statistically significant (0.55 vs 0.68). Patients with ischemic mitral regurgitation had a lower ejection fraction (0.50) compared to those with rheumatic or other etiologies (0.67).

NYHA classification

The effect of the preoperative New York Heart Association Classification (figure 14-8) was statistically significant at p = .001 between Class III (80% 6-year survival) and Class IV (44% 6-year survival). Preoperatively, more patients in Class IV had coronary artery disease than had isolated mitral valve disease. Postoperatively there was a significant shift downward in classification, but many of the Class IV patients remained in Class III postoperatively. Overall, the number of patients remaining in Class III and IV was high. Approximately 10% of all patients had an intra-aortic balloon in place, and both early and late mortality was prohibitively high in this subset (figure 14-9). At 4 years, only about 20% of patients with an intra-aortic balloon remained alive, compared to 80% survival in patients not requiring the use of an intra-aortic balloon.

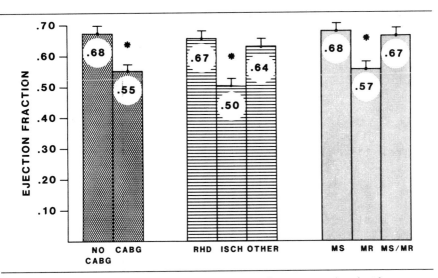

Figure 14-7. Preoperative left ventricular ejection fraction for patients with and without coronary artery bypass (CABG); ischemic (ISCH), rheumatic (RHD) and other etiologies of mitral valve disease (OTHER); and for patients with mitral stenosis (MS), mitral regurgitation (MR) or both (MS/MR).

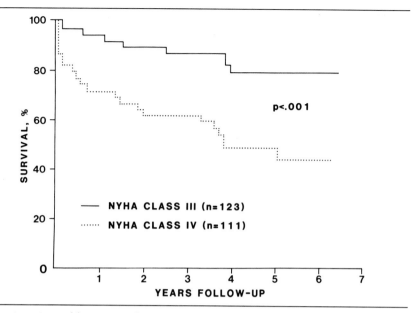

Figure 14-8. Survival by New York Heart Association (NYHA) Classes III and IV.

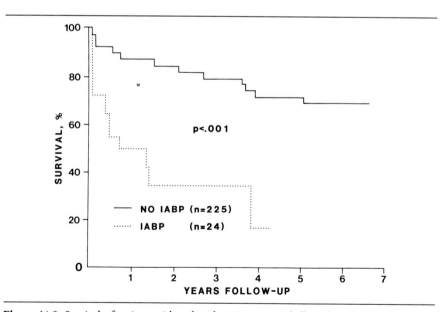

Figure 14-9. Survival of patients with and without intra-aortic balloon (IABP).

Hypothermia and cardioplegia

At the time these two changes were made, a change also occurred in our patient population. With the availability of hypothermic, hyperkalemic cardioplegia, referring cardiologists have become more likely to procrastinate in the belief that no patient will become inoperable. As a result, patients have been older and more commonly in NYHA Class IV; they have had associated coronary artery disease more often, and of greater extent when present; they more frequently have had mitral regurgitation and an ischemic etiology of the mitral valve disease; and they have had a lower ejection fraction preoperatively.

Because of these changes, early mortality for mitral valve replacement during the era of cardioplegia was significantly greater when coronary artery disease was present than when not present (15.9% vs. 4.4%; p < .05) (table 14-2). Before the use of cardioplegia, in contrast, there had been no difference in early mortality between patients with and without coronary artery disease (10.6% vs. 8.0%). Utilizing multivariate analysis and controlling for the changes in patient population that have occurred since 1978, it was found that the use of systemic hypothermia and cardioplegia in patients with associated coronary disease improved early survival, although this effect did not reach statistical significance [6].

The results are similar for late mortality: patients without coronary artery disease had a 4.9% per patient-year late mortality and patients with coronary artery disease had a 12.4% per patient-year late mortality despite the use of cardioplegia. This difference is again due to the change in patient populations.

AORTIC VALVE REPLACEMENT

A dramatic improvement was observed (table 14-3) in patients with coronary artery disease, whose early mortality decreased from 20% to 3.1% (p < .05) with the use of cardioplegia and ST. JUDE MEDICAL valves for the high-risk patients. An improvement was also observed in early mortality in patients without associated coronary disease, but this did not achieve statistical significance. Late mortality was

Table 14-2. Mitral valve replacement

	Cardioplegia	Early #	Early Rate*	Late #	Late Rate**
O Coronary disease	+	4/90	4.4%†	12/86	4.9† (244)
	−	12/150	8.0%	53/128	6.4 (826)
Coronary disease	+	18/113	15.9%†	27/93	12.4† (217)
	−	7/66	10.6%	24/58	7.4 (326)

* % < 30 days postoperatively
** % per patient-year
† p < .05
( ) Patient years of follow-up
Lost to follow-up: 13/419

Table 14-3. Aortic valve replacement.

	Cardioplegia	Early		Late	
		#	Rate*	#	Rate**
Ō Coronary disease	+	2/99	2%	5/97	2.4% (212)
	−	3/41	7.3%	8/37	4.3% (186)
Coronary disease	+	3/97	3.1%†	12/94	5.8% (208)
	−	5/25	20%†	3/19	3.5% (85)

* % < 30 days postoperatively
** % per patient-year
† p < .05
( ) Patient years of follow-up
Lost to follow-up: 2/262

slightly, but not significantly, higher in patients with coronary disease, probably reflecting a compensatory effect of CAB surgery.

DOUBLE VALVE REPLACEMENT

Results for patients with double valve replacement (table 14-4) are similar to those for patients with aortic valve replacement. In the presence of coronary artery disease, the use of cardioplegia has decreased the early mortality from 33% to 0% (p < .05). Late mortality for patients with and without coronary disease is similar.

OVERALL EXPERIENCE

Examining the early and late mortality in all 825 patients undergoing valve replacement with or without CAB (table 14-5), several distinct patterns emerge. The proportion of patients having associated coronary artery disease requiring concomitant revascularization increased from 29% (100 out of 344) to 48% (228 out of 472) after the institution of cardioplegic arrest in 1978. The presence of

Table 14-4. Double valve replacement

	Cardioplegia	Early		Late	
		#	Rate*	#	Rate**
Ō Coronary disease	+	3/55	5.5%	8/50	5.7% (140)
	−	6/44	13.6%	14/35	8.9% (158)
Coronary disease	+	0/15	0†	2/15	5.0% (40)
	−	3/9	33%†	3/6	18.8% (16)

* % < 30 days postoperatively
** % per patient-year
† p < .05
( ) Patient years of follow-up
Lost to follow-up: 5

Table 14-5. All replaced valves

	Cardioplegia	Early #	Rate*	Late #	Rate**
Ō Coronary disease	+	11/253	4.3%†§	27/240	4.5† (606)
	−	22/244	9.0%§	78/208	6.4 (1215)
Coronary disease	+	22/228	9.6%†	41/204	8.7† (472)
	−	15/100	15.0%	30/83	7 (426)

* % < 30 days postoperatively
** % per patient-year
† $p < .05$
§ $p < .05$
( ) Patient years of follow-up
Lost to follow-up: 20

coronary disease increased operative mortality before the use of cardioplegia (from 9.0% to 15%) and after its use (from 4.3% to 9.6%; $p < .05$). Despite the increased operative risk in patients with coronary disease, the use of cardioplegia reduced early mortality from 15% to 9.6% (this became statistically significant after changes in the mitral valve population were accounted for). The use of cardioplegia also reduced early mortality in patients without associated coronary disease (9.0% to 4.3%, $p < .05$), probably reflecting a beneficial effect on preservation of global ventricular function and myocardial energy stores. Coronary artery disease, despite revascularization, was associated with an increased late mortality even after the use of cardioplegia, probably due to the progression of atherosclerosis in the grafts and/or native circulation.

CONCLUSION

In recent years, coronary artery disease has been encountered with increasing frequency in patients requiring valve replacement. These patients have a higher operative and late mortality, despite revascularization. Patients with mitral valve and coronary artery disease, especially those with ischemic mitral regurgitation, are at particularly high risk of early and late death. The use of hypothermic cardioplegia has dramatically reduced early mortality for patients undergoing aortic or double valve replacement and concomitant coronary artery bypass grafting. Its use has also reduced (but not significantly) early mortality in patients undergoing mitral valve replacement and coronary artery bypass grafting, after changes in patient population were taken into account.

The use of cardioplegia also benefited the lower risk group of patients undergoing valve replacement without associated coronary disease, reducing early mortality from 9.0% to 4.3% ($p < .05$). This may reflect better preservation of global ventricular function and myocardial energy stores.

Improvements in methods and delivery of myocardial protection are needed in order to reduce the exceptionally high early mortality in patients with ischemic mitral regurgitation requiring valve replacement.

Increased attention needs to be directed at the causes and prevention of progressive atherosclerosis in patients requiring valve replacement and revascularization, if late mortality is to be reduced.

REFERENCES

1. Chaux A, Gray RJ, Sustaita H, et al: Single valve replacement using porcine xenografts: Hemodynamic performance, incidence of thromboembolic complications and analysis of survival as compared to other non-biologic prostheses, in Sebening F, Klovekorn WP, Meisner H, et al (eds): *Bioprosthetic Cardiac Valves,* Munchen, Deutsches Herzzentrum, 1979, pp 243–254.
2. Chaux A, Gray RJ, Matloff JM, et al: An appreciation of the new St. Jude valvular prosthesis. J Thorac Cardiovasc Surg 1981; 81:202–211.
3. Gray RJ, Shell WE, Conklin C, et al: Quantification of myocardial imaging during coronary artery bypass grafting. Circulation 1978;58:1,38.
4. Hearse JD, Stewart DA, Brambridge MV: Cellular protection during myocardial ischemia: The development and characterization of a procedure for the induction of reversible ischemic arrest. Circulation 1976;54(2):193.
5. Czer L, Matloff J, Gray R, et al: Mitral valve replacement wit coronary artery disease, in Duran C, Angell WW, Johnson AD, et al (eds): *Recent Progress in Mitral Valve Disease.* London, Butterworths, 1984.
6. Czer LSC, Gray RJ, DeRobertis M, et al: Mitral valve replacement: Impact of coronary artery disease and determinants of prognosis after revascularization. Circulation 1984;70(Suppl 1):I-198.

PART III. DISCUSSION

DONALD B. DOTY AND EUGENE M. BAUDET, MODERATORS

GRAFT PREPARATION

DONALD B. DOTY: I am sure that all of us would like to question Dr. Cooley on some technical aspects of his presentation on annuloaortic ectasia. I have a couple of questions to initiate the discussion. You mentioned the favorable qualities of the velour sewing ring. Why not a velour graft packed with albumin or clotted with plasma?

DENTON COOLEY: We have had so much difficulty in developing an impervious graft that I have never seen a way of avoiding postoperative bleeding with a velour graft in a patient who is undergoing cardiopulmonary bypass with full heparinization. My experience is that 90% will bleed excessively, no matter what you do. It may be that with collagen impregnation of grafts, that situation will change. Under those circumstances, I would prefer to use a velour graft, but until that happens, I think we are better off continuing with the so-called low porosity, flexible, woven graft with impregnation of plasma.

DONALD B. DOTY: The reason I ask is that my own impression has been that the low porosity graft clotted with albumin or plasma isn't as tight as a velour that has concentrated albumin "cooked" into it. These grafts become tight and there is little bleeding.

DENTON COOLEY: I haven't had any experience with that technique. I have avoided it believing that our past experience would be repeated if we went that route. But you have apparently found that the albumin will render the graft impervious in patients with cardiopulmonary bypass?

DONALD DOTY: It will render it tighter than woven. The favorable qualities you mentioned of the velour enable a nice anastomosis around the coronary arteries.

DENTON COOLEY: That is a very interesting observation which I may try, also.

123

ANASTAMOSIS

DONALD B. DOTY: Another question, Dr. Cooley, pertains to the technical aspects of the coronary anastomosis, and the potential for hemorrhage later around coronary ostia. You mentioned that a 2 cm cephalad displacement of the coronary ostia was the criteria for reimplantation. Is there ever a patient who has such a big aneurysm and lateral displacement that you can't pull the ostia back to the graft?

DENTON COOLEY: I'm not absolutely certain what you mean. I have said that we think a minimal displacement of 2 cm is necessary to allow easy approximation of the coronary ostia in the graft. If there is less than a 2 cm displacement, you probably ought to do a supracoronary anastomosis of the graft, leaving the coronary ostia intact below the aortic anastomosis. If it's more than 2 cm then it's relatively easy to do the anastomosis without having the threat of subsequent hemorrhage, which you cannot get to if you try to perform coronary anastomosis closer to the annular anastomosis.

DONALD DOTY: Suppose we have a 10 cm diameter aneurysm and the tube graft is farther from the aortic wall than 2 cm?

DENTON COOLEY: I would remind you that the anulus is never bigger than 27 mm.

DONALD DOTY: Correct, but supposing we had a 27 mm anulus and a 30 mm tube coming out so the distance between the edge of the tube and the coronary arteries may be more than 2–3 cm.

DENTON COOLEY: Some believe that is an important consideration, Dr. Doty; and I know that there are those who use a loop of tube graft between the two coronary ostia and place this side-to-side into the aortic graft. We have not found that to be necessary. If the aneurysm were calcified and you could not pull the coronary vessels into the graft without tension, then such a maneuver might be appropriate. However, in the absence of calcification, the coronary vessels are usually rather mobile and the graft fits in very satisfactorily.

DONALD DOTY: Are there any techniques to reinforce the coronary ostia or do you just use sutures?

DENTON COOLEY: We've tried pledgets in the anulus and pledgets in the coronary ostia and have always come back to just using continuous sutures in both locations. With such a technique we have not had a bleed or a break down up to this point.

SUTURING TECHNIQUE

QUESTION: Dr. Cooley, do you use the continuous suture in this circumstance only for hemostasis or do you do all your aortic valve replacements with a continuous suture?

DENTON COOLEY: We only use the continuous suture for annuloaortic ectasia procedures. If there is aortic stenosis with calcification in the anulus, we always use interrupted sutures in our institution. In some patients with aortic regurgitation predominating and an enlarged anulus we do use a continuous suture.

PRECLOTTING

DONALD B. DOTY: One other question about preclotting. Your slide showed you dipping the graft into the albumin solution. Are there any problems with getting that albumin on the mechanical prosthesis and then turning it egg-white with autoclaving? This can become a very "sticky" coating on the valve poppets.

DENTON COOLEY: Well, I don't think so. You probably should remove it with the suction tip or with a cloth. You know, albumin is rather expensive and I'm very cost-conscious; I think albumin costs $75 or $80 for a small bottle, and therefore I prefer the homologous plasma, which is free. Also, our Jehovah's Witness patients won't allow the use of albumin.

VALVE REPLACEMENT IN GERIATRIC PATIENTS

EUGENE M. BAUDET: Are there any further questions or comments about these papers? About double valve replacemenet? About the paper on valve replacement in the geriatric patient?

JACK M. MATLOFF: I have a question if there are no other questions. Dr. Nicoloff, did I hear you say that some of the older mitral recipients tend to have a higher incidence of thromboembolism?

DEMETRE NICOLOFF: Yes.

JACK M. MATLOFF: Are some of those events due to the intrinsic effects of aging, that is due to intrinsic cerebrovascular disease and other factors? As you know, it is common in older people to have dizzy spells after surgery, and many of them had the spells before surgery, as well. Is it your impression that these are clearly thromboembolic events, as differentiated from other causes of stroke?

Another question I have has to do with the general etiology of the valve disease, particularly mitral valve disease, in patients 70 years of age and older, as opposed to those 50 and younger. In the latter, I would presume there is a larger cohort of rheumatics that should predetermine a different natural history after surgery.

DEMETRE NICOLOFF: Right. I think, as Dr. Fisk tried to point out in his talk, one makes the immediate assumption any cerebrovascular accident in a patient who has a prosthesis, is due to the prosthesis. It may not be. What one has to use as a background is how many 70-year olds who have cardiac disease without a prosthesis have these accidents. What is the control level of cerebrovascular accidents in this age group? I don't think we can arrive at that figure easily because the control group would have to be 70-year olds with heart disease; and then you would have to address the matter of whether the patient has atrial fibrillation, a large atrium or a myopathic ventricle. What you can compare is 70-year olds who have had an aortic valve replaced. However, we found that the incidence of thrombo-emboli in patients with aortic valve replacement is no different for a 70-year old than it is for the 60-to-69-year old. In contrast, I would think if we see a higher incidence in the 70-year old with mitral valve disease, it must have something to do with the mitral valve prosthesis or the pathology of the left atrium.

JACK M. MATLOFF: We have just looked at the results of surgery in patients over 80-years old. The stimulus for this was to try to understand what was going to happen when DRG's become effective; so we initiated a project to evaluate people at different ages to see what their courses had been, how they do and how that might be affected by reimbursement under the DRG's. The first group were patients over 80 years of age. We found that although they were sicker preoperatively and had more early morbidity, the intermediate-term outcome was similar to that in the younger age groups when one makes comparisons with age-adjusted cohorts without cardiac surgery. This supports in part what you are saying.

RICHARD GRAY: I think the common thread that runs through my presentation and Dr. Nicoloff's and to a certain extent with Dr. Matloff's, is that patient selection plays a very important part in the outcome of these various series of patients, whether it's mitral or aortic valve replacement or whatever else might have been done to them. If you can recall instances where 80-year olds are proposed for surgery, unless they have very compelling symptoms, surgery would not be considered. To a certain extent, patients who are older, have in many cases, more unstable symptoms. There are more compelling indications for surgery if the patient has coronary disease than if the patient has valve disease. By and large you don't operate on a NYHA Class II 80-year old who has the need for one valve replacement.

EUGENE M. BAUDET: Are there any questions or comments concerning the paper of Dr. Matloff?

VALVE REPLACEMENT AND CORONARY ATHEROSCLEROSIS

QUESTION: Yes, one question. Dr. Matloff clearly demonstrated the higher instance of mortality in patients with coronary artery bypass and mitral valve replacement. In this group of patients, the question is, have you isolated those with true ventricular aneurysms and those with ischemic papillary muscle dysfunction in terms of their relationship to mortality?

JACK M. MATLOFF: That is a difficult proposition. We have looked at the data and included patients who had aneurysmectomy, bypass and valve replacement along with those who had only valve replacement and bypass. Including or excluding that group really does not change the overall impression. This is primarily because there are not a great number of those patients around. Among the patients in the group of ischemic mitral valve disease, the outlook of those with aneurysms is very, very poor. This should not be a great surprise because they are the patients with the most advanced coronary disease and the most depressed ventricular function.

The concept of mitral valve dysfunction from ischemic papillary muscles is difficult to deal with. We almost never see a patient with significant mitral regurgitation and functional papillary muscle dysfunction who doesn't have an infarct of the tip of the papillary muscle as the basis for the mitral regurgitation. I think that true papillary muscle dysfunction with a viable but ischemic papillary muscle must be a very rare phenomenon. It is an extremely unusual situation when you can revascularize the patient and their mitral regurgitation will disappear. More often than not, when we have an aneurysm and the papillary muscle is involved, it's the whole papillary muscle that is infarcted. It is not a matter of papillary muscle dysfunction. That's not the consideration. If the papillary muscle is not directly involved, but is adjacent to the area that's been infarcted, that also creates a problem; if you resect the aneurysm, you're going to interfere with papillary muscle function when you close the heart. So I think that with aneurysm, the degree of pathology is far more advanced than just the tip of the papillary muscle in a functional papillary muscle ischemic syndrome. Thus, the results between patients with true papillary muscle dysfunction and those with aneurysms are totally different.

IV. CARDIAC VALVE REPLACEMENT IN PEDIATRIC PRACTICE: EXPERIENCE WITH THE ST. JUDE MEDICAL® VALVE

15. ST. JUDE MEDICAL® VALVE REPLACEMENT IN INFANTS AND CHILDREN

A. MICHAEL BORKON, BRUCE A. REITZ, JAMES S. DONAHOO, TIMOTHY J. GARDNER

Abstract. Cardiac valve replacement with ST. JUDE MEDICAL® valves was undertaken in 27 infants and children ages 3 weeks to 17 years, with an average age of 9 years. Valve implant sites were 12 aortic, 14 mitral and 1 pulmonic. Six aortic valve replacements were with 19 mm aortic valves; only 1 required anulus enlargement. Due to the small size of the mitral anulus, a 19 mm aortic valve was used in 3 children. Follow-up was 100% for a mean of 2.3 years per patient. Seven children (5 mitral and 2 aortic) took aspirin for anticoagulation with 1 valve thrombosis and 2 deaths. The number of children over age 5 taking warfarin was 18 with 1 emboli, 1 hemorrhage, no valve thrombosis and 1 death. The number of patients event-free at 5 years was 76%.

INTRODUCTION

Cardiac valve replacement in infants and children presents technical challenges and postoperative considerations that often differ from the adult population undergoing valve replacement [1]. Bioprosthetic valve substitutes, because of their low thrombogenicity and lack of requirement for warfarin anticoagulation, were thought to be superior alternatives to mechanical heart valves. Unfortunately, initial enthusiasm for bioprosthetic valve replacement in children has been severely dampened by demonstration of accelerated tissue deterioration [2]. In addition, porcine aortic valve bioprostheses have been hemodynamically inefficient, often requiring concomitant aortic anulus enlargement to overcome this drawback. In the hope of finding a more suitable cardiac valve substitute for the pediatric age group, we began to use the ST. JUDE MEDICAL prosthesis in 1979 [3].

METHODS

The ST. JUDE MEDICAL valve has been used in 27 consecutive infants and children undergoing cardiac valve replacement at Johns Hopkins Hospital. Excluded from this group were patients who required conduit valve reconstruction where a bioprosthesis was employed. The techniques of valve replacement have been published elsewhere [3]. Of the 27 children, there were 17 boys and 10 girls with an average age of 9 years. All were under 17 years of age at the time of operation. Eight patients were less than 3 years old (figure 15-1). The youngest was a 3-week-old infant with L-transposition who underwent replacement of a regurgitant left sided atrioventricular valve. Aortic valve recipients tended to be older than mitral valve patients with an average age of 9 and 6 years, respectively. Postoperative evaluation and follow-up was conducted at our institution or by the child's pediatrician. Follow-up was 100%. The total duration of follow-up was 58 patient-years; the mean follow-up was 2.3 years per patient.

The preoperative weight for all of the children ranged from 3.7 to 77 kilograms (figure 15-2). Five infants were less than 10 kilograms at the time of operation. All underwent mitral valve replacement. Overall, 14 patients received mitral valves; while aortic valve replacement was carried out in 12. In addition, 1 patient underwent pulmonary valve replacement 5 months after repair of pulmonary atresia with a nonvalved conduit. Fourteen of the 27 (50%) had undergone at least 1 prior heart operation (table 15-1).

Among children requiring aortic valve replacement, congenital aortic stenosis was the most common pathologic condition (table 15-2). There were 10 patients in this group, 9 of whom had undergone previous valvotomy or valve replacement. Residual regurgitation or obstruction were indications for reoperation. One child

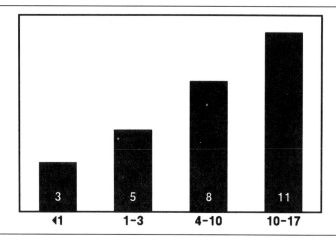

Figure 15-1. Age range (years) of patients undergoing valve replacement with the St. Jude Medical valve.

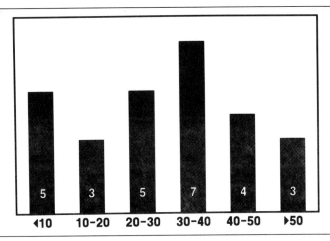

5	3	5	7	4	3
◀10	10-20	20-30	30-40	40-50	▶50

Figure 15-2. Preoperative weight (kilograms) of 27 patients undergoing St. Jude Medical valve replacement.

required reoperation 1 year after a 17 mm BJÖRK-SHILEY® valve had been inserted for congenital aortic stenosis. Postoperative cardiac catheterization revealed an unacceptably high residual gradient across the prosthesis, and it was replaced with a 21 mm ST. JUDE MEDICAL valve. On the other hand, the indications for mitral valve replacement were diverse (table 15-3). Two children required mitral valve replacement in conjunction with correction of a single ventricle.

Table 15-1. Previous operations

Aortic valvotomy	8
AV canal repair	2
VSD & AR repair	1
Starr-Edwards mitral valve	1
Björk-Shiley aortic valve	1
Pulmonary atresia repair	1
Ligation anomalous coronary artery	1

AV = atrioventricular
VSD = ventricular septal defect
AR = aortic regurgitation

Table 15-2. Aortic valve replacement

Congenital aortic stenosis	9
VSD & aortic regurgitation	1
Björk-Shiley valve obstruction	1
Rheumatic aortic stenosis	1

VSD = ventricular septal defect

Table 15-3. Mitral valve replacement

Congenital regurgitation	2
AV canal	2
Marfan's syndrome	2
Single ventricle	2
Rheumatic regurgitation	1
Cardiomyopathy	1
Starr-Edwards valve obstruction	1
Parachute valve	1
Anomalous coronary artery	1
Mitral valve obstruction to LV outflow	1

AV = atrioventricular

The range of valve sizes implanted is demonstrated in figure 15-3. Six children underwent aortic valve replacement with a 19 mm aortic valve. Only 1 child required enlargement of the aortic anulus to facilitate insertion of the valve. The spectrum of valve sizes used in the mitral position was variable. Due to the small size of the mitral anulus, a 19 mm aortic valve was used in 3 children.

RESULTS

There were 2 hospital deaths (7.5%). One occurred in a 3.7 kilogram, 3-week-old infant following replacement of an incompetent left-sided atrioventricular valve associated with L-transposition of the great vessels. Although the child recovered from the operation and had a normally functioning valve, death occurred 5 weeks

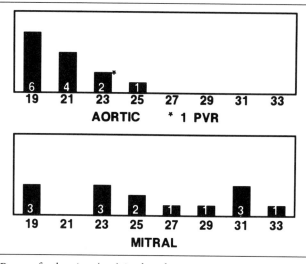

Figure 15-3. Range of valve sizes (mm) implanted.

later from pneumonia. The other death occurred in an 18-month-old infant after operation for severe mitral regurgitation and left ventricular failure due to an anomalous left coronary artery. Death resulted from postoperative left ventricular failure.

Late deaths have occurred in 3 of 25 hospital survivors (12%). One child, a 13-year-old girl, died as a result of severe left ventricular failure with a normally functioning prosthesis. Another infant who was 1 year of age at the time of operation died suddenly at home 2 months following the procedure. Unfortunately, an autopsy could not be obtained, and it is impossible to exclude reporting this as a valve-related death. Valve thrombosis resulted in 1 death. It occurred in a 3½-year-old boy 2 months following mitral valve replacement and correction of a single ventricle. In this instance, valve thrombosis was believed to have been precipitated by an episode of dehydration. Reoperation at an outside hospital confirmed thrombosis of the mitral valve. All surviving patients are asymptomatic.

Because warfarin anticoagulation in young children is fraught with difficulty and frequent complications, patients under the age of 5 have routinely been placed only on aspirin. Seven children (5 mitral and 2 aortic valve recipients) are currently receiving this therapy (table 15-4). There have been no thromboemboli or major bleeding complications. However, 2 late deaths have occurred in this group and may be related to valve thrombosis. The majority of patients (18) have been maintained on warfarin anticoagulation with therapeutic levels ranging between 1.5 and 1.8 times control values. In this group, there has been 1 cerebral embolus and 1 psoas muscle hematoma that resulted in femoral nerve paralysis. There was also 1 late death that was the result of progressive left ventricular failure. One patient in this series required reoperation for paravalvular regurgitation.

The overall 5-year actuarial survival for 25 children surviving operation is illustrated in figure 15-4. Since none of the patients receiving aortic valves has died, the curve reflects deaths occurring in the mitral valve group.

Figure 15-5 depicts an event-free analysis of children who have survived operation. Seventy-six percent of the children have been free of any major event for up to 5 years following operation. When analyzed according to valve position, it is apparent that patients following aortic valve replacement have had relatively few complications (figure 15-6). On the other hand, mitral valve recipients had a probability of only 65% of being free from any major event for up to 5 years.

Table 15-4. Anticoagulation

	No.	Mean age	Total follow-up	Embolus	Hemorrhage	Valve thrombobis	Death
Aspirin	7	5.5	20.4	0	0	1	2
Warfarin	18	14.3	37.4	1	1	0	1

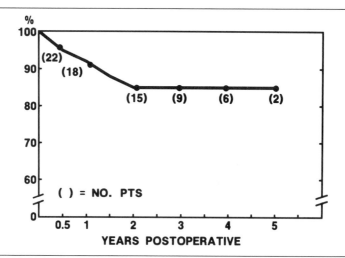

Figure 15-4. Five-year actuarial survival for 25 hospital survivors.

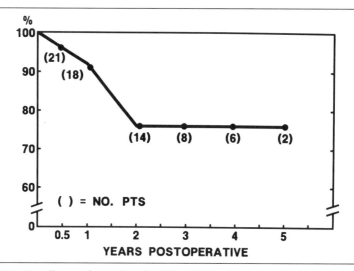

Figure 15-5. Overall event-free analysis for 25 hospital survivors.

SUMMARY

The ST. JUDE MEDICAL prosthesis demonstrates excellent hemodynamic function and provides satisfactory performance in the pediatric population. Children receiving an aortic valve substitute tended to have fewer late complications then mitral valve recipients. Aortic anulus enlargement procedures were rarely required in our experience. While we currently employ aspirin therapy for patients less than 5 years of age or when the risk associated with warfarin therapy outweighs its

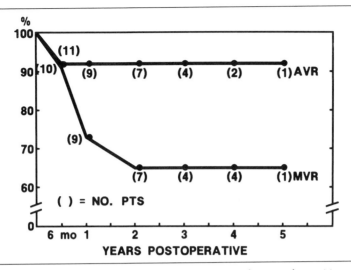

Figure 15-6. Event-free analysis for 25 hospital survivors according to valve position.

benefit, older patients should be managed with warfarin. In addition, warfarin anticoagulation probably should be used in children less than 5 years of age who are undergoing mitral valve replacement and who may be identified to be at high risk for thrombemboli or valve thrombosis. We believe that the St. Jude Medical valve is currently the most appropriate cardiac valve substitute in the pediatric population.

REFERENCES
1. Gardner TJ, Roland JMA, Neill CA, Donahoo JD: Valve replacement in children. A fifteen year perspective. J Thorac Cardiovasc Surg 1982; 83:178–185.
2. Dunn JM: Porcine valve durability in children. Ann Thorac Surg 1981; 32:357–368.
3. Donahoo JS and Gardner TJ: Early and intermediate experience with the St. Jude mechanical cardiac valve prosthesis in infants and children. Southern Medical Journal 1982; 75:1538–1543.

16. PEDIATRIC USE OF THE ST. JUDE MEDICAL® PROSTHESIS

ROBERT M. SADE, FRED A. CRAWFORD, JR, HARVEY I. PASS, JOHN M. KRATZ

Virtually all of the chapters in this book to this point have emphasized that every patient with a mechanical valve prosthesis should be on warfarin anticoagulation. We have developed experimental, clinical data over the past five years that supports the proposition that such anticoagulants are not always needed.

Earlier [1], we reviewed all the published reports of valve replacement with mechanical prosthesis in children. The mortality rates were very high, ranging from 26% to 48%. The complication rates were also high, including thromboembolism at 9.1%, despite the use of anticoagulation, and major bleeding episodes due to anticoagulation were at 9.9%. In our own series of 25 patients with mechanical prostheses, the overall mortality rate was 33%, and 50% of the long-term survivors had thromboembolism, hemorrhage or endocarditis [1].

Because of the worldwide experience and our own experience we began in 1975 to use what seemed to be a very logical prosthesis for children: the porcine bioprosthesis. We hoped to negate the complications of anticoagulation in these children by avoiding it altogether. Over the next four years we implanted 24 porcine valves in children and found the results far superior to our group of children with mechanical prosthesis. In the latter group, only 54% were alive and free of major complications one year after operation, compared with 85% of the children with porcine prosthesis [1].

Enthusiasm for the use of porcine valves in children was short-lived, however, because soon after the publication of that paper, reports from several institutions suggested that early calcification may be a problem in children [2–4]. We saw our first calcified porcine valve within a year after our recommendation of the porcine valve for children was published. Good actuarial data are now available regarding the longevity of the porcine bioprosthesis in children, which shows these prostheses can be expected to fail at a rate of 60% by four years after aortic valve replacement (AVR), and 60% by five years after mitral valve replacement (MVR) [5].

Fortunately, the ST. JUDE MEDICAL® valve became available around that time. Because of its all-carbon construction and its demonstrated excellent hemodynamic function, it appeared to have the promise of low thrombogenicity. Thus, we began to use this prosthesis for valve replacement in children, without anticoagulation, in March 1979. We felt justified in not using COUMADIN® because of the high incidence of complications in children who are taking that drug [1].

To the present, we have implanted the ST. JUDE MEDICAL valve in 42 patients. Of those patients, 4 infants with associated complex congenital lesions died in the hospital, and 5 patients have been treated with COUMADIN because their surgeon preferred it. One patient was lost to follow-up. Over the past five years, we have followed 33 children without anticoagulation or antiplatelet agents of any kind, with the exception of 6 (MVR) patients who have been maintained on aspirin by their surgeon.

The 18 boys and 15 girls were aged 8 months to 21 years (13.9 $\pm$ 2.5, mean $\pm$ SEM). The valves replaced were 16 aortics and 9 mitrals, 3 double valves and 5 pulmonary valves, one in a conduit and 4 free in the outflow tract following repair of complex malformations.

RESULTS

Follow-up has been 1 to 58 months (30.2 $\pm$ 2.6), with 857 months of aggregate risk for these patients. The 2 late deaths were due to a ventricular arrhythmia that occurred 5 weeks postoperatively, and an acute exacerbation of leukemia, 18 months after valve replacement. The clinical response to valve replacement has been very good, with all patients improving in functional Class, and all being in Class I or II (figure 16-1).

There have been 5 late complications, including a 7-year-old girl who had leaflet entrapment by a small bit of unresected mitral valve tissue. She did well after reoperation and excision of the tissue. A 15-year-old boy developed prosthetic endocarditis with aortic root abscess, because of his failure to seek treatment and antibiotic therapy for a dental abscess. His aortic root was replaced with a composite graft containing a ST. JUDE MEDICAL valve and his coronary arteries were reimplanted. Two years after his operation, the patient is doing well. A paravalvular leak developed in a 16-year-old girl after mitral valve replacement, and this problem was alleviated at reoperation by a mattress suture repair of the leak. A 4-year-old girl had thrombosis of a pulmonary prosthesis, requiring replacement with a tissue valve, and she is now doing well. A 17-year-old boy had an acute myocardial infarction, which cleared within a few days. Cardiac catheterization a

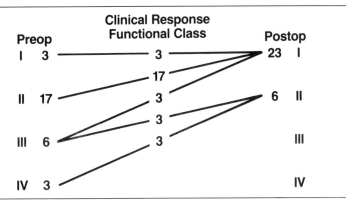

Figure 16-1. Functional class in 29 patients followed more than 3 months after valve replacement with St. Jude Medical valve, without warfarin anticoagulation.

week after the episode showed normal coronary arteries; nevertheless, we attribute this incident to a coronary thromboembolism.

DISCUSSION

Two important related, but separate questions arise in regard to this series of patients: 1) How will we know when these children should be anticoagulated? 2) At what age should they no longer be considered children and should be anticoagulated at that time? The answer to the first question is provided by statisticians. With our own data and data from two published studies with a combined total of 550 patients [6,7] using probabilities calculated from the binomial distribution, they have indicated that when 4 aortic thromboembolic episodes or 6 mitral episodes occur, our results will be significantly worse ($p < 0.05$) than the published series of patients who have been anticoagulated [6,7]. The single instance of aortic thromboembolism was well within these limits, as was the absence of thromboembolism in the mitral group. We recognize that it is not entirely appropriate to compare a group of non-anticoagulated children with a group of anticoagulated adults, but until a prospectively randomized study of patients with and without anticoagulation is done, we will have to be satisfied with these imperfect historical comparisons. We will not anticoagulate our patients until the record of thrombosis and thromboembolism becomes significantly worse than that of reported series of anticoagulated adults; at this time we plan to avoid anticoagulation indefinitely. There will certainly come a time when our patients will no longer be classified as children, but as adults. However, it may well be that the risk of thromboembolism will remain low for these patients as they grow into adulthood.

Cardiac valve replacement with the ST. JUDE MEDICAL valve is safe and effective in children. Our experience, to date, suggests anticoagulants may safely be avoided in this group of patients, and our data provide ample justification for avoiding anticoagulation in any patient under the age of 21 who has received a ST. JUDE MEDICAL valve.

REFERENCES

1. Sade RM, Ballenger JF, Hohn AR, et al: Cardiac valve replacement in children. Comparison of tissue with mechanical prosthesis. J Thorac Cardiovasc Surg 1979; 78:123–127.
2. Kutsche LM, Oyer P, Shumway N, et al: An important complication of Hancock mitral valve replacement in children. Circulation 60:1979; Suppl 1:98–103.
3. Silver MM, Pollock J, Silver MD, et al: Calcification in porcine xenograft valves in children. Am J Cardiol 1980; 45:685–689.
4. Williams DB, Danielson GK, McGoon DC, et al: Porcine heterograft valve replacement in children. J Thorac Cardiovasc Surg 1982; 84:446–450.
5. Dunn JM: Porcine valve durability in children. Ann Thorac Surg 1981; 32:357–368.
6. Nicoloff DM, Emery RW, Arom KV, et al: Clinical and hemodynamic results with the St. Jude Medical cardiac valve prosthesis. J Thorac Cardiovasc Surg 1981; 82:674–683.
7. Lillehei CW: Worldwide experience with the St. Jude Medical valve prosthesis. Clinical and hemodynamic results. Contemp Surg 1982; 20:17–30.

17. MITRAL VALVE REPLACEMENT IN A CHILD USING THE ST. JUDE MEDICAL® VALVE

JOHN W. MACK

Although mitral valve replacement is performed with reluctance in children, many patients with congenitally abnormal valves experience severe hemodynamic and clinical compromise and are candidates for valve replacement. Following insertion of a prosthetic mitral valve they can demonstrate dramatic improvement.

CASE REPORT

The patient for presentation is a boy with no stigmata of Down's syndrome who was noted to have a heart murmur early in life. The electrocardiogram showed left axis deviation. He developed congestive heart failure and was placed on digoxin and diuretics. At fourteen months cardiac catheterization was performed, which revealed an incomplete atrioventricular canal defect (A-V canal) with marked mitral insufficiency and a large left-to-right shunt at the atrial level.

Because of persistent heart failure and failure to thrive, he underwent elective repair of his cardiac defect at 18 months of age. The surgical findings included a large ostium primum atrial septal defect with a complete cleft in the mitral valve, which was quite dysplastic. There was no ventricular septal defect. The cleft was repaired conservatively, and the atrial septal defect was closed with a pericardial patch.

There were no perioperative complications; however, the child continued to have mitral insufficiency with congestive heart failure. Six months following surgery he was not growing, had moderate congestive heart failure and continued to have cardiomegaly and pulmonary congestion on his chest x-ray (figure 17-1).

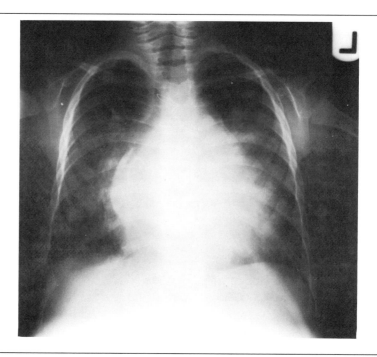

Figure 17-1. Chest x-ray prior to valve replacement showing cardiomegaly and pulmonary vascular congestion.

Recatheterization showed no residual shunt; however, there was 4+ mitral regurgitation with an enlarged left atrium. The mitral valve was thickened and shortened so that it did not coapt, and the mitral anulus was small (figure 17-2).

At two years of age, he underwent mitral valve replacement with a 19 mm ST. JUDE MEDICAL® valve. He was placed on aspirin and dipyridamole for its antiplatelet adhesive effect and was continued on digoxin and diuretics. He made an uneventful recovery demonstrating excellent relief of symptoms. During the year following valve replacement, cardiomegaly improved significantly (figure 17-3) and he has grown impressively.

The patient's 36-month evaluation showed him to be in the 50th percentile for weight, and the 20th percentile for height, whereas he had been well below the 5th percentile for both prior to mitral valve replacement. He was happy and active and had no tachypnea or tachycardia. A two-dimensional echocardiogram revealed a normal-sized, properly functioning left ventricle and a normally functioning prosthetic valve.

DISCUSSION

In our experience, significant mitral insufficiency occurring early after repair of A-V canal defects is not uncommon when there is marked deformity of the mitral

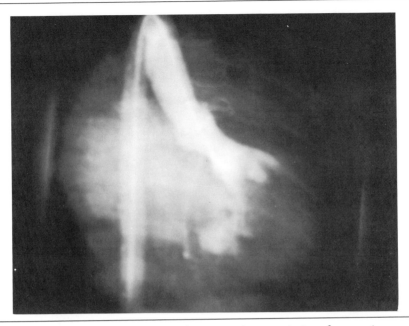

Figure 17-2. A left ventricular angiogram showing massive regurgitation of contrast into a large left atrium. The mitral anulus is small and the leaflets are short and thickened.

valve. In our patients, persistent mitral regurgitation was more common after repair of incomplete A-V canals than with complete. In addition, there are other congenital mitral valve anomalies not amenable to repair that may require valve replacement during infancy or early childhood.

One of the most important considerations in children with severe mitral valve disease is the timing of valve replacement. The limited growth potential of the mitral anulus, inability to significantly enlarge the mitral anulus, the small prosthetic valve sizes required during infancy and the difficulties with anticoagulation in childhood are all reasons to defer insertion of a prosthetic valve in a child for as long as possible. However, the alternatives must be considered. The hemodynamically normal patient with an artificial valve, who is growing and developing normally, is much easier for both physician and family to care for than the chronically ill child with refractory congestive heart failure. We favor earlier mitral valve replacement after having a bad experience with a teenage boy who had valve replacement deferred until an adult size valve could be inserted. The result was a poorly functioning left ventricle and a fatal outcome at surgery.

We feel that the ST. JUDE MEDICAL valve is the prosthesis of choice for mitral valve replacement in children for several reasons. Bioprosthetic valves on the left side of the heart deteriorate early, making them unacceptable. Of the mechanical valves, the ST. JUDE MEDICAL valve probably has the lowest

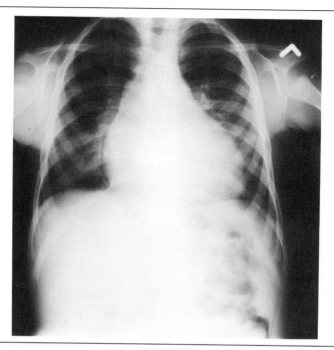

Figure 17-3. Chest x-ray 3 months after mitral valve replacement showing marked improvement in cardiomegaly and vascular congestion.

thrombogenicity and the best hemodynamics in small sizes of any currently available valve. An additional advantage of the ST. JUDE MEDICAL valve is that it does not interfere with two-dimensional echocardiographic study of the heart. Since there are no metal components in the ST. JUDE MEDICAL valve, the echos are not scattered. This allows the pediatric cardiologist to evaluate cardiac anatomy and function, as well as prosthetic valve function, when following these patients postoperatively.

In conclusion, we agree that the ST. JUDE MEDICAL valve is the valve of choice in children undergoing valve replacement on the left side of the heart.

18. THROMBOEMBOLISM IN CHILDREN WITH ST. JUDE MEDICAL® VALVES MAINTAINED ON ASPIRIN AND PERSANTINE®

STUART L. BOE, KATHLEEN W. MCNICHOLAS, HENRY F. OLIVIER, FAUSTINO N. NIGUIDULA, GEORGE J. MAGOVERN, GERALD M. LEMOLE

Abstract. Twenty-five consecutive pediatric patients underwent the insertion of 27 ST. JUDE MEDICAL® valves in a nonrandomized clinical trial. All were managed with aspirin and PERSANTINE® postoperatively. Five thromboembolic events (TE) were observed in the 25 patients during a total of 199 patient-months of follow-up. This represents a 20% TE incidence and extrapolates to 30.1 TE events per 100 patient-years. Based on these data, all children are now placed on COUMADIN® therapy. We recommend COUMADIN anticoagulation in all children with the ST. JUDE MEDI-CAL valve and suggest a cooperative multicenter trial to help resolve the issue.

INTRODUCTION

Reports of early heterograft valve failure in children have lead to a resurgence of usage of mechanical valves in the mitral and aortic positions [1–3]. This resurgence has brought with it a renewed acquaintance with the difficulties of anticoagulating pediatric valve patients. These difficulties and previous reports suggesting the adequacy of antiplatelet adhesive agents in the absence of COUMADIN anticoagulation led to a clinical trial at the Deborah Heart and Lung Center (DHLC) using solely aspirin (ASA) and Persantine in patients with the ST. JUDE MEDICAL valve [4–7].

CLINICAL METHODS AND MATERIALS

Twenty-five consecutive pediatric patients undergoing valve replacement were entered into the study over a 22-month period (table 18-1). All patients receiving

Table 18-1. Clinical trial profile

Time: February 1982 to November 1983
Patients: 25 Pediatric
Valve: 27 St. Jude Medical
Anticoagulation: All treated with aspirin and Persantine

valves were included in the trial. The 13 female and 12 male patients had an age range of 5 to 20 years with an average of 12.3 ± 5.2 years (SD). Fourteen patients (64%) had previous cardiac operations.

Twenty-seven valves were placed in 25 patients. Fourteen patients received mitral prostheses, 10 patients received aortic prostheses and 1 patient had tricuspid, mitral and aortic valves inserted (table 18-2).

The clinical diagnoses for which the valves were placed are noted in table 18-3. Each patient underwent cardiac catheterization before surgery at DHLC. Aortic valve patients had nuclear wall motion studies with pre-exercise and postexercise ejection fractions calculated prior to surgery. Significantly falling ejection fractions with exercise were considered important in making the clinical decision for earlier operative intervention.

Aortic valve replacement (AVR) was carried out most commonly for aortic regurgitation, with or without concomitant stenosis. Two patients had AVR after previous ventricular septal defect (VSD) repair with aortic valvuloplasty. Three patients with aortic valvular insufficiency of the right coronary leaflet and concomitant VSD underwent AVR. These patients each had previous VSD closure and aortic valvuloplasty where feasible. One of these 3 had tetralogy outflow tract reconstruction at the time of original surgery. Two patients had previous aortic commissurotomy with subsequent restenosis leading to valve replacement. One AVR was done with aortic root replacement for Marfan's syndrome and another had stenosis of a previously placed porcine valve.

Mitral valve replacement (MVR) was done in 4 patients with L-transposition of the great arteries (L-TGA). Two of these patients had previous operations. Four children with complete atrioventricular canal (AVC) underwent MVR. Two of

Table 18-2. Patient age and valve profile

Pediatric	
Total	25
Female	13
Male	12
Age range	5 to 20 years
Average age	12.3 ± 5.2 (SD)
St. Jude Medical valves	
Mitral	14
Aortic	10
Mitral/aortic/tricuspid	1

Table 18-3. Preoperative diagnosis and clinical results for 25 patients implanted with St. Jude Medical valves

	No.	Reop	TE	Deaths
AVR for:				
Congenital AR	3	1	2	
VSD, AI	2	2	1	
Postaortic commissurotomy	2	2		
Postrepair tetralogy	1	1		
Aortic root for Marfan's	1	−		
Porcine valve stenosis	1	1	−	−
	10	7	3	0
MVR for:				1 early
L-TGA	4	2	1	2 late
AVC	4	2		
RHD	2		1	
Porcine valve stenosis	2	2		
Congenital MR	2	1	−	−
	14	7	2	3
TVR + MVR + AVR for:				
RHD	1			1 late

these 4 had previous reconstruction. The single patient with triple valve replacement had severe rheumatic valvulitis with pulmonary hypertension and tricuspid insufficiency.

Our usual cardiac surgery protocol was maintained in these patients. Perioperative antibiotics (KEFLIN® 25 mg/kg each 6 hours) were given, and central venous and radial or femoral arterial lines were placed in each patient. Mediansternotomy was accomplished in the usual manner in males and also in females with previous longitudinal skin incisions. A transverse, bilateral, inframammary incision was used in all females done per primum or in those with a previous transverse incision. The superior flap was developed anterior to the pectoralis fascia to the level of the sternal notch and subsequent median sternotomy performed.

Patients were perfused via the ascending aorta and dual vena cava cannulae inserted through a single right atrial incision. In some reoperations the right iliac artery was exposed through a retroperitoneal incision when necessary for immediate cannulation. The left ventricle was vented via the foramen ovale or through its apex. Membrane oxygenators were used in all cases. After aortic cross clamping and systemic perfusion with moderate hypothermia, crystalloid cardioplegia was used at 4° C.

The maximum valve prosthetic size was selected and oriented as described previously [8,9]. Polyester 2-0 pledgeted sutures were used in all cases for intra-annular placement. Transthoracic catheters were tunneled through the right ventricle into the pulmonary artery and used in combination with right atrial lines for determining cardiac output by thermodilution technique after the patients were weaned from bypass. SWAN-GANZ® catheters were used in a smaller number of patients. Sternal closure was done with No. 4 polyester suture after placing temporary epicardial pacing leads and drainage tubes. A suction drain was utilized under the superior flap when the transverse inframammary incision was used.

The 25 patients were followed postoperatively with hemodynamic and ventilatory monitoring and observed for evidence of valve-related complications. After extubation, patients were started on liquids, and ASA and PERSANTINE therapy was begun. ASA was given at a dose of 6 mg/kg up to a maximum of 325 mg once a day. PERSANTINE was given in a dose of 25 mg each day to children under 12 years and 50 mg each day for those older than 12.

RESULTS

Twenty-seven valves were placed in 25 patients. One operating room (OR) death was recorded and 3 late deaths were reported with 96% early survival (one month) and 84% overall survival. The operative death occurred in a 14-year-old female with L-TGA who had previously undergone a Mustard operation with subsequent severe mitral insufficiency and congestive heart failure (CHF). She underwent MVR but could not be discontinued from cardiopulmonary bypass.

Two late deaths occurred at 5 and 19 months postoperatively in a 15-year-old male with previous operation for L-TGA with MVR and in a 6-year-old female with previous L-TGA and MVR. Each had end-stage CHF unresponsive to aggressive medical management. The fourth death was in a 19-year-old male with severe rheumatic valve disease. He died of unmanageable CHF 2 months after triple valve replacement. No evidence of valve malfunction or endocarditis was found in these patients.

Wound infections were absent in these 25 patients, including females with transverse inframammary incisions. All of the transverse incisions healed in a very cosmetically acceptable manner. Those reoperated upon had similar results with no delay in wound healing.

Patients were observed for evidence of thromboembolic (TE) events within the hospital and during outpatient clinic visits. Parents and physicians were contacted directly or by questionnaires in cases where discharged patients had returned to their country of origin. One hundred percent follow-up was achieved.

Five patients were observed to have TE events during this brief follow-up period (table 18-3). Two separate events were recorded in 1 AVR patient. The AVR patient group follow-up was from 1 to 20 months, with a total of 73 patient-months (table 18-4). Thromboembolic events were recorded in 3 of these 10 patients. These occurred in 2 patients within 2 weeks postoperatively and in a third patient at 2 months postoperatively. Transient visual field cuts were noted in the first 2 patients and the third had unilateral visual field blurring. All 3 events were transient and completely resolved within 24 hours. Each patient was teenaged and capable of giving a detailed history and accurately and reliably responding to the consulting ophthalmologist during visual examination. The first patient also

Table 18-4. Length of patient follow-up and time of thromboemboli for 25 patients with St. Jude Medical valves

Follow-up Range 1 to 20 Months	
AVR	73 Patient-months
	3 TE events
	2 at 1 month, 1 at 2 months
MVR	123 Patient-months
	2 TE events
	1 at 6 months, 1 at 1 year
TVR + MVR + AVR	3 Patient-months
	0 TE events
TOTAL	199 Patient-months
	5 TE events

reported a subsequent visual field change 48 hours after resolution of the first event. This also cleared, without permanent deficit.

The MVR group had 123 patient-months of follow-up with 2 TE events, one at 6 months and the other at 12 months postoperatively. The first TE produced visual field deficits. The second patient, a 5-year-old female, sustained a left hemiplegia with incomplete resolution reported at the end of the follow-up period. No TE events were observed during the follow-up of the triple valve patient, who expired 3 months after operation.

Five documented TE events were noted in 199 patient-months or 16.6 patient-years. This extrapolates to 30.1 TE events per 100 patient-years (30% per patient-year). It also represents 5 TE events in 25 patients for a 20% incidence. After analysis of this data and the determination of a clearly unacceptable TE rate, ASA and PERSANTINE were discontinued in all patients and each was placed on COUMADIN with patient/control prothrombin time ratios of 1.5 to 1.8.

DISCUSSION

The major challenges of prosthetic valve replacement in children are similar to those in adults: minimizing the risks of anticoagulation and the frequency of thromboemboli and selecting a valve with the best hemodynamic performance and the longest durability. Valvuloplasty remains our first choice in children whenever possible, as reoperation with increased mortality persists as an inevitable problem whenever valve replacement occurs [10,11].

The initial enthusiasm toward using heterograft tissue valves in children has been tempered by reports of high tissue calcification rates with valve failure rates of 60% at 4 years in some series [12–19]. We now use the ST. JUDE MEDICAL valve primarily, based on its low physical profile, hemodynamic characteristics and the reported low TE rate [20–23]. We make exception and use heterograft valves in the pulmonic or tricuspid positions if no left sided mechanical valves are used, as the heterograft valves have an acceptable longevity on the right side [14].

While the status of mechanical valves without COUMADIN anticoagulation in children may not be resolved, the evidence in adults strongly supports the use of COUMADIN over other agents. A three-fold decrease in TE event rates has been noted using COUMADIN [24,25]. Although ASA was shown in one study to be equally as effective as COUMADIN in protecting adults from heterograft thromboemboli, caution usually leads to the use of COUMADIN in adult hetero-graft mitral valve patients who are not in sinus rhythm [26].

The frequency of complications from COUMADIN in children is not docu-mented nearly as well as in adults. It is unclear if it is higher than the 1 to 2% per year rate reported in adults [27]. The actual follow-up, repeated phlebotomy and frequent testing in a growing active child, is clearly more difficult than in an adult. The pediatric patient on COUMADIN may have to sustain "hard to understand" physical restrictions during an active growth period by protective parents and physicians. The difficulty of follow-up is enhanced at DHLC where the open-door, no-patient-cost policy has brought patients from all corners of the world. Ensuring safe and therapeutic levels of anticoagulation in these patients remains a formidable problem after they return home.

Given the difficulty of monitoring these patients' prothrombin levels and reports suggesting the adequacy of thromboembolism control with ASA and Persantine alone, we undertook a trial using only these two drugs. A randomized trial was not attempted because of the small number of pediatric valves inserted and the length of time anticipated to acquire adequate numbers in each group. It was recognized that a multicenter trial may be necessary to include enough patients to answer the question within a reasonable length of time.

Our results demonstrate the inadequacy of ASA and PERSANTINE at the stated doses to control thromboembolism from mechanical prostheses in these patients. The 20% patient incidence of TE or extrapolated 30.1 TE events per 100 patient-years is several-fold higher than rates reported in adults. It may be that higher doses of ASA and Persantine are necessary. However the doses used are similar to those in other reports using ASA and Persantine.

We also draw attention to reports of 3 cases of leaflet entrapment by thrombus in children and adults with ST. JUDE MEDICAL valves managed without COUMADIN.[28,29] While we had no evidence of prosthetic leaflet malfunction in the children in our trial, we note the report of Moulton detailing a fatal thrombosis of an aortic ST. JUDE MEDICAL prosthesis in an adult despite adequate COUMADIN anticoagulation [30].

The five patients with emboli were examined closely for characteristics predis-posing to TE including arrhythmias, congestive heart failure (CHF), history of infarction, endocarditis of rheumatic or bacterial origin and the findings of a large left atrium or thrombus at the time of surgery. No history of infarction, CHF or bacterial endocarditis was present in any patient with thromboembolism. All were in documented sinus rhythm, except possibly the MVR patient with a late embolus at 12 months. Her episode of thromboembolism occurred while at home in eastern Europe; her rhythm was not determined at the time, although she was in sinus rhythm at discharge. No left atrial thrombi were recorded at the time of surgery in the MVR patients. Previous surgery was present in 64% of the entire patient population, and in 2 of the 3 AVR patients and in 1 of the 2 MVR patients with thromboemboli. The early MVR patient with a thromboembolic event was the only 1 of 5 with rheumatic endocarditis.

Complications from COUMADIN may partially be iatrogenic, caused by over-zealous anticoagulation. The previous goal of patient/control prothrombin ratios of 2.0 to 2.5 may not be more therapeutic than a ratio of 1.5 to 1.8 and probably is associated with more bleeding complications. For this reason we strive for a ratio in the latter range (18 to 20 seconds with a control of 12 seconds). No anticoagu-lant-related difficulties from emboli or bleeding have occurred in these patients at these ratios after switching them from ASA and PERSANTINE to COUMADIN. Subramanian stresses the relative safety of COUMADIN in children when the patient, parents and pediatrician are closely involved [31].

SUMMARY AND CONCLUSIONS

From this small group of 25 pediatric patients with the ST. JUDE MEDICAL valve and ASA and PERSANTINE therapy in a nonrandomized trial, the follow-ing findings were noted:

1. ASA and PERSANTINE did not provide acceptable protection against throm-boemboli, with a rate of 30.1 TE events per 100 patient-years or a 20% patient incidence during this short follow-up.
2. In contrast to previous reports, thromboembolic events were associated with AVR more often than with MVR, although the difference is not statistically significant (p > 0.05).
3. The transverse inframammary incision provided superior cosmetic results when used in female patients undergoing primary or reoperative mediansternotomy with no wound complications observed.
4. Pediatric patients are quite capable of reporting neurologic changes when an adequate history is taken.

We conclude that all children with the ST. JUDE MEDICAL valve prostheses should be placed on COUMADIN except in unusual circumstances or if they are participants in a large multicenter randomized trial to determine the efficacy of ASA and PERSANTINE versus COUMADIN for thromboembolism prevention in patients with mechanical valves. We believe that such a study will be necessary to fully resolve the issue.

REFERENCES

1. Gardner TJ, Roland JMA, Neill CA, et al: Valve replacement in children: A fifteen year experience. J Thorac Cardiovasc Surg 1982; 83,178–185.

2. Donahoo JS, Gardner TJ: St. Jude Medical valve prostheses in infants and children. S Med J 1982; 75,1538–1540.
3. Human G., Jaffe HS, Fraser CB, et al: Mitral valve replacement in children. J Thorac Cardiovasc Surg 1982; 83,873–877.
4. Lomeo A, Patene L, Gentile M, et al: Aortic valve replacement with St. Jude valve without long term anticoagulants: A prospective study, in DeBakey ME (ed): *Advances in Cardiac Valves: Clinical Perspectives,* New York, Yorke Medical Books, 1983, pp 170–172.
5. Pass HI, Sade RM, Crawford FA, et al: St. Jude Prostheses without anticoagulation in Children. Am J Card 1982; 49,1035.
6. Smith JM, Cooley DA, Ott DA, et al: Aortic valve replacement in preteenage children. Ann Thorac Surg 1980; 29,512–518.
7. Geha AS: Valve replacement in children. Ann Thorac Surg 1980; 29,500–501.
8. Baudet EM: Cardiac valve replacement in children with St. Jude Medical prosthesis, in DeBakey ME (ed): *Advances in Cardiac Valves: Clinical Perspectives,* New York, Yorke Medical Books, 1983, pp 149–155.
9. Nicoloff DM, Arom KV, Lindsay WG, et al: Techniques for implantation of the St. Jude valve in the aortic and mitral positions, in Debakey ME (ed): *Advances in Cardiac Valves: Clinical Perspectives.* New York, Yorke Medical Books, 1983, pp 191–196.
10. Williams WG, Pollock JC, Geiss DM, et al: Experience with aortic and mitral valve replacement in children. J Thorac Cardiovasc Surg 1981; 81:326–333.
11. Matthews RA, Park SC, Neches WH, et al: Valve replacement in children and adolescents. J Thorac Cardiovasc Surg 1977; 73:872–878.
12. Geha AS, Laks H, Stansel HC et al: Late failure of porcine valve heterografts in children. J Thorac Cardiovasc Surg 1979; 78:351–364.
13. Wada J, Yokoyama M, Hashimoto A, et al: Long term followup of artificial heart valves in patients under 15 years old. Ann Thorac Surg 1979; 29:519–520.
14. Dunn JM: Porcine valve durability in children. Ann Thorac Surg 1981; 32:357–368.
15. Williams WG, Pollock JC, Geiss DM, et al: Experience with aortic and mitral valve replacement in children. J Thorac Cardiovasc Surg 1981; 81:326–333.
16. Fiddler GI, Gerlis LM, Walker DR, et al: Calcification of glutaraldehyde-preserved porcine and bovine xenograft valves in young children. Ann Thorac Surg 1983; 35:257–261.
17. Walker WE, Duncan JM, Frazier OH, et al: Early experience with the Ionescu-Shiley pericardial xenograft valve: Accelerated calcification in children. J Thorac Cardiovasc Surg 1983; 86: 570–575.
18. Crupi G, Gibson D, Heard B, et al: Severe late failure of a porcine xenograft mitral valve: Clinical, echocardiographic and pathological findings. Thorax 1980; 35:210–212.
19. Cuicio CA, Commerford PJ, Rose AG, et al: Calcification of glutaraldehyde-perserved porcine xenografts in young patients. J Thorac Cardiovasc Surg 1981; 81:621–625.
20. Lillehei CW: Worldwide experience with the St. Jude Medical valve prosthesis: Clinical and hemodynamic results. Contemp Surg 1982; 20:17–32.
21. Wortham DC, Tri TB, Bowen TE: Hemodynamic evaluation of the St. Jude Medical valve prosthesis in the small aortic annulus. J Thorac Cardiovasc Surg 1981; 81:615–620.
22. Nicoloff DM, Emery RW, Arom KV, et al: Clinical and hemodynamic results with the St. Jude Medical cardiac valve prosthesis. J Thorac Cardiovasc Surg 1981; 82:674–683.
23. Chaux A, Gray RG, Matloff JM, et al: An appreciation of the new St. Jude valvular prosthesis. J Thorac Cardiovasc Surg 1981; 81:202–211.
24. Moggio RA, Hammond GL, Stansel HC, et al: Incidence of emboli with cloth-covered Starr-Edwards valve without anticoagulation and with varying forms of anticoagulation. J Thorac Cardiovasc Surg 1978; 75:296–299.
25. St. John Sutton MG, Miller GAH, Oldershaw PJ, et al: Anticoagulants and the Bjork-Shiley prosthesis: Experience of 390 patients. Br Heart J 1978; 40:558–562.
26. Nunez L, Aguado MG, Celemin D, et al: Aspirin or Coumadin as the drug of choice for valve replacement with porcine bioprosthesis. Ann Thorac Surg 1982; 33:354–358.
27. Horstkotte D, Korfer R, Seipel L, et al: Late complications in patients with Bjork-Shiley and St. Jude Medical heart valve replacement. Circulation 1983; 68 (Supp II):11–175—11–184.
28. Nunez L, Iglesias A, Sotillo J: Entrapment of leaflet of St. Jude Medical cardiac valve prosthesis by miniscule thrombus: Report of two cases. Ann Thorac Surg 1980; 29:567–569.

29. Sharma A, Johnson DC, Cartmill TB: Entrapment of both leaflets of St. Jude Medical aortic valve prosthesis in a child. J Thorac Cardiovasc Surg 1983; 86:453–454.
30. Moulton AL, Singleton RT, Oster WF, et al: Fatal thrombosis of an aortic St. Jude Medical valve despite "adequate" anticoagulation. J Thorac Cardiovasc Surg 1982; 83:472–473.
31. Subramanian S: Use of the St. Judge Medical prosthesis in children, in DeBakey ME (ed): *Advances in Cardiac Valves: Clinical Perspectives.* New York, Yorke Medical Books, 1983; pp 129–137.

PART IV. DISCUSSION

EUGENE M. BAUDET AND DONALD B. DOTY, MODERATORS

DONALD B. DOTY: I am sure that after hearing these papers there are some areas of controversy that should be directly approached. Are there any questions?

ANTICOAGULATION IN CHILDREN

QUESTION: At what age would you start to use anticoagulation therapy after prosthetic valvular replacement?

ROBERT M. SADE: We do not believe there is any magic time as to when a patient is no longer a child and becomes an adult. We intend to follow this particular series of children indefinitely without anticoagulation; and later on, the incidence of thromboembolism may start to increase. We will determine whether to start anticoagulation therapy based on the statistics at the time. However, although thromboembolism can occur at any time in the history of a prosthetic valve, there is some data to suggest that an increased incidence occurs in the first couple of years after a valve is implanted. So it may be that once these children are past the first 2 or 3 years after implantation, the risk of thromboembolism will remain small, forever. Therefore, we do not have any particular time when we plan to put them all on anticoagulants. We are going to wait and see what the clinical results tell us to do.

A. MICHAEL BORKON: We have taken a different approach in that children, when they reach 5 to 7 years of age depending on their relative risk for potential hemorrhage have been started on low enough doses of COUMADIN® to maintain their prothrombin times about 1.5 times control. We have done this in the majority of instances, particularly in mitral valve replacements.

QUESTION: Were any of your patients in atrial fibrillation postoperatively and was this associated in any way with the occurrence of thromboembolism?

ROBERT M. SADE: If we had a patient with atrial fibrillation, that patient would have been given COUMADIN. All of our patients were in sinus rhythm as are most children. If we had one who wasn't, we would anticoagulate that patient.

LAWRENCE H. COHN: I think that is a very important point to be made because I think there is a big difference. Most children are not in atrial fibrillation.

RICHARD N. EDIE, M.D. PHILADELPHIA, PENNSYLVANIA: Do you have any hints for orientation of prosthetic valves in the pulmonic position? And, when you removed the valve in the pulmonic position because of thrombosis, did you replace it with another ST. JUDE MEDICAL® valve or with another type of valve?

ROBERT M. SADE: The pulmonary valve was replaced with a porcine valve. I am not sure that using a ST. JUDE MEDICAL valve in the pulmonary position is wise. All the published data suggest very strongly that the probability of a pulmonary or tricuspid bioprosthetic valve failing early in a child is very small. The bioprostheses behave differently in children on the right side of the heart than on the left side. It seems very likely that both tricuspid and pulmonary bioprostheses will last for at least 10 years, possibly substantially longer. So we are likely in the future to use a bioprosthesis in the pulmonary position.

QUESTION: I would like to ask the speakers who, in their opinion, is a child in terms of cardiac valve replacement, because in the literature the variation in cited ages is from 12 to 20 years. I believe that after 15 years of age a child becomes an adult.

ROBERT M. SADE: I do not know the answer to that question. As I said before, I do not know when a child is no longer a child. However, this may be a moot point; what we should be discussing may be whether any patient with a ST. JUDE MEDICAL valve needs COUMADIN anticoagulation. Dr. Crawford is going to present the rest of our series of 200 additional patients with ST. JUDE MEDICAL valve replacements at our institution. Those data are going to suggest that this may be the time to do a prospectively randomized study of adult patients, and, in fact, perhaps the whole spectrum of patients, with ST. JUDE MEDICAL valves to determine whether anticoagulant therapy is indicated. His data will suggest that the complication rate and mortality rate from COUMADIN anticoagulation alone may exceed the complication rate in nonanticoagulated patients at any age with ST. JUDE MEDICAL valves. Such a study should be done as a prospective, randomized investigation, which is, of course, an extremely rare event in the field of valve surgery.

DONALD B. DOTY: I think you probably all want to have the opportunity to ask Dr. Baudet, as long as he is here, what the status of valves is in the Fontan–Baudet operation. We saw one valve here in the atrioventricular position next to the ventricle in the Hopkins series.

EUGENE M. BAUDET: We consider mitral insufficiency in tricuspid atresia or a univentricular heart as a contraindication to the operation. In the experience of Dr. Fontan with this operation, there is only one case of mitral replacement before repair of tricuspid atresia that had a bad result. So we have had no experience of concomitant mitral valve replacement before the Fontan procedure for univentricular heart and tricuspid atresia.

SHAHBUDIN RAHIMTOOLA: I guess I have to take issue, Dr. Sade, with some of your statements. You suggested this might happen by saying you are going against the current practice trends. I do not practice pediatric cardiology, but I think I do understand data and statistics. I cannot counter your beliefs because your beliefs are your own. However, you recall what happened, according to your beliefs, to all children who received bioprostheses. But as far as the ST. JUDE MEDICAL valve and the data you have presented us, I think that from a statistical consideration it is violating some of the fundamental principles of statistical analysis to generalize from adults to children because you are comparing apples to pears. No amount of statistical manipulation is going to compensate for a such comparison. Why do you feel this valve is totally safe? I would like to remind you that among your patients, four have undergone reoperation and, thus, have already had two open heart surgeries and one has had a myocardial infarction. None of this leads me to believe that what you are proposing is a solution or an appropriate answer to the problems you face. I guess I am not convinced by your basic methodology, and therefore, I am not sure that you will arrive at the end point that you are seeking.

ROBERT M. SADE: Please do not put words in my mouth. I did not say this was the ideal valve. I did not say that it was the best possible thing to do for children. I am merely saying, based on our series, and it is probably the best data that we have, that it is just as safe for us to treat an adult with a ST. JUDE MEDICAL valve without anticoagulation as it is to treat a child with anticoagulation. That is not to say that it is perfectly safe. I did not say that, and I do not think that anybody would. There are complications and risks with any kind of valve replacement. The job of surgeons is to find the safest possible way to do this kind of surgery and not to delude ourselves into thinking anything we do is perfect or completely safe. The least risk is what we are trying to achieve. The risk of anticoagulation itself is very considerable. That needs to be put into any equation when considering whether or not to anticoagulate any given patient. I don't know why your results are different from ours. I think such differences may be related to the kind of follow-up you have, the kind of detail you go into when you're talking to patients, and how thoroughly you take a history. There are a lot of possible explanations. I think that Dr. Rahimtoola and I can agree on one thing, perhaps, and that is we certainly don't know now and we won't ever know, whether it's reasonable to treat pediatric patients with Persantine and aspirin, with aspirin alone, without any antithrombotic agents or with COUMADIN. Until we have a properly done prospective, randomized study, there is simply no way of knowing, what we're doing with these drugs. I think it's going to be a very important thing for us to do that at some time in the future.

DEMETRE NICOLOFF: I believe we have the longest experience with a ST. JUDE MEDICAL valve in a child. We put it in about 6 years ago and at that time we were faced with whether we were going to put this child on anticoagulants or not. We took the very conservative approach as we did with all the ST. JUDE MEDICAL valves. We did anticoagulate that child, and so far have anticoagulated all the children. We have 14 children with valves in place. There has been one thromboembolic event—in a boy with an ascending aortic aneurysm with a bicuspid valve that dissected. So we placed a ST. JUDE MEDICAL valve and a woven graft in the aorta. This occurred about 3 months after surgery. His protime was normal. He is now completely asymptomatic, so it was a very transient event. There have been no other instances of thromboembolism. It is a problem to keep these children on anticoagulants and to draw the blood, but I think the pediatricians, when they look back and see that there have been no thromboemboli and no major problems with the anticoagulants in this small group of 14 patients, they put up with the problems of anticoagulating children. It is a small, early series.

ROBERT M. SADE: One of the things that we see in both the adult and the pediatric experience is the diversities of outcomes, particularly with respect to the thromboembolism and thrombosis. I think two comments must be in order here. One is that these are relatively small numbers of events. These are not large population studies where we can be very secure about the meaning of each of the individual events. For instance, we did not find a statistical association with atrial fibrillation, preoperative thromboembolism or any of the predictive factors; and we probably will not, until we have more events upon which to actually make a concerted statistical analysis. The second comment I have is that there must be differences we are not recognizing in the types of patients operated upon and their status in other respects after surgery. Dr. Fisk very nicely elaborated all of the nonprosthetic factors that can contribute to the occurrence of postoperative emboli; and some of these yet undefined factors must go into making the wide, diverse, results that we see. I think I'd have to agree with the comment about needing some kind of basis for a comparison. We can't rely on comparisons between multiple centers. The study really has to be done at one or two centers that have a comparable basis to arrive at such conclusions.

RICHARD GRAY: I used to think that people from the South couldn't talk fast, but Dr. Sade has done a good job. The question I would like to ask is, do you have an explanation for why there is an increased incidence of bleeding complication in your reported patient population, since your aim is to have only mildly anticoagulated patients?

ROBERT M. SADE: I have no reason to explain why our patients have had more anticoagulant-related complications. We have anticoagulated at a lower level than we have with all previous valves. I have no argument with the data presented here this morning, but in our series we have had more problems and more serious difficulties from anticoagulation than we have had from valve-related events.

QUESTION: Dr. Sade, what was your dose of aspirin, again?

ROBERT M. SADE: It was roughly equivalent to one aspirin a day for a patient of 70 kg. We taper that down for the younger patients based on relative size.

ALTERNATIVES TO VALVE REPLACEMENT

DONALD B. DOTY: Are there further questions on this interesting and unsolved subject?

DENTON COOLEY: I would like to address Dr. Borkon and Dr. Sade. I see that you both have a rather large series of valve replacements by comparison to what we have and a much larger pediatric practice. I wonder if you have other alternatives for patients with valve incompetence and valve stenosis, in the time period in which you are reporting? How many patients underwent valvuloplasty or valvotomy during this period or is valve replacement the procedure of choice?

A. MICHAEL BORKON: In our aortic group, 9 out of 10 individuals had at least 1 prior valvotomy, if not 2, and 1 patient had 3 valvotomies prior to valve replacement. In the mitral valve group, as in many centers, we will do everything we possibly can to the regurgitant valve to try to restore its competence, before valve replacement. We see very few young children with rheumatic-related mitral stenosis. We have had several parachute mitral valves but they have required valve replacement. Unfortunately, many do come to reoperation even after initial attempts at *sparing* operations.

ROBERT M. SADE: I agree with that. I think conservative treatment to preserve a reasonably functioning natural valve is the operation of choice. But sometimes we are forced to do a valve replacement. A majority of the aortic valve replacements in this series were for aortic insufficiency; and except for aortic insufficiency associated with ventricular septal defects, I do not know a good operation to preserve the valve in aortic insufficiency. There were only 9 patients who had isolated mitral valve disease. Very few of the rest of the patients had primary operations done to replace the valve; most had conservative operations initially, and this was a second or subsequent procedure. Many of our patients had a previously implanted porcine valve replaced with a ST. JUDE MEDICAL prosthesis.

JOSEPH J. AMATO, M.D. NEWARK, NEW JERSEY: We tend toward conservatism, and we do mostly valvuloplasties if we can. However, in the past 5 years, our experience has included 16 valve replacements in children. We have had 3 nonvalve-related deaths; and therefore, we have been following 13 patients who have been on COUMADIN. We have had a policy of using COUMADIN anticoagulation in all children greater than the age of 10. These children have had no thromboembolic events and there have been no hemorrhagic incidents. Therefore, we really feel that this is the way to go in children.

VALVE SIZING

DR. CLARENCE S. WELDON, M.D., ST. LOUIS, MISSOURI: Could I just make a comment about replacing prostheses in children? In the aortic position, you can do one of two things. You can either put a large valve in the first time and do this by performing an aortoventriculo-plasty, or you can put a small valve in and do the aortoventriculoplasty the next time you operate. It doesn't really matter. It's possible to change an aortic valve with an aortoven-triculoplasty, a ventral one, quite easily—just as easy as it is to redo any other aortic operation. On the other hand, the atrioventricular position presents a special problem. It's very hard to get a bigger valve in the second time around because there's so much fibrosis in the atrioventricular groove that you can't put in a valve much bigger than you did the first time. If you are going to put atrioventricular valves in small children, who have a lot of growth potential, and you expect the atrioventicular valve ring to grow so you can put a bigger one in the second time, you can't do it. Therefore, it behooves you to put a big one in the first time.

DONALD B. DOTY: Well, we have heard some very conflicting reports and opinions during this discussion that are obviously not going to be easily resolved. What this discussion has done is to make us aware of the very important area of anticoagulation and to indicate that if a multicenter prospective randomized study is needed, it is in the pediatric population.

V. INTERMEDIATE FOLLOW-UP OF PATIENTS WITH ST. JUDE MEDICAL® PROSTHESES: 52 TO 72 MONTHS

19. A 52-MONTH EXPERIENCE WITH THE ST. JUDE MEDICAL® CARDIAC PROSTHESIS AT THE MEDICAL UNIVERSITY OF SOUTH CAROLINA

FRED A. CRAWFORD, JR, JOHN M. KRATZ, ROBERT M. SADE, MARTHA P. STROUD, DAVID M. BARTLES

In the mid and late 1970s, the porcine heterograft became the most frequently used valvular prosthesis at the Medical University of South Carolina. This prosthesis began to be less attractive, however, as we, like many others, noted a progressive increase in failure rates due to early calcification. Because of the possibility of improved flow characteristics and of decreased thromboembolic complications, a clinical trial with the ST. JUDE MEDICAL® valve was initiated in April 1979.

Since April 1979, over 300 patients have undergone valve replacement with the ST. JUDE MEDICAL prosthesis at the Medical University of South Carolina. This chapter considers only those patients who have undergone isolated aortic or mitral valve replacement with or without coronary artery bypass surgery between April 1979 and August 1983[1].

PATIENTS AND METHODS

In this interval, 118 patients underwent *isolated aortic valve replacement*. Age ranged from 7 to 84 years with a mean of 49.1 years. Ninety patients have undergone *mitral valve replacement* with age ranging from 6 to 78 years with a mean of 44.5 years. Associated coronary artery bypass surgery was performed in 23.7% of the aortic valve group and 7.8% of the mitral valve group.

Operative techniques included standard cardiopulmonary bypass with moderate hypothermia, crystalloid potassium-induced cardioplegia and topical myocardial cooling. All valves were inserted with interrupted mattress sutures backed with TEFLON® felt pledgets. Valve sizes ranged from 19 mm to 31 mm in the aortic position with 71% of the aortic replacements being size 23 mm or smaller. Mitral valves ranged from 23 mm to 33 mm. Adults were anticoagulated with COUMADIN® to a prothrombin time from 1.5 to 1.8 normal. Follow-up was 97.6% complete and ranged from 1 to 54 months with a mean of nearly 2 years.

RESULTS

In the aortic group, 3 patients died in the postoperative period for an operative mortality of 2.5% (table 19-1). There have been 9 late deaths, and the actuarial survival at 42 months is 86.7 $\pm$ 3.8%. Of the 9 late deaths, 2 were due to anticoagulant related complications. Three patients have had thromboembolic episodes, all transient and occurring within the first 12 months after surgery for a linearized rate of 1.6% per patient-year. The probability of remaining free of thromboembolism at 42 months is 96.9 $\pm$ 1.8%. Important anticoagulant-related complications occurred in 13 patients (6.9% per patient-year). Four patients developed prosthetic valve endocarditis. Two patients developed paravalvular leakage unrelated to prosthetic valve endocarditis. The probability of remaining free of all valve-related complications in the aortic position is 59.4 $\pm$ 9.7% at 42 months largely because of the significant number of anticoagulation-related problems. The probability of remaining free of reoperation is 96 $\pm$ 2.0% at 42 months. Of the

Table 19-1. Aortic mortality and complication rates and actuarial data at 42 months for 106 patients

	No. patients	Percent (simple)
Mortality		
operative	3	2.5
late deaths	9	

	No. events	Percent per patient-year
Complications		
thromboembolic episodes	3	1.6
anticoagulant related	13	6.9
paravalvular leakage	2	
valve mechanical failure	0	
thrombosis	0	

	Percent (actuarial)
Actuarial data at 42 months	
survival	86.7
thromboembolism	96.9
free of all valve-related complications	59.4
free of reoperation	96.0

106 long-term survivors, 102 have improved at least one or more New York Heart Association functional Classes, and the mean change in functional Class from preoperative to postoperative is 3.1 $+$ 0.7 to 1.2 $+$ 0.4 (p $<$ 0.001).

In the mitral group, 4 patients died in the postoperative period for an operative mortality of 4.4% (table 19-2). There have been 4 late deaths, and the actuarial survival at 42 months is 89.3 $+$ 3.8%. Two late deaths were due to anticoagulant-related complications, 1 to a stroke and 1 to progressive cardiomyopathy. Two patients have sustained thromboembolic complications, both occurring within the first 12 months following surgery for a linearized rate of thromboembolic episodes of 1.2% per patient-year. The probability of remaining free of thromboembolism at 42 months is 97.2 $+$ 2.0%. Anticoagulant-related complications have occurred in 4 patients (2.4% per patient-year). One patient has developed paravalvular leak. The probability of remaining free of all valve-related complications in the mitral position is 81.2 $+$ 5% at 42 months and of being free of reoperation is 97.2 $+$ 2.0%. Of the 82 long-term survivors in the mitral group, 81 have improved one or more functional Classes, and the mean improvement from preoperative to postoperative is 3.2 $+$ 0.7 to 1.3 $+$ 0.5 (p $<$ 0.001).

No mechanical failure of the ST. JUDE MEDICAL valve has occurred in either position, and no patient has developed thrombosis of the valve.

Table 19-2. Mitral mortality and complication rates and actuarial data at 42 months for 82 patients

	No. patients	Percent (simple)
Mortality		
operative	4	4.4
late deaths	4	

	No. events	Percent per patient-year
Complications		
thromboembolic episodes	2	1.2
anticoagulant related	4	2.4
paravalvular leakage	1	
valve mechanical failure	0	
thrombosis	0	

	Percent (actuarial)
Actuarial data at 42 months	
survival	89.3
thromboembolism	97.2
free of all valve-related complications	81.2
free of reoperation	97.2

DISCUSSION

The ST. JUDE MEDICAL valve has become our mechanical prosthesis of choice because of favorable hemodynamic results that are associated with marked clinical improvement and low thromboembolic rates. Because the incidence of anticoagulant-related complications is higher in our series than that of thromboembolism, we believe it may be appropriate to consider a prospective trial of alternate methods of anticoagulation in those patients in sinus rhythm undergoing aortic valve replacement with the ST. JUDE MEDICAL prosthesis. The experience of others with significant anticoagulant-related complications provides further support for such a proposal. Given the excellent clinical response of patients, anticoagulant-related complications remain the primary concern that we have in patients undergoing valve replacement therapy with this prosthesis.

REFERENCE

1. Crawford FA, Kratz JM, Sade RM, et al: Aortic and mitral valve replacement with the St. Jude Medical prosthesis. Ann Surg 1984; 199(6):753–761.

20. A 57-MONTH EXPERIENCE WITH THE ST. JUDE MEDICAL® CARDIAC PROSTHESIS AT HAHNEMANN UNIVERSITY HOSPITAL

ELDRED D. MUNDTH

Our experience with the ST. JUDE MEDICAL® prosthetic valve was initiated in late 1978 because of our increasing concerns over the significant incidence of thromboembolic events and valve thrombosis of the BJÖRK-SHILEY® valve and of degenerative, component failure with the porcine valve, necessitating reoperation.

The data for this study was collected from October 1978 to June 1983, a 57-month period. There were a total of 376 patients in this series with 417 valve implants. Table 20-1 indicates the distribution of valve replacement procedures: 117 isolated aortic valve replacements, 131 mitral valve replacements, 31 double valve replacements and 97 various combined coronary bypass and valve replacement procedures.

The overall operative hospital mortality was 9.5% (table 20-2). We analyzed the risk of surgery according to preoperative risk. The lower risk operative mortality was 3%, and the higher risk operative mortality was 17%. The clinical parameters that were used to define high risk were:

1. preoperative ejection fraction less than 30% either by left ventricular angiographic technique and/or radionuclide studies;
2. cardiac index of less than 2.0 L/min/m² associated with left ventricular segmental wall contractile abnormalities;
3. systolic pulmonary artery pressure over 60 mm Hg associated with a significantly lowered cardiac output;
4. acute myocardial infarction within three weeks preoperatively;

Table 20-1. Distribution of valve replacement procedures

Study period	57 months
Patients	376
Valve implants	417
Isolated AVR	117
Isolated MVR	131
AVR + MVR	31
Valve replacement + CAB or other procedure	97

AVR = aortic valve replacement
MVR = mitral valve replacement
CAB = coronary artery bypass

Table 20-2. Operative mortality

Operative mortality	9.5%
Low-risk operative mortality	3.0%
High-risk operative mortality	17.0%
Major complications	8.8%
Minor complications	5.0%

5. acute bacterial endocarditis with hemodynamic deterioration at the time of surgery; or
6. reoperative surgery with any of the above criteria.

Major complications occurred perioperatively in approximately 9% and minor complications in approximately 5%.

The valve-related complications in the overall series were 12.7% (table 20-3). Known thromboembolic complications (TE) were 2.4%. Suspected, but not proven thromboembolic events totalled 2%. The low 1% incidence of TE per 100 patient-years, including both the documented as well as suspected events, was quite

Table 20-3. Percentage of valve-related complications per 100 patient-years

Overall	12.7%
Thromboembolic	
Known	2.4% (7)
Suspected	2.0% (6)
Prosthetic endocarditis	1.7% (5)
Paravalvular leak	
Significant	1.4% (4)
Insignificant	5.1% (15)
Valvular stenosis or other	0.3% (1)

low compared with our previous experience with other prosthetic valves. There was a significant incidence of infection postoperatively. Five patients (1.7%) in this series developed prosthetic endocarditis and the significant paravalvular leaks (1.-4%) that occurred were in some of these patients. There was only one questionable valve-related problem of mechanical dysfunction. Unfortunately, there is not documentation of whether this was true valvular dysfunction.

Postoperative survival was evaluated over a mean of 1.7 years in 376 patients (table 20-4). There were 5.3% late deaths (> 30 days postoperatively) yielding an attrition rate of approximately 3.1% per year (table 20-4).

The functional status in follow-up was evaluated in 292 patients (86%) (table 20-5) over a mean of 2.6 years. Postoperatively, 87% were in New York Heart Association (NYHA) Class I. Mild or moderate symptoms (NYHA Class II) were present in 12%, and there were very few patients remaining in higher functional classifications. The great majority of patients were relieved of any symptoms of failure or angina.

ISOLATED AORTIC VALVE REPLACEMENT

The operative mortality was 0.8% in the overall group of patients. There were no deaths in the low operative risk category (table 20-6). In the high-risk category, operative mortality was 2.7%. There were 3.4% late deaths or, 2.1% per patient-year. The mean follow-up period in this group was 1.6 years, varying from six months to 3 years.

The thromboembolic complication rate was approximately 2% per patient-year with isolated aortic valve replacement. The only complications were in patients who had questionable anticoagulation at the time of the thromboembolic event. Actuarial cumulative survival at 3 years was 94%. The percentage of patients asymptomatic or in NYHA Class I was 87%.

Table 20-4. Postoperative survival (> 30 days)

Survival follow-up	92%
Mean follow-up	1.7 years
Late deaths (≥ 30 days)	5.3%
	3.1% per year

Table 20-5. Functional status postoperatively of 292 patients

Follow-up	86% (292)
NYHA Class I or asymptomatic	87%
NYHA Class II	12%
NYHA Classes III and IV	3.1%
Free of shortness of breath	87%
Free of angina	98%

NYHA = New York Heart Association

Table 20-6. Results of isolated aortic valve replacement in 117 patients

Operative mortality	0.8%
low risk	0.0%
high risk	2.7%
Late deaths	3.4%
Mean follow-up	1.6 years
Valve related complications	16.3%
Thromboembolic complications	4.1% (4)
Prosthetic endocarditis	0.0%
Parvalvular leak	
significant	2.0% (2)
insignificant	10.2% (10)
Actuarial survival at 3 years	94.0%
NYHA Class I or asymptomatic	87%
NYHA Class II	12%
NYHA Class III & IV	1%

NYHA = New York Heart Association (98 patients)

ISOLATED MITRAL VALVE REPLACEMENT

For 131 isolated mitral valve replacement patients, the overall hospital mortality was 8% (table 20-7). In the low-risk category the operative mortality was 3.3%, and for the high-risk patient the operative mortality was 14%. The complication rate for mitral valve replacement was 18%. There was a 4.2% per patient-year late death rate, somewhat higher than for isolated aortic valve replacement. There was an incidence of 12% valve-related complications with a thromboembolic complication rate of 4% or approximately 2% per patient-year. At three years, 78% of the patients were surviving. The functional status of 100 patients was determined over a mean follow-up period of 1.6 years.

DOUBLE VALVE REPLACEMENT

Double valve replacement was carried out in 31 patients. There was a very substantial operative mortality rate because many of these patients were in a high-risk category preoperatively. There was a very favorable flat curve for cumulative survival of over 80% up to a 3 year period of follow-up.

Table 20-7. Results of isolated mitral valve
replacement in 131 patients

Operative mortality	8.0%
low risk	3.3%
high risk	14.0%
Late deaths	7.5%
Mean follow-up	1.6 years
Valve-related complications	12.0%
Thromboembolic complications	
known	2.0% (2)
suspected	4.0% (4)
Prosthetic endocarditis	3.0% (3)
Paravalvular leak	
significant	1.0% (1)
insignificant	2.0% (2)
Actuarial survival at 3 years	78%
NYHA Class I or asymptomatic	81%
NYHA Class II	13%
NYHA Class III & IV	6%

NYHA = New York Heart Association (100 patients)

COMBINED PROCEDURES

For combined procedures of valve replacement and coronary bypass, the operative mortality depended upon the preoperative risk category that had a great influence upon immediate operative risk. In those patients who survived surgery, during a 3 year period of follow-up, there was excellent overall survival. For mitral valve and coronary bypass graft procedures, we noted a significant operative mortality. This is related to the fact that many of these patients had mitral regurgitation as a result of ischemic heart disease with poor left ventricular function. One expects a fairly high mortality rate for these combined procedures. Cumulative survival is quite good if the patient is operated on at an appropriate time in the course of the disease.

CONCLUSION

In summary, we have had a good experience with the ST. JUDE MEDICAL cardiac prosthetic valve and do consider it as the prosthetic mechanical valve of choice. We do anticoagulate all patients unless specific anticoagulant complications occur. The only case of valve thrombosis occurred in a drug addict who would not take COUMADIN®. That patient eventually died of bacterial endocarditis from use of drugs. Where anticoagulation is contraindicated we tend to use porcine tissue valves but are still somewhat concerned about the long-term durability of that particular valve type.

21. INCIDENCE OF COMPLICATION WITH THE ST. JUDE MEDICAL® PROSTHESIS: A 58-MONTH STUDY AT HAMOT MEDICAL CENTER

GEORGE J. D'ANGELO, G. F. KISH, P. G. SARDESAI, W. S. TAN

Abstract. From April 1979 to January 1, 1984 (58 months), 220 patients received ST. JUDE MEDICAL® cardiac valve prostheses (106 aortic, 101 mitral, 13 double). Incidents of nonfatal thromboembolism occurred in 2 of 202 late survivors (0.4% per patient-year). Six patients (1.2% per patient-year) sustained anticoagulation-related complications, 3 of which were fatal and 3 nonfatal. There was one incident of paravalvular leakage (0.2% per patient-year) and no incidents of hemolysis, valve thrombosis or valve infection.

Mechanical prosthetic valves have established long-term durability but the incidence of thromboembolism has been less satisfying. Therefore, the search for the perfect valve continues.

The choice of replacing a cardiac valve with a prosthetic valve is based upon its hemodynamics, durability, thromboembolic propensity and hemolytic potential. The hemodynamic assessment of the ST. JUDE MEDICAL valve demonstrates that it performs well in the aortic, mitral and tricuspid positions. The central bileaflet flow design leads to minimal gradients even in the small valves, which make it ideal for use in children. The purpose of its all-pyrolytic construction is to decrease the incidence of thromboembolism.

MATERIALS AND METHODS

The ST. JUDE MEDICAL valve has been used at our institution, the Hamot Medical Center, since April 1979. From April 1979 to January 1, 1984, 233 valves were implanted in 220 patients. Their ages ranged from 7 to 85 years (mean age of 57). Single valves (106 aortic, 101 mitral) with or without concomitant cardiac procedures were placed in 207 patients. Thirteen patients received double valves. The operative mortality ($\leq$ 30 days) was 8.2% (18/220) for the series (table 21-1).

The total follow-up was 464 patient-years, with a mean follow-up of 2.3 years and a maximum of 4.8 years. Twenty-five patients had other prosthetic valves that required replacement.

ANTICOAGULATION

All patients were started on COUMADIN® by the third postoperative day except for one patient who could not tolerate anticoagulation. She previously had a mechanical valve that required explantation because of a high pressure gradient. She was begun on aspirin on the third postoperative day and has remained on it for a period of 51 months. The prothrombin time of all patients is regulated between 20% to 30% activity.

Patients who sustained complications of anticoagulation therapy, or were difficult to control, had warfarin discontinued and were begun on antiplatelet adhesive agents. Eleven are presently on either dipyridamole and aspirin or aspirin alone (table 21-2) for a period of 8 to 51 months.

Table 21-1. Patient distribution

No. of patients	220
Age range (years)	7–85 (mean 57)
Previous cardiac operations	25 (11.3%)
Concomitant cardiac operations	51 (23.2%)
Operative mortality	18 (8.2%)

Table 21-2. Patients not receiving anticoagulation

Patient	Valve	Rhythm	Drug	Duration (months)
L.B.	Mitral	AF[1]	D[3] & A[4]	30
G.M.	Mitral	AF	D & A	11
C.W.	Mitral	AF	D & A	9
H.B.	Aortic	Reg[2]	None	22
C.D.	Aortic	Reg	D & A	10
F.H.	Aortic	Reg	D & A	33
M.M.	Aortic	Reg	D & A	6
L.R.	Aortic	Reg	D & A	29
D.S.	Aortic	Reg	D & A	19
J.T.	Aortic	Reg	D & A	8
K.W.	Aortic	Reg	A only	51

[1]AF = atrial fibrillation
[2]Reg = regular
D[3] = dipyridamole
A[4] = aspirin

FOLLOW-UP

Complete follow-up of all survivors was obtained by patient contact or report by the family physician.

RESULTS

Thromboembolism

Nonfatal thromboembolism occurred in 2 of the 202 late survivors (0.4% per patient-year). A transient episode occurred 2 months postoperatively in a patient with a mitral valve prosthesis. The other incident occurred after an aortic valve replacement at 3 months; this patient continues to have a minimal residual neurologic deficit (table 21-3).

Hemolysis

Although LDH is not an accurate measurement for the degree of hemolysis, when a high value is coupled with an abnormal reticulocyte count and a low RBC, it does indicate a significant degree of hemolysis.

All patients had an LDH value taken preoperatively (normal = 110–225 U/L). In 144 patients (71%) this test was performed postoperatively from 3 months to 3 years. In 37 of 144 patients the value was normal both before and after valve replacement; 47 of 144 patients had normal values preoperatively but abnormal results postoperatively; and 60 of 144 patients had abnormal values before surgery, which remained elevated after surgery (table 21-4). One patient who had a prior mechanical mitral valve (BJÖRK-SHILEY®) removed because of multiple episodes of thromboembolism had a LDH value of 1200 U/L immediately postopera-

Table 21-3. Complications

	No of patients	Percent per patient-year
Due to anticoagulation	6	1.2
Thromboembolism	2	0.4
Hemolysis	0	0.0
Paravalvular leak	1	0.2
Valve thrombosis	0	0.0
Valve infection	0	0.0

Table 21-4. LDH (N=110–225 U/L) in 144 patients postoperatively

LDH value	Patients
Normal before and after	37
Normal before but increased postoperatively	47
Abnormal before	60

tively; this decreased to a value of 671 U/L with a red blood count of 4.04 million and a hematocrit of 38.6.

COMPLICATIONS FROM ANTICOAGULATION

Six patients (1.2% per patient-year) sustained complications due to anticoagulation. Three were fatal and an equal number were nonfatal. The fatalities were the result of intracerebral hemorrhage and subdural hemorrhage (table 21-5).

LATE DEATHS

Two late deaths were cardiac related, but none were valve related. There was a total of 16 late deaths (7.9%) in the 202 late survivors (table 21-5).

COMMENT

Our results with the ST. JUDE MEDICAL valve prosthesis compare favorably with other centers utilizing either mechanical or bioprosthetic valves. The excellent durability and hemodynamic function of the valve are proven. Our study demonstrates the low incidence of thromboembolism.

A question that should be addressed is whether the newer methods of prevention of thromboembolism should be instituted in place of the conventional use of warfarin therapy. In our experience, anticoagulation complications pose a greater risk than did thromboembolism. Should we not consider a coordinated study by several centers to begin an antiplatelet drug regimen of dipyridamole and aspirin after a limited period of warfarin in those patients with regular rhythm?

The low incidence of thromboembolism associated with use of the ST. JUDE

Table 21-5. Causes of late death

Cardiac related	
Myocardial infarction	1
Cardiac failure	1
Total	2
Related to anticoagulation	
Cerebral hemorrhage	2
Subdural hemorrhage	1
Total	3
Others	
GI bleeding	1
Aplastic anemia	1
Renal failure	3
Pneumonia	3
CA of brain	1
CA of stomach	1
Rupture of colon diverticulum	1
Total	11

MEDICAL valve, in addition to excellent durability, hemodynamic design and flow pattern, make it the mechanical valve of choice.

REFERENCES

1. Janusz MT, Miyagishima RT, Tutassura H, et al: Experience with the Carpentier-Edwards® porcine valve prosthesis in 700 patients. Ann Thorac Surg 1982; 34:625–634.
2. Pelletur C, Chaitman BR, Baillot R, et al: Clinical and hemodynamic results with the Carpentier-Edwards® Porcine Bioprosthesis. Ann Thorac Surg 1982; 34:612–625.
3. Angell WW, Angell JD, Kosek JC: Twelve-year experience with glutaraldehyde-preserved porcine xenografts. J Thorac Cardiovasc Surg 1982; 83:493–503.
4. Ionescu MI, Smith DR, Hasan SS, et al: Clinical durability of the pericardial xenograft valve: Ten years' experience with mitral replacement. Ann Thorac Surg 1982; 34:265–278.
5. Daenen W, Navelstein A, van Cauwelaert P, et al: Nine years' experience with the Björk-Shiley® prosthetic valve: Early and late results of 932 valve replacements. Ann Thorac Surg 1983; 35:651–664.
6. Hill JD, La Follette L, Szaruicki RJ, et al: Risk-benefit analysis of warfarin therapy in Hancock mitral valve replacement. J Thorac Cardiovasc Surg 1982; 83:718–724.
7. Miller DC, Oyer PE, Stinson EB, et al: Ten to fifteen year reassessment of the performance characteristics of the Starr-Edwards® Model 6120 mitral valve prosthesis. J Thorac Cardiovasc Surg 1983; 85:1–21.
8. Cheung D, Flemma RJ, Mullen DC, et al: Ten-year follow-up in aortic valve replacement using the Björk-Shiley® prosthesis. Ann Thorac Surg 1981; 32:138–146.

22. MITRAL VALVE REPLACEMENT WITH ST. JUDE MEDICAL® PROSTHESES: A 60-MONTH STUDY OF 350 CASES AT CENTRE HOSPITALIER UNIVERSITAIRE

HENRI DUPON, J. L. MICHAUD, D. DUVEAU, PH. DESPINS, M. TRAIN

Abstract. Between March 1979 and March 1984, 350 patients underwent valve replacement with the ST. JUDE MEDICAL® (SJM) cardiac valve prosthesis in the mitral position. Operative mortality for the entire group was 4.3% and for single mitral valve replacement (MVR), 3.1%. There was 98% follow-up from 6 to 60 months with a mean follow-up of 31 months. Warfarin (COUMADIN®) anticoagulation was recommended for all patients. There were no cases of mechanical failure. The incidence of thromboembolism was 0.57% per patient-year. Thrombosis of a prosthesis occurred in 3 patients (0.34% per patient-year). Clinically significant hemolysis occurred in 5 patients with paravalvular leaks following MVR. Late mortality was 8.3% during a follow-up of 865 patient-years. There were 10 cases (36%) of cardiogenic causes, and 2 cases of sudden death not documented. Symptoms consistent with NYHA Class I or II were reported in 283 patients (94.3%). The actuarial survival curve for all patients shows an 84% survival at 5 years. This experience indicates that the ST. JUDE MEDICAL valve offers an excellent alternative for the surgeon when choosing a mechanical valve.

INTRODUCTION

From March 1971 to March 1979, the BJÖRK-SHILEY® cardiac valve prosthesis was used routinely in the mitral position in our clinic. Hemodynamic performance was satisfactory; safety and durability were good; and mechanical failure or prosthesis-induced hemolysis did not occur. But our cardiologists observed too many thromboembolic events. We became more aware of this major problem in 1977 when the ST. JUDE MEDICAL (SJM) valve, which was designed to overcome this problem, was introduced. This was the reason we decided to use the SJM valve in March 1979.

This report documents our experience with mitral valve replacement (MVR) with the SJM prosthesis from March 1, 1979 to March 1, 1984 (60 months), involving 350 consecutive patients and 98% follow-up.

MATERIALS AND METHODS

This study included 153 males and 197 females. Mean age was 55.6 years with a range of 7 to 77 years and 137 (39%) from 60 to 77 years (see figure 22-1).

Mitral valves were implanted in 350 patients (figure 22-2). MVR was performed in 252 patients of whom 9 also had coronary artery bypass (CAB) and 13 also had tricuspid annuloplasty. Double valve replacement was carried out in 93 patients:

- 91 had MVR with a SJM valve and aortic valve replacement (AVR) with a BJÖRK-SHILEY valve.
- 2 had MVR and tricuspid valve replacement (TVR) with SJM valves.

Triple valve replacement was carried out in 5 patients with MVR and TVR with SJM valves and AVR with a BJÖRK-SHILEY valve.

The predominant lesion (table 22-1) was mitral regurgitation in 130 patients. Combined stenosis and regurgitation was the cause for replacement in 105 patients

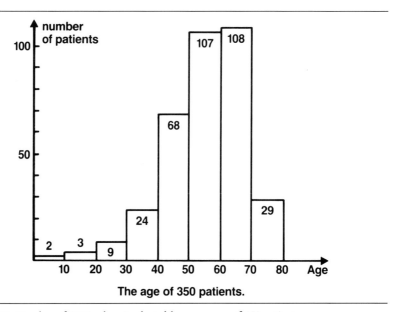

Figure 22-1. Number of SJM valves implanted by age range of 350 patients.

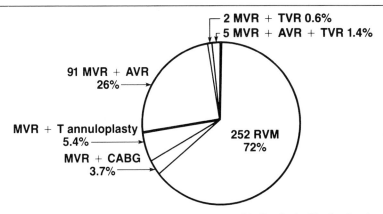

MVR : mitral valve replacement with St. Jude Medical valve.
AVR: aortic valve replacement with Björk-Shiley valve.
T: tricuspid
TVR: tricuspid valve replacement with SJM valve.
CABG: coronary artery bypass

Figure 22-2. Distribution of surgical procedures in 350 cases of SJM mitral valve implants.

and mitral stenosis, in 97. Fourteen SJM valves were used for endocarditis (1 for a heterograft), 2 for obstructive cardiomyopathy with mitral regurgitation, 1 for endomyocardial fibrosis and 1 to replace a BJÖRK-SHILEY mitral valve for thrombosis.

SURGICAL TECHNIQUE

A similar surgical technique was used in each case. The prostheses were implanted with interrupted mattress sutures (00-Ticron). Pledgets were used only if warranted by the anatomic situation.

Table 22-1. Incidence of anatomical lesions as cause for mitral valve replacement with SJM valves

Type	No. of patients	Percent
Mitral stenosis	97	27.7
Mitral insufficiency	130	37.1
Mitral disease	105	30.0
Endocarditis	14	04.0
Obstructive cardiomyopathy	2	0.57
Endomyocardial fibrosis	1	0
Björk-Shiley valve thrombosis	1	0
Total	350	

In the first group (142 patients) the mitral prosthesis was implanted so that the leaflets were parallel to the natural mitral leaflets. This placement is referred to as the anatomical position. In a second group (208 patients), the prosthesis was positioned so the leaflets were perpendicular to the natural mitral leaflets in what Eugene Baudet has termed the perpendicular or antianatomical position.

The number of prostheses according to size is shown in figure 22-3. Sizes 29 and 31 mm comprised 60%.

All patients, regardless of heart rhythm, underwent postoperative anticoagulation therapy. As soon as bleeding in the drains was no longer significant, patients were administered heparin subcutaneously (3 mg/kg/24 hr in 3 equally divided injections). All patients were given warfarin (COUMADIN) beginning 8 days postoperatively (table 22-2).

RESULTS

Total operative mortality at ≤ 30 days (table 22-3) was 4.3% or 15 of 350 patients. Among the 252 patients receiving isolated MVR, there were 8 deaths (3.1%); for the 91 patients undergoing DVR there were 6 deaths (6.6%); and for the 5 TVR there was 1 death.

None of the deaths was valve related. Eight died of low cardiac output. Two of these 8 were in NYHA Class IV and had emergency MVR for acute ischemic mitral regurgitation, 1 of which occurred perioperatively. One patient died of ventricular rupture, 1 of arrhythmia, 1 of sudden death (determined at autopsy),

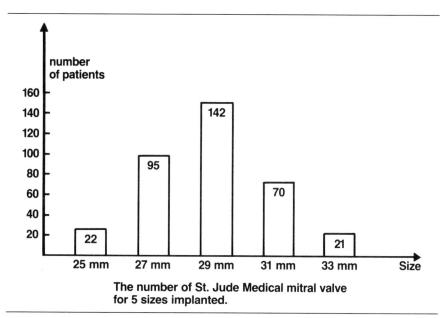

The number of St. Jude Medical mitral valve for 5 sizes implanted.

Figure 22-3. Distribution of number of mitral valves implanted by valve size.

Table 22-2. Anticoagulation protocol

*6th and 8th postoperative hour = subcutaneous haparin therapy: 3 mg/kg/24 hr. in
  3 equally divided injections (calcium heparin)
*8th to 10th postoperative day: warfarin sodium (Coumadin®)

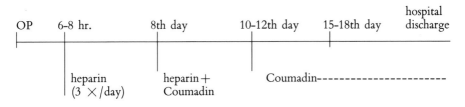

Patient coagulation tests = control × 1.5 or 2

Table 22-3. Operative mortality ≤ 30 days

Procedure	No. of patients	No. of deaths	Percent
MVR	252	8	3.1
MVR + AVR	91	6	6.6
MVR + TVR	2	–	–
MVR + AVR + TVR	5	1	20.0
Total	350	15	4.3

MVR = mitral valve replacement with SJM valve
AVR = aortic valve replacement with Björk-Shiley valve
TVR = tricuspid valve replacement with SJM valve

2 of cerebral or gastrointestinal hemorrhage, 1 of respiratory insufficiency and 1 of peritonitis (table 22-4). There were no valve-related postoperative deaths.

All patients undergoing cardiac valve replacement from March 1, 1979 to March 1, 1984 were contacted during January and February 1984 and a questionnaire was completed by the local physician. When questions about patient problems arose from the questionnaire, the local physician was contacted for details.

Late results are for 335 survivors, 328 of whom could be followed-up (98%). Seven could not be contacted. Follow-up information was obtained for 6 to 60 months with a mean of 31 months for a total of 865 patient-years or 10,380 patient-months.

Late deaths occurred in 28 cases (8.3%), 16 occurring during the first postoperative year. Table 22-5 lists the main causes of late deaths. Only 10 cases were of cardiac origin (36%): 5 congestive heart failure, 2 valve thrombosis, 1 arrhythmia, 1 atrioventricular block and 1 renal insufficiency secondary to low cardiac output. Two sudden deaths were not documented. Four complications of anticoagulation

Table 22-4. Operative mortality

Low cardiac output (2 emergency MVR)	8
Left ventricular rupture	1
Arrhythmia	1
Sudden death	1
Respiratory insufficiency	1
Hemorrhagic death	
cerebral	1
gastrointestinal	1
Peritonitis	1
Total	15 (4.3%)

Table 22-5. Late mortality

Cause	No. of patients	Percent
Cardiogenic causes		
heart failure	5	
renal insufficiency secondary to low cardiac output	1	
valve thrombosis	2	
AV block	1	
arrhythmia	1	
Total	10	36
Infection		
peritonitis	1	
endocarditis	3	
pneumonia	1	
Total	5	18
Complication of anticoagulation	4	14
Sudden death	2	7
Miscellaneous		
cancer	1	
hepatitis	2	
accident	1	
suicide	2	
senile dementia	1	
Total	7	25

(cerebral or gastrointestinal hemorrhage) and 5 infections (3 endocarditis, 1 peritonitis and 1 pneumonia) occurred. Total mortality was 43 of 350 patients (12.3%) for a maximum follow-up of 5 years. The actuarial survival curve for all patients shows an 84% survival at 5 years (figure 22-4).

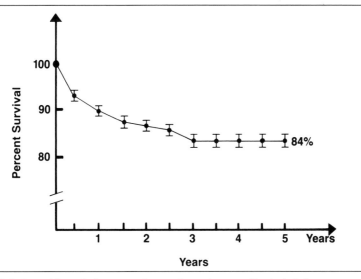

Figure 22-4. Actuarial survival curve to 5 years (operative mortality included).

FOLLOW-UP

Surveillance of anticoagulant treatment was strict. In 335 patients, the mean range of prothrombin rate was 0.31, but in 38 patients (11%) it was over 0.40. The prothrombin rate was irregular in 10%.

The incidence of thromboembolism (table 22-6) has been the major problem for mechanical valves. In 335 patient, 5 thromboembolic events were observed: 1

Table 22-6. Incidence of thromboembolism and valve thrombosis*

	No. of events	Percent per patient-year
Thromboembolism		
arterial embolism of an eye at 16 months	1	
transient aphasia without paralysis	2	
hemiplegia (without anticoagulant)	1	
transient hemiplegia (without anticoagulant)	1	
Total	5	0.58
Valve thrombosis		
deaths (at 2 months and 10 months)	2	
successful reoperation (at 10 months)	1	
Total	3	0.34
Combined total events	8	0.90

*All patients were not well anticoagulated (prothrombin rate > 0.50) or were without anticoagulation.

embolism of a retinal artery causing hemianopsia, 2 incidents of transient aphasia associated with 1 transient hemiplegia, 1 hemiplegia and 1 transient hemiplegia. There were 3 transient thromboembolic events without sequelae. These events were observed in 5 MVR, 3 done for mitral stenosis and 2 for mitral regurgitation, 1 of which was associated with AVR. Valve sizes were 27, 29, 30, 33 mm (2). The incidence was 5 in 865 patient-years (0.54% per patient-year or 5 in 10,380 patient-months (0.48 per 1000 patient-months).

The incidence of valve thrombosis is another, frequently emergent, problem. Valve thrombosis occurred in 3 patients at 2, 10 and 10 months after MVR; 2 patients had mitral stenosis and 1 mitral regurgitation (valve sizes 27, 29 and 27 mm, respectively). In 2 cases, acute pulmonary edema was unimproved by emergency fibrinolytic treatment. One reoperated patient is still alive at this writing. The incidence of valve thrombosis was 3 in 865 patient-years (0.34% per patient-year) or in 10,380 patient-months (0.20 per 1000 patient-months).

The total incidence of thromboembolism and valve thrombosis was 8 in 865 patient-years (0.9% per patient-year) or 8 in 10,380 patient-months (0.77 per 1000 patient-months).

All eight patients experiencing thromboembolism were in atrial fibrillation and poorly anticoagulated; the prothrombin rate was over 0.50 and occasionally 0.80 in 6 patients. Of three patients who were not anticoagulated at the time, 2 had valve thrombosis, 1 of whom died, and 1 had transient hemiplegia.

Overall, the number of thromboembolic events or valve thrombosis was very low. Because of their occurrence over a 5-year period, an actuarial curve of these events would be nearly flat. It is noteworthy that the no events occurred in SJM implanted patients who were correctly anticoagulated. These results were considerably better than those obtained with the BJÖRK-SHILEY valve.

COMPLICATIONS ACCORDING TO ORIENTATION

In 142 patients with valves implanted in the anatomical position, 2 valve thromboses and 3 thromboembolic events occurred. In the 208 patients with valves implanted perpendicular to the septum, 2 valve thromboses and 2 thromboembolic events occurred (table 22-7). It is impossible to conclude that risk is greater when

Table 22-7. Complications by valve orientation

Cause	Anatomical (142 patients)	Perpendicular (208 patients)
Paravalvular leakage	2	6
Hemolysis*	1	4
Sudden death	1	2
Valve thrombosis	2	1
Thromboembolism	3	2

*All cases caused by valve dysfunction (paravalvular leak).

the valve is implanted in the anatomical position. In fact, these events occurred in poorly anticoagulated patients. Among the other complications were: 2 paravalvular leaks in the 142 patients with SJM valves in the anatomical position; 6 paravalvular leaks in the 208 patients with SJM valves in the perpendicular position; and 5 cases of hemolysis caused by valve dysfunction (paravalvular leaks).

FUNCTIONAL RESULTS

Improvement by New York Heart Association Classification (NYHA) is shown in figure 22-5. Before valve replacement, 3 patients reported symptoms consistent with NYHA Class I, 83 with NYHA Class II, 145 with NYHA Class III, 69 with NYHA Class IV (overall, 71.3% NYHA Class III and IV).

After valve replacement, 157 patients reported symptoms consistent with NYHA Class I, 126 NYHA Class II, 13 with NYHA Class III, 4 with NYHA Class IV (overall, 94.3% NYHA Class I and II). This 94.3% incidence is a manifestation of the excellent hemodynamic performance of the SJM cardiac valve.

ECHOCARDIOGRAPHIC STUDY

An analysis of the influence of valve positioning on its functional properties as observed by echocardiography was reported at the Third International Heart Valve Symposium sponsored by St. Jude Medical, Inc., at Scottsdale, Arizona in 1982.

Our study was carried out in 69 patients divided into 2 homogenous groups of 38 SJM valves in the anatomical position and 31 SJM valves in the perpendicular. Data show the opening valve amplitude is the only parameter influenced by valve positioning (p < 0.01). This amplitude is maximum in the perpendicular position, regardless of cardiac rhythm. In this position we never observed asynchronous closure of the posterior leaflet, nor fluttering of this leaflet in atrial fibrillation.

We recommend implantation of the mitral SJM valve in the perpendicular position; since this study was carried out, all SJM mitral prostheses have been implanted in this position.

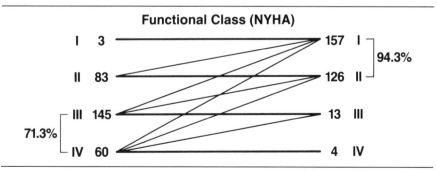

Figure 22-5. Number of patients in New York Heart Association (NYHA) Classification preoperatively and postoperatively.

CONCLUSION

The hemodynamic qualities of the SJM prosthesis have been clearly demonstrated. Its intermediate durability seems satisfactory. No mechanical failures have been observed over 5 years. The cases of hemolysis were due to paravalvular leaks; there has been no clinical hemolysis related to the prosthesis.

Our choice of prosthesis was determined by the desire to reduce thromboembolic risk. With the SJM valve there is little thrombogenic risk if anticoagulant treatment is carried out with great care under strict surveillance. Our clinical experience indicates that the SJM valve offers an excellent alternative in the mitral position.

23. A 60-MONTH EXPERIENCE WITH THE ST. JUDE MEDICAL® PROSTHESIS AT CEDARS-SINAI MEDICAL CENTER

RICHARD J. GRAY, AURELIO CHAUX, LAWRENCE S.C. CZER, MICHELE DEROBERTIS, JACK M. MATLOFF

INTRODUCTION

Use of the ST. JUDE MEDICAL® cardiac valve was begun as a limited trial in high-risk subsets of valve recipients in March 1978. As of March 1984, we have implanted 442 valves in 382 patients. There has been increasing clinical utilization of this prosthesis in many other centers since the valve's FDA approval. However, the responsibility of the original clinical investigators is to continually review and analyze the experience with the earliest recipients of this prosthesis to address the as yet unanswered question about its long-term durability. Accordingly, we recently analyzed the clinical results of our patients with a maximum of 5 years follow-up and a minimum of one year follow-up.

METHODS

The clinical results in 215 patients receiving 256 valves who were operated between March 1978 and June 1982 are the basis for this report. The mean follow-up period is 34 months. The follow-up procedure consisted of annual questionnaires, supplemented with an interview either conducted in person or by telephone for those persons who had moved away from the vicinity of the medical center. One percent of patients were lost to follow-up (2 out of 215).

Single aortic valve replacement was performed in 73 patients, single mitral valve replacement in 89, double ST. JUDE MEDICAL valve replacement (aortic and mitral) in 35, multiple valve replacement in 18. This last category of patients includes those with two prosthetic implants, one of which was not a ST. JUDE MEDICAL valve or in whom the location was other than aortic and mitral.

Concomitant myocardial revascularization was performed in 48% of all patients, which included 56% of both the isolated aortic and mitral groups, 29% of the double valve recipients and 11% of the multiple valve recipients. The etiology of the valve disease was rheumatic in 50% of our overall patient population. The average age was 62 $\pm$ 13 years (mean $\pm$ standard deviation), 36% of whom were male. The majority of patients had advanced symptomatology: 48% were NYHA Class III and 48% were Class IV. Preoperative angiographic left ventricular ejection fraction was less than .35 in 11% of patients and between .35 and .55 in 25% of patients. Thus, 36% of patients had a modestly or severely impaired left ventricle.

RESULTS

Mortality

Table 23-1 summarizes the early (≤ 30 days) and late mortality in the four major patient subgroups. Single aortic valve replacement and double valve replacement was associated with the lowest early mortality, 2.7% and 2.9%, respectively. In contrast, mortality for mitral and multiple valve replacement was 11.2% and 11.1% respectively. The overall early mortality was 7%. Late mortality is also illustrated for each of the patient cohorts and averages 15.8%. Similar to early mortality, single aortic and double valve replacement were associated with the lowest late mortality of 12.3% and 11.4%, respectively, followed by mitral valve replacement with 18.0%, and multiple valve replacement with 27.8% mortality. These results are shown in actuarial form in figure 23-1. The outcome of patients with single aortic valve replacement and double valve replacement is similar throughout the follow-up interval and is superior to both the mitral valve or multiple valve recipients ($p < .05$). It should be noted that a major difference in the survival curves is imparted by the relatively high early mortality experienced by these latter two cohorts of patients.

Symptomatic Status

Table 23-2 illustrates the functional classification before and after surgery in the 164 late survivors. Preoperatively 87 patients were functional Class III and 68 were functional Class IV compared with late postoperative status when only 19 were

Table 23-1. Mortality after implantation of St. Jude Medical heart valves

	Early (≤ 30 D)	Late (> 30 D)
Aortic (N=73)	2.7%	12.3%
Mitral (N=89)	11.2%	18.0%
Double (N=35)	2.9%	11.4%
Multiple (N=18)	11.1%	27.8%
TOTAL (N=215)	7.0%	15.8%

N = number

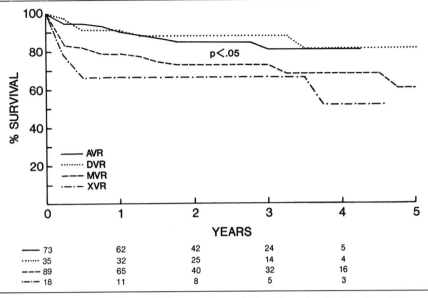

Figure 23-1. Likelihood of survival after St. Jude Medical cardiac valve implantation. AVR = aortic valve replacement; DVR = double valve replacement; MVR = mitral valve replacement; XVR = multiple valve replacement.

Class III and 7 were Class IV. Ninety percent of patients improved by one or more functional classifications. Ten patients were unchanged and 6 worsened by one or more classification levels.

Thromboembolism

Single thromboembolic events occurred in 8 patients. These were transient in 7 but resulted in a permanent hemiparesis and visual field defect in the remaining patient.

Table 23-2. Functional New York Heart Association Class (survivors)

			I	II	III	IV
			102	36	19	7
	I	2	1	1	0	0
PREOP	II	7	6	0	0	1
	III	87	57	19	7	4
	IV	68	38	16	12	2

Note: Patients within diagonal dashed lines had no change in functional class after surgery; those to the left of the dashed lines were improved by one or more levels; those to the right were worse by one or more levels after surgery.

The highest incidence, 4 events, was in the category of single mitral valve replacement with a linearized rate of 2.3% per patient-year. Double valve recipients experienced an incidence of 2.8% per patient-year and aortic valve replacement had a rate of 0.6% per patient-year. All but 14 late survivors were on chronic warfarin therapy. Anticoagulation was stopped in 14 patients because of hemorrhagic complications; all were restarted on either aspirin or dipyridamole. In those patients on warfarin, the thromboembolic rate was 2.0% per patient-year in contrast to 3.6% per patient-year in the 14 patients not so treated.

Several preoperative and postoperative factors were analyzed, seeking predictors of postoperative thromboembolism. This was accomplished by calculation of relative risk ratios, computed from the incidence of thromboembolism in the presence of the risk factor compared to the incidence in the remaining population without that factor. In descending order of importance, four characteristics, associated with an elevated relative risk ratio were: 1) the presence of left atrial thrombus or performance of left atrial thrombectomy at the time of valve replacement surgery; 2) non-use of warfarin-type anticoagulation; 3) preoperative thromboembolism; and 4) postoperative atrial fibrillation. The relative risk ratio varied from 4.4:1 for the highest risk predicator (left atrial thrombus or performance of thrombectomy) downward to 1.8:1 for postoperative atrial fibrillation.

One additional patient experienced aortic valve thrombosis approximately 3 years after implantation. This patient, who was poorly controlled with warfarin anticoagulation, presented with congestive heart failure and underwent successful reoperation. The explanted valve showed a small amount of thrombus material at both pivot guards, immobilizing both leaflets in a semi-open position.

Paravalvular leak was diagnosed in two patients early after surgery, both of which were associated with early postoperative infectious endocarditis. Both underwent successful reoperation. Another patient experienced an early postoperative erosion of the atrioventricular ring and succumbed on the second postoperative day.

Overall, a total of 13 valve-related complications occurred resulting in a linearized event rate of 2.9% per patient-year.

There have been no early or late material or mechanical valve failures.

Biocompatibility

Hematocrit, serum LDH and peripheral blood smear were obtained in 50 long-term survivors of either single aortic or single mitral valve replacement at an average of 2.5 years after surgery. The mean hematocrit, after either aortic or mitral valve replacement, was 42 $\pm$ 5 vol%. Serum LDH (expressed as percent of upper limits of normal) for aortic valve replacement was 103 $\pm$ 25% and for mitral valve replacement, 117 $\pm$ 30%. No schistocytes were seen on peripheral blood smear.

Chromium[51]-tagged red blood cell survival studies were performed in 19 aortic valve recipients at least one year after their surgery. Six patients with ST. JUDE MEDICAL valves were compared to 7 patients with BJÖRK-SHILEY® prostheses and 6 patients with HANCOCK® prostheses. The average red blood cell survival for the ST. JUDE MEDICAL and BJÖRK-SHILEY recipients were identical at 26.3 days and statistically similar to the 6 patients with biological valves whose survival was 28.0 days. In this small group of patients there were no differences in average hematocrit, serum LDH, bilirubin, haptoglobin or iron binding capacity.

SUMMARY

After 1 to 5 years of follow-up in 215 patients with 256 valves, the clinical results with ST. JUDE MEDICAL valve replacement appear to be excellent. This has been particularly rewarding in that the initial use of the valve was limited to subsets of patients who had been identified from our prior experience to be at high risk. The overall thromboembolic event rate is 1.8% per patient-year. No clinically significant hemolysis is seen and only one valve-related death occurred early postoperatively. Data now emerging are establishing the ST. JUDE MEDICAL bileaflet prosthesis as a safe and durable valve substitute. There has been no instance of primary structural failure.

24. A 60-MONTH EXPERIENCE WITH THE ST. JUDE MEDICAL® PROSTHESIS AT UNIVERSITY HOSPITAL, BRUGMANN

JEAN-LOUIS LECLERC, FRANCIS WELLENS, FRANK E. DEUVAERT, MARTINE ANTOINE, JACQUES DEPAEPE, GEORGES PRIMO.

The success of heart valve replacement depends on several conditions. Refinements in patient selection, in surgical technique, in the availability of valve substitutes and in postoperative care have markedly reduced operative mortality.

Clinical improvement is easy to document in the majority of valve substitutes, both mechanical and biological. The superiority of one valve substitute over another depends on long-term durability, incidence of valve-related complications and hemodynamic performance.

The ST. JUDE MEDICAL® prosthesis was evaluated according to these requirements at our institution from 1978 through 1983. Patient follow-up extended from 2 years to 5.4 years.

STUDY PARAMETERS

The ST. JUDE MEDICAL prosthesis is the only mechanical valve used at our institution and represents 90% of all implantations. Porcine bioprostheses are used in 10% of patients, mostly the elderly (70 + years of age).

From October 1978 to December 1983, 1144 patients underwent ST. JUDE MEDICAL (SJM) valve replacement with a total of 1302 prostheses. Distribution by position is detailed in table 24-1 Combinations of different valve substitutes were used with ST. JUDE MEDICAL valves in a few individuals and these were excluded from the follow-up.

In order to establish a minimum postoperative evaluation of 2 years, this

Table 24-1. Cardiac valve replacement with St. Jude Medical prostheses from October 1978 to December 1983

	No. of patients	No. of valves
AVR	504	504
MVR	483	483
AVR + MVR	142	284
AVR + MVR + TVR	1	3
MVR + TVR	13	26
AVR + PVR	1	2
Total	1144	1302

follow-up analysis reviews only the patients operated on prior to December 31, 1981 (table 24-2). A total of 741 valves were implanted in 628 patients. By implant position the number of patients were: aortic valve replacement (AVR) = 269; mitral valve replacement (MVR) = 244; AVR + MVR = 98; AVR + MVR + tricuspid valve replacement (TVR) = 1; MVR + TVR = 12; TVR = 3; AVR + pulmonary valve replacement (PVR) = 1.

Patient population by age and sex is given in table 24-3 Additional procedures are listed in table 24-4. An appreciable number of patients had a previous cardiac surgical procedure. Indications for reoperation were tissue valve failure in the majority of cases.

Table 24-2. Number of patients operated on prior to December 31, 1981 for heart valve replacement with the St. Jude Medical valve

	No. patients	No. valves
AVR	269	269
MVR	244	244
AVR + MVR	98	196
AVR + MVR + TVR	1	3
MVR + TVR	12	24
TVR	3	3
AVR + PVR	1	2
Total	628	741

Table 24-3. Patient population with St. Jude Medical prostheses

Position	Age	Male (%)	Female (%)
AVR	10 to 78 yr. (mean 54)	71	29
MVR	5 mo. to 74 yr. (mean 53)	31	69
AVR + MVR	9 to 73 yr. (mean 54)	49	51

Table 24-4. Valve replacement with combined procedures

Procedure	AVR	MVR	Multiple replacements
CABG (1)	16	2	2
CABG (2)	15	6	1
CABG (3)	1	1	–
CABG (4)	–	1	–
Mitral commissurotomy	5	–	–
Tricuspid annuloplasty	1	11	8
Resection subaortic stenosis	1	–	1
Atrial septal defect closure	–	3	–
Ventricular septal defect closure	1	1	1
Pacemaker	2	1	1
Ascending aortic aneurysm	5	–	–
Patent ductus arteriosus	–	1	–

CABG = coronary artery bypass graft
AVR = aortic valve replacement
MVR = mitral valve replacement

Anticoagulation with acenocoumarol was routinely prescribed from the second postoperative day.

RESULTS

Mortality

None of the early deaths ($\leq$ 30 days postoperative) was valve related. Causes of early death are listed in table 24-5. Analysis of late mortality (table 24-6) indicates that progressive heart failure was the most common cause of death, occurring primarily during the first 6 to 12 months postoperatively. Postoperative cardiac catheterization did not reveal valve dysfunction. Autopsies confirmed that fatality was due to impaired ventricular function. One occurrence of valve thrombosis in the mitral position was fatal 2 months after surgery. Ineffective anticoagulation was documented in this case.

Three fatalities were related to thromboembolic episodes and three other late deaths were proved to be of hemorrhagic origin. Figure 24-1 shows that 14% of

Table 24-5. Early deaths ($\leq$ 30 days)

Position	No.	%	Causes
AVR	4	1.5	renal, respiratory failure
MVR	7	2.8	low cardiac output, renal, respiratory failure, infection
AVR + MVR	6	6.1	low cardiac output, respiratory failure, gastrointestinal bleeding, sudden death
MVR + TVR	2	17	low cardiac output

Table 24-6. Late mortality with the St. Jude Medical prosthesis

Causes	AVR	MVR	AVR + MVR
Heart failure	3	12	4
Arrhythmia	–	–	–
Sudden death	5	3	1
Stroke (TE)	–	1	2
Valve thrombosis	–	1	–
Hemorrhagic death	–	–	–
Cerebral hemorrhage	–	2	–
Gastrointestinal hemorrhage	–	–	1
Sternal infection	–	1	–
Allergic shock	–	1	–
Tracheal stenosis	–	1	–
Neoplasia	6	1	–
Total	14	23	8

late mortality can be considered as valve related. This includes 3 cerebrovascular accidents (CVA), 1 valve thrombosis and 3 hemorrhagic deaths.

Durability
No structural failures occurred in the series.

Thrombogenicity
Incidence of thromboembolic complications (TE) is detailed in table 24-7: AVR = 1.4% per patient-year; MVR = 3.3% per patient year; AVR + MVR = 3.1% per patient-year.

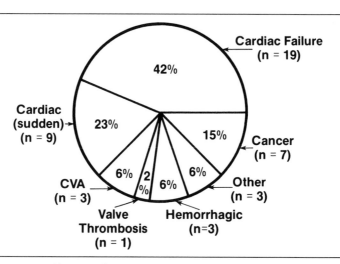

Figure 24-1. Causes of late mortality.

Table 24-7. Thromboembolic complications for 2 to 5 years followup

	AVR	MVR	AVR + MVR
No. of patients	265	237	92
Patient-years of follow-up	646	624	285
No. of TE events	9	21	9
Emboli per 100 patient-years	1.4	3.3	3.1

Valvular occlusion due to thromboembolic material or pannus overgrowth was observed on 4 occasions (table 24-8). Occurrence after insertion of the prosthesis was variable from 6 weeks to 3 years. Three patients were successfully reoperated on as emergencies. The diagnosis of valvular occlusion must be based on:

- patient history of progressive shortness of breath and angina,
- valve sounds that diminish and may even disappear or new murmurs that are audible at auscultation,
- cinefluoroscopy, which allows rapid, noninvasive verification of leaflet motion.

Anticoagulation

In a group of 18 patients, anticoagulant treatment was not started or was discontinued because of hemorrhagic complications (table 24-9). Thromboembolic events occurred only in the aortic group during a follow-up of 248 months. These included 2 transient ischemic attacks and 1 valve thrombosis requiring emergency reoperation.

Results in elderly

Although we theoretically prefer to implant a tissue valve in the elderly (70 + years of age), we have a fair proportion of patients in this age group with ST. JUDE MEDICAL valves implanted for a small aortic root. This age group represents 10% of all patients operated on between October 1978 and December

Table 24-8. Valvular occlusion of St. Jude Medical prostheses

	Age	Delay (mo.)	Anticoag	Outcome
AVR (2/265)	10	14	none	reop SJM
	43	36	Coumadin®	reop SJM
MVR (2/237)	53	1.5	Coumadin	death
	59	27	Coumadin	reop CE

anticoag. = anticoagulation
reop = reoperation
SJM = St. Jude Medical
CE = Carpentier-Edwards®

Table 24-9. Results of no anticoagulation with the St. Jude Medical prosthesis

Position	Reasons	Follow-up	TE events
AVR (12)	hemorrhage hemodialysis age Jehovah Witness	248 months	2 TIA 1 valve occlusion
MVR (4)	hemorrhage geographic	76 months	—
AVR + MVR (2)	hemorrhage	60 months	—

TIA = transient ischemic attach

1983. No death in this age group was valve related, including anticoagulant-related events.

CONCLUSION

Experience with the ST. JUDE MEDICAL prosthesis has been very gratifying in the majority of patients followed up to 60 months after surgery. Hemodynamic performance is excellent and mechanical failure was absent. Thromboembolic complications compared favorably with other valves; but, unfortunately, since such complications have not been eliminated, an effective and well-controlled anticoagulation regimen is mandatory.

After 6 years of utilization, the ST. JUDE MEDICAL prosthesis continues to be our cardiac valve substitute of choice.

25. A 72-MONTH CLINICAL EXPERIENCE WITH THE ST. JUDE MEDICAL® CARDIAC VALVE PROSTHESIS AT NEWARK BETH ISRAEL MEDICAL CENTER

ISAAC GIELCHINSKY, MARK S. HOCHBERG, S. MANSOOR HUSSAIN, VICTOR PARSONNET, DANIEL FISCH, JOHN C. NORMAN

The clinical experience with the ST. JUDE MEDICAL® cardiac valve prosthesis at the Newark Beth Israel Medical Center has recently been reviewed. This institution was one of the original investigational centers for that valve.

PATIENT POPULATION

From January 1978 through February 1984, a total of 149 patients underwent valve replacement with the ST. JUDE MEDICAL cardiac valve prosthesis. The male to female ratio in this patient series was 67:82 with a mean age of 56 $+$ 1.1 SEM years (range 18 to 79 years). The primary diagnoses in these patients were: rheumatic heart disease, 57 (38%); ischemic heart disease, 50 (34%); bacterial endocarditis, 13 (9%); and congenital heart disease, 29 (19%).

Preoperatively, 11 patients (7%) were in New York Heart Association (NYHA) Class II, 64 (43%) were Class III, and 74 (50%) were in Class IV. Twenty-three (15.4%) were considered to be high-risk patients preoperatively: 4 because of cardiogenic shock, 6 because of acute bacterial endocarditis with congestive heart failure and 6 with end-stage congestive heart failure. Intra-aortic balloon pump counterpulsation was required in 35 (23.5%) with the following breakdown: preoperative, 4 (2.7%); intraoperative, 24 (16.1%); and postoperative, 7 (4.7%).

A total of 171 valves were implanted in these 149 patients (table 25-1). Eighty-two were single valve replacements, 17 were double valve replacements, 45 were single valve replacements with concomitant coronary artery bypass surgery and 5 were double valve replacements with coronary artery bypass surgery. There were

Table 25-1. Valve distribution of 171 St. Jude Medical heart valves implanted in 149 patients

Position	No.	Procedure	No.
AVR	87	SVR	82
Repeat AVR	4	SVR & CAB	45
MVR	74	DVR	17
Repeat MVR	5	DVR & CAB	5
TVR	1		
Total	171	Total	149

AVR = aortic valve replacement
MVR = mitral valve replacement
TVR = tricuspid valve replacement
SVR = single valve replacement
CAB = coronary artery bypass
DVR = double valve replacement

87 primary aortic valve implants and 4 repeat aortic implants; 74 had primary mitral valve replacements and 5 had repeat mitral implants. The 1 tricuspid implant was the third valve replacement of a patient who was a chronic intravenous drug abuser.

RESULTS

With regard to morbidity and mortality, there were 8 (5.4%) operative deaths and 28 (18.8%) late deaths (table 25-2). One patient expired following discharge because he refused to maintain his discharge medications, including COUMA-DIN®. Seventeen patients (14%) were lost to follow-up. Thus, long-term follow-up was achieved in 96 patients (85%) for a total of 75 patient-years (range 1–65 months).

The overall valve-related complication rate in this series was low (table 25-3). There was one episode of thromboembolism, one case of paravalvular leak, and one case of prosthetic endocarditis, for a complication rate of 1.3% per patient-year each.

We also experienced one case of structural failure (1.3% per patient-year) during aortic valve replacement in a 73-year-old woman who had aortic stenosis

Table 25-2. Morbidity and mortality

	No.	%
Operative deaths	8	5.4
Late deaths	28	18.8
Lost to follow-up	17	14.0
Long-term follow-up*	96	85.0

*Total patient-years = 75; range 1–65 months

Table 25-3. Complication rates for 96 patients implanted 1 to 65 months for a total of 75 patient-years

	Events	% Events
Thromboembolism	1	1.3
Paravalvular leak	1	1.3
Prosthetic endocarditis	1	1.3
Structural failure*	1	1.3
Complications of anticoagulation and anemia due to hemolysis	2	2.6
Total	6	8.0

*during surgery

and was in NYHA Class IV. A 19 mm ST. JUDE MEDICAL valve was inserted. Once all the sutures were applied and we attempted to remove the valve holder, the valve housing came out along with the holder. A 19 mm BJÖRK-SHI-LEY® valve was inserted. Subsequent to this event, we have never experienced a problem with the sewing ring.

The total valve-related complication rate, including complications of anticoagulation and anemia due to hemolysis, was 8% per patient-year (6 events).

CONCLUSION

With 72 months of follow-up after valve replacement with the ST. JUDE MEDICAL cardiac valve prosthesis there was a low rate of structural failure and thromboembolism (1.3% per patient-year each). Our experience supports the continued use of this prosthesis.

26. A 72-MONTH EXPERIENCE WITH THE ST. JUDE MEDICAL® PROSTHESIS AT THE MINNEAPOLIS HEART INSTITUTE AND UNITED HOSPITALS, ST. PAUL, MINNESOTA

WILLIAM G. LINDSAY, DEMETRE NICOLOFF, KIT V. AROM, WILLIAM F. NORTHRUP, III, THOMAS E. KERSTEN

Our current study of the ST. JUDE MEDICAL® heart valve began in October 1977 when the first ST. JUDE MEDICAL valve was implanted clinically. Subsequently, these patients have been followed through October 3, 1983.

PATIENT POPULATION

There were 680 patients: 359 male and 321 female. The age distribution was 6 months to 87 years. Aortic valve implants totaled 361, of which isolated aortic valve implants (AVR) were 218, AVR implants with coronary artery bypass (CAB) were 129 and AVR with other procedures were 14. Mitral valve implants totaled 264, of which isolated mitral implants (MVR) were 178, MVR implants with CAB were 71 and MVR with other procedures were 15. Double valve replacements totaled 55, of which isolated double valve replacements (DVR) were 40, DVR and CAB were 12 and DVR combined with other procedures were 3.

Valve distribution shows the most commonly used aortic sizes to be 23 mm to 25 mm (75%) and the most common mitral sizes to be 27 mm to 31 mm (80%). The smallest sizes were placed in children. In the youngest patient, a double valve implant was performed utilizing two 19 mm ST. JUDE MEDICAL valves and a combination of Manougian's and Konno's techniques [1,2].

FOLLOW-UP

Follow-up was ongoing, and was accomplished by questionnaire, telephone interviews and office visits, resulting in a combined 95% follow-up for 6 years.

MORTALITY

Among the 680 patients, operative mortality was 6.6% (45). Of the 45 operative deaths, 26 were due to cardiac failure, 8 to renal failure, 3 to respiratory failure, 4 to cerebrovascular accidents and 4 to uncontrolled sepsis. Operative mortality for AVR in 218 patients was 3.7%. Operative mortality for AVR and CAB was 1.6%. When AVR was combined with other procedures, such as left ventricular aneurysm resection, the operative mortality was considerably higher (14.3%). Mortality among patients with elective MVR was 7.9%. When MVR was done in association with CAB it was 15.5% and with other procedures it was 33%.

Overall late mortality among the 95% (635) of patients followed 6 years was 7.7% (49). Late mortality among aortic and mitral valve patients was similar: AVR = 6.2%; AVR and CAB = 6.3%; MVR = 7.9; MVR and CAB = 6.7%. Patients with higher late mortality were those patients who had poor ventricular function, including left ventricular aneurysms. Patients with DVR had a 15.8% late mortality and this increased slightly with DVR and CAB to 18.2%.

COMPLICATIONS

All postoperative valve patients were maintained on COUMADIN®. Complications due to excessive bleeding, including hematoma and hematuria, were: AVR = 4.6% per patient-year (30); MVR = 2.2% per patient-year (11); and DVR = 2.0% per patient-year (1).

Thromboembolism

The overall incidence of thromboembolism after AVR was 1.4% per patient-year and for mitral valves was 2.4% per patient-year. Approximately 97% had no evidence of thromboembolic events in the 6 year follow-up period. Probability of being free from a major neurological deficit from any embolic episode was 99%.

Thrombosis

Three patients experienced a clotted leaflet. Because the ST. JUDE MEDICAL valve has two leaflets, catastrophic failure did not occur and the patient often had time for reoperation. One thrombus occurred in a male patient with a mitral valve implant. One leaflet was clotted. This patient subsequently died of a number of unrelated problems. A second patient had a clotted tricuspid valve and died of that complication. The third patient was our youngest patient, a 6-month-old infant with a double valve replacement. The baby, who was on aspirin and PERSANTINE® developed a clotted single leaflet. The baby was treated with urokinase, which resulted in dissolution of the clot and normal functioning of the aortic valve. The child is now doing well and is maintained on COUMADIN.

SURVIVAL

Overall survival at 6 years with 95% follow-up was 86.2%. Survival by operation was: AVR = 89.9%; AVR and CAB = 92.2%; MVR = 84.8%; MVR and CAB = 79.9%; DVR = 80%; and DVR and CAB = 75%.

CONCLUSION

In summary, 680 patients have undergone 735 ST. JUDE MEDICAL valve replacements in a wide variety of conditions and operations. No mechanical failures occurred in this 6-year period. This 6-year study with 95% follow-up represents the longest known follow-up of the ST. JUDE MEDICAL valve.

REFERENCE

1. Kersten T, Bessinger B, Stone F, et al: Combined techniques for double valve replacement in the infant. Abstracted, The Society of Thoracic Surgeons, Twentieth Annual Meeting 1984; 108.
2. Kersten TE, Nicoloff DM: Double-valve replacement in the infant. Bulletin of the Minneapolis Heart Institute, Summer 1984;2(1):11–12.

27. A 72-MONTH EXPERIENCE WITH THE ST. JUDE MEDICAL® PROSTHESIS AT THE TUCSON MEDICAL CENTER

CHRISTOPHER T. MALONEY

Early *in vitro* studies of the ST. JUDE MEDICAL® valve prosthesis demonstrated superior hemodynamic and mechanical characteristics. We were intrigued with these findings, primarily because of the obvious hemodynamic disadvantages of the other valves available at that time. Since January 1978 the ST. JUDE MEDICAL prosthesis has been our valve of choice, although other mechanical and tissue valves have been widely used, mainly due to patient and physician request.

PATIENT POPULATION

Between January 5, 1978 and December 1983, 131 patients received 141 ST. JUDE MEDICAL heart valves. The group was 43% male and 57% female. The average age was 60 years with a range of 22 to 85 years. This older age group reflects similar American reports, as distinguished from European studies, which report a somewhat younger group. All patients who had undergone cardiac valve replacement were contacted during January 1984 by questionnaire, telephone or office visit. Information was obtained on 126 patients, resulting in a 95.5% active follow-up.

METHODS AND PROCEDURES

The usual methods of cardiopulmonary bypass, including hypothermia to 28°C, cold potassium cardioplegia and a membrane or bubble oxygenator were used. Where indicated, coronary revascularization routinely was done first with additional cardioplegia infused to the coronary artery via the bypass. Interrupted suture technique was preferred. The frequency of implant by site was: aortic (AVR)

49.6% (65), mitral (MVR) 40.5% (53) and multiple 9.9% (13), (10 double, 3 tricuspid). Of AVR patients, 34% underwent combined procedures, usually with concomitant coronary artery revascularization. Very careful attention was paid to complete revascularization when warranted. Nine patients had previous valve surgery performed. Three had mitral valve commissurotomies, four had calcific degeneration of porcine heterografts and two STARR-EDWARDS® cloth-covered prostheses were removed due to hemolytic anemia. Associated procedures included coronary artery bypass, ascending aortic replacements, with and without coronary revascularization, and mitral commissurotomy.

The small aortic anulus seen in many elderly patients was quite appropriately managed with size 19 mm and 21 mm ST. JUDE MEDICAL valves, as opposed to tissue valves where a size 19 mm and 21 mm would show significant gradients. Annular enlargement procedures were not performed. Ninety-four percent of our patients were discharged on COUMADIN®. It was felt that in the remaining patients, the risk of anticoagulation outweighed the risk of thrombosis. Patients were instructed to keep their prothrombin time at 1.5 times normal control values, achieving an activity level between 19 and 21 seconds. Despite a vigorous education program, disparities in prothrombin control still occur. On follow-up, we found a great disparity in anticoagulation, reflecting physicians' varying desires for anticoagulation in patients with valvular heart disease.

RESULTS

Functional status

All patients who were in New York Heart Association (NYHA) Class IV preoperatively were compared with their postoperative Class. Over 60% of patients receiving single aortic valve implants improved to Class I and 80% to Class I or II (figure 27-1). Over 80% of all patients receiving either single aortic valve replacements or single mitral valve replacements improved from Class IV to Class I or II.

Mortality

Thirty-day operative mortality was 7% in AVR and 15% in MVR, including isolated valves and combined procedures. This latter increased mortality reflects the poor left ventricular function seen in many patients with mitral valvular disease. Late survival at 2.5 years was 75.8% for isolated AVR and 75.3% for isolated MVR (figure 27-2). The combined figure was also 75.3%.

Thromboembolism

Thromboembolism remains the prime complication for valvular heart surgery patients. At 3 years, 97.3% of patients with AVR and 96.4% of all AVR and MVR patients combined, were free of thromboembolism (figure 27-3). From the follow-up questionnaire, 4 patients were identified as having strokes postoperatively. However, there were no sequelae or clinical evidence that this was true. One young

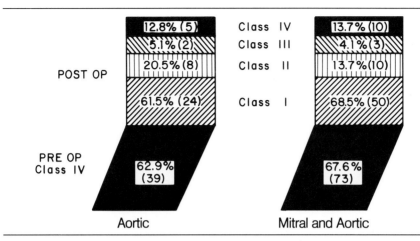

Figure 27-1. Preoperative and postoperative New York Heart Functional Classification for patients receiving St. Jude Medical heart valves.

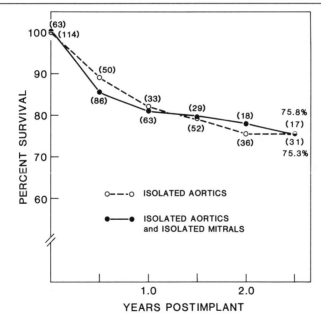

Figures include intraoperative deaths and complications. Numbers in parentheses are the number of patients entering this interval.

Figure 27-2. Actuarial survival by percent of patients.

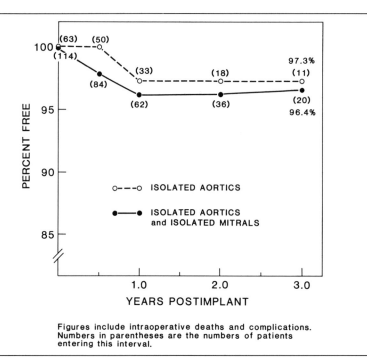

Figure 27-3. Percent of patients free of thromboembolism.

female patient was discharged without anticoagulation and approximately one year postoperatively she experienced numbness in her hand. She was hospitalized and her valve was found to be functioning properly; but she developed a transient ischemic attack (TIA) while hospitalized. She was subsequently anticoagulated and for the past four years has been functional Class I with no further evidence of a TIA.

Thrombosis

Two patients had complete thrombosis of their valves following sudden cessation of COUMADIN (table 27-1). One of these patients had an aortic and mitral valve replacement; he had a sudden withdrawal of COUMADIN anticoagulation. Within a week the patient was brought to the emergency room in pulmonary edema. He was brought immediately to the operating room where both valves were found to be completely clotted. The clots were removed from around the prosthetic valves. The patient has done extremely well postoperatively and remains in NYHA Functional Class I. A second patient had an aortic valve replacement and a single coronary artery bypass. He was fully anticoagulated at discharge and was doing very well for 22 months when he also had his COUMADIN rapidly withdrawn. Three days later, the patient had a syncopal episode, but this was not investigated.

Table 27-1. Complications

	AVR	MVR	DVR
Early Deaths < 30 days	6	9	0
Late Deaths > 30 days	8	2	0
Thromboembolism	1	3	1
Hemolysis	0	0	0
Prosthetic Failure	0	0	0
Paravalvular Leak	0	0	0
Hemorrhagic Complications	0	1	0
Explant	0	0	1
Thrombosis	1	0	1

A week following the syncopal episode, he was brought to the hospital DOA. Autopsy showed the valve to be completely clotted.

Other complications

We experienced no evidence of prosthetic structural failure, hemolysis, paravalvular leak, endocarditis or thrombosis in the appropriately anticoagulated patients.

CONCLUSIONS

In summary, we feel that the ST. JUDE MEDICAL valve prosthesis offers superior hemodynamic characteristics with low gradients in small sizes and low turbulence. These hemodynamic and flow characteristics almost certainly contribute to the low incidence of thromboembolism in this and other series. Patients with prosthetic valves are best anticoagulated with COUMADIN alone, but the risk of anticoagulation must be weighed. Once COUMADIN therapy is instituted, it should be continued for life; sudden cessation may prove fatal. With these findings, we continue to believe that the ST. JUDE MEDICAL prosthesis is the valve of choice for valvular replacement in cardiac surgery.

PART V. DISCUSSION

SHAHBUDIN RAHIMTOOLA, MODERATOR

VALVE THROMBOSIS

SHAHBUDIN RAHIMTOOLA: While questions are being formulated, we should address and come to a conclusion for some of the questions that have been asked earlier. One of the first ones that was asked by Dr. Larry Cohn yesterday was whether valve thrombosis occurs in the ST. JUDE MEDICAL® prosthesis; and, secondly, if it occurs, what is its incidence? Professor Baudet, you have a large experience. Would you comment?

EUGENE M. BAUDET: The valve thromboses we have observed have been fatal in 1 mitral and in 1 double valve, both without anticoagulation. In these 2 cases, 1 death was sudden. For the second patient the ST. JUDE MEDICAL valve was replaced by a BJÖRK-SHILEY® valve and the patient died 1 month later from thrombosis of the BJÖRK-SHILEY valve. There are 4 cases of aortic valve thrombosis. All 4 cases were without anticoagulation. None of these patients developed a dramatic emergency status, because in every case there was only one leaflet blocked by the thrombus. Three out of 4 patients have been "fibrinized" successfully. However, 2 patients have had additional surgery. In 1 case, the residual clot was removed by septectomy because the valve was in an orientation parallel to the septum with a grossly hypertrophied septum that seemed to interfere with leaflet motion. In the second case, the patient has been operated on secondarily without evidence of dysfunction prior to surgery, to reorient the valve in the aortic root. So, I think in the aortic position, there is time to undertake medical and then surgical therapy. In contrast, as our experience shows, mitral thrombosis may be a much more emergent situation.

SHAHBUDIN RAHIMTOOLA: Do any of the panel members disagree? I think then, Larry, we have an answer to your question; the panel agrees that valve thrombosis occurs, the incidence of this is small and one of the predominant factors is no anticoagulation or poor anticoagulation therapy. By *poor* I am including inappropriate or inadequate anticoagulation therapy. It is not necessarily sudden and fatal with an exception or two, Professor Baudet?

EUGENE M. BAUDET: No patient died after valve thrombosis in the aortic position. All patients initially have been treated medically.

SHAHBUDIN RAHIMTOOLA: Any other questions from the audience?

CARL GILL, M.D., CLEVELAND, OHIO: Out of about 200 ST. JUDE MEDICAL valve replacement patients, we have had one aortic valve that clotted and was replaced successfully; another valve in a right-sided atrioventricular valve replacement was clotted and replaced successfully. I heard yesterday about one pulmonary valve that occluded and today another tricuspid valve that occluded. I wonder if any members of the panel have had or are aware of other right-sided valve thrombotic occlusions?

EUGENE M. BAUDET: Personally, I have never had the opportunity of seeing such a valve in right side, but I think that Dr. LeClerc had this opportunity.

JEAN-LOUIS LECLERC: Yes, 2 or 3 years ago, we did a series of 12 or 13 double, tricuspid and mitral valve replacements. Our experience is that the ST. JUDE MEDICAL valve has a high tendency to clot in the right side and we no longer recommend use of any mechanical device on the right side. We have had the same experience before with other mechanical devices as well.

ORIENTATION

ARTHUR LURIE, M.D., RENO, NEVADA: Could each panelist kindly tell us how they orient the ST. JUDE MEDICAL valve in the aortic and mitral position, and tell us if there are any unique factors in the implantation of this valve versus others?

WILLIAM G. LINDSAY: Sometimes orientation is predetermined by the calcium or the anatomy of the intrinsic valve, either aortic or mitral; but in the mitral position we tend to position the pivot guards in the natural commissures. We place a pivot guard of the aortic valve in the center of the left coronary cusp. This is changed somewhat if there is a lot of calcium, but these positions appear, at least to us technically, to be the most pliable.

CHRISTOPHER T. MALONEY: In the mitral position, we don't have any particular orientation. In the aortic position, we try, like Dr. Lindsay, to place the pivot guard in area of least fibrosis. It reminds me of a number of years ago when I heard a very interesting paper on the orientation of the BJÖRK-SHILEY valve in the mitral position. The physician gave a very detailed scientific dissertation as to why the valve should be orientated in just that particular position. Dr. Björk was in the audience and was asked to comment. He enjoyed the paper very much, but he indicated that he orientated the valve in just the opposite direction.

JACK M. MATLOFF: For those surgeons who do a fair number of aortic valve replacements, and this is particularly true of the aortic valve, I think you have to be reasonably aggressive about removing the calcium. If one is careful and comes down on the junction of the anulus and the aortic root, you can virtually remove all of the calcium, including that which extends down onto the mitral valve. I think when one is aggressive in removing the calcium, and I don't mean so aggressive that you are outside the confines of the aorta, you really won't have a problem in seating the valve. On the other hand, if you leave large pieces of calcium there, you will have problems no matter how you orientate the valve, and that is a truism for most valve substitutes.

GEORGE J. D'ANGELO: In the aortic position, we orient the valve with the leaflets perpendicular to the septum and align the leaflets in the mitral position to correspond to the normal leaflet position.

SHAHBUDIN RAHIMTOOLA: I would assume that Dr. Gray leaves this decision entirely to Dr. Matloff.

RICHARD J. GRAY: No, not entirely. Those of us interested in imaging the valve after surgery have some considerations as to how the valve is oriented. One of the most important ways to image the valve after surgery, we have found, is by cinefluoroscopy, which admittedly is difficult unless the patient's valve is very carefully orientated toward the x-ray tube. You must look at the valve with the leaflets end-on. You cannot see them well if you see them front-on, so to speak; you must see them end-on. So, with respect to the orientation of the patient's anatomical structures, the elongation of the aorta and so forth, one would have to adjust the valve orientation somewhat to achieve the best end-on view—by viewing the patient in some degree of obliquity from the front to the back through the chest. That's actually more of a request than the way it is done; but that is important for imaging the patient after surgery.

Now there is another consideration to Dr. Matloff's comment that it isn't a critical decision. We do have new equipment that allows for digital enhancement of standard cinefluoroscopic images. The particular type of equipment we use is called the Adak System and it allows us to see the sewing ring of the valve, which is virtually not visible by standard fluoroscopy. We can see it extremely well with this technique, but we have to position the patient properly with respect to the valve orientation to see the leaflets, which requires special patient positioning. However, in most institutions where such image enhancement is not available, we must consider valve and patient orientation to facilitate postoperative, noninvasive, assessment of valve function.

SHAHBUDIN RAHIMTOOLA: I am going to take the chairman's privilege and change direction at this time, because I think the other two members of the panel have already told us in their presentation how they orient the valve.

ANTICOAGULATION

JOSEPH LOCICERO, III: I have a question for Professor Baudet. You have a number of patients that you said were without anticoagulation. Do you mean totally without aspirin, PERSANTIN®, and COUMADIN? And were these patients on COUMADIN and then withdrawn?

EUGENE M. BAUDET: As mentioned in my presentation, most of these patients come from the first year of my experience and they were either without any anticoagulant or with aspirin alone. Most of these patients without initial anticoagulation are placed on anticoagulation after the first experience of embolism. But, it remains that there are a certain number of patients who are not on anticoagulation because they are young, are old, or have discontinued anticoagulants on their own.

SHAHBUDIN RAHIMTOOLA: There are several reasons why anticoagulation is not used. I think you have touched on the next most important topic we should now address, and that is thromboembolism and anticoagulant therapy. Let us start off by seeing if we can get an agreement: (1) that thromboemboli do indeed occur with the ST. JUDE MEDICAL valve; and (2) whether there is evidence that anticoagulant therapy reduces this risk.

I am going to make a statement from all the presentations I heard in this particular session, that indeed, thromboemboli do occur with the ST. JUDE MEDICAL valve. Do the panelists disagree with that? I see there is no disagreement. This is not utopia; this valve will not insure against emboli.

I think we now have to touch on the difficult question of anticoagulation therapy. It is not difficult for me personally; but I guess it is a difficult issue for others. Let us ask each of the panelists whether they feel, on a routine basis, where there is no contraindication to anticoagulant therapy, that patients with the ST. JUDE MEDICAL prosthesis should receive anticoagulant therapy with COUMADIN-type drugs?

WILLIAM G. LINDSAY: Yes, we feel that emboli do occur with the ST. JUDE MEDICAL valve; but the incidence is extremely low, as we pointed out. We do favor anticoagulants in all patients who have no contraindication to COUMADIN therapy, and we start all patients on that. There are some patients with aortic valves, whose incidence of embolism is lower: if these patients develop a problem with bleeding or COUMADIN, including a COUMADIN sensitivity, they are treated only with aspirin and PERSANTINE. But yes, we do favor anticoagulation with COUMADIN as a matter of choice.

CHRISTOPHER T. MALONEY: I can reiterate what Dr. Lindsay just said. Also, we all know that patients with normal valves can have thromboembolic episodes from nonvalvular locations in the heart. So, we anticoagulate all our patients unless there is a very significant contraindication to do so.

JEAN-LOUIS LECLERC: Yes, we also recommend anticoagulation for all patients. In a small group of 12 patients observed for 248 months of follow-up, we had 3 complications including 2 TIA's (transient ischemic attacks) and 1 thrombosed valve. This thrombosed valve occurred in a child of 10 years. After the ST. JUDE MEDICAL valve implantation she was put on anticoagulants, but because of a cerebral hemorrhage, the treatment was discontinued before the child was discharged. The child was okay for 14 months, but she came back with a thrombosed valve that required an emergency reoperation. After a new ST. JUDE MEDICAL valve was put in, she was again put on COUMADIN treatment.

RICHARD J. GRAY: Well, I agree that thromboembolism does occur. Based on that, we have, and I think must, continue to recommend COUMADIN anticoagulation. There may be a subset of patients with absolutely no thromboembolic risk factors, particularly in the aortic position, who may have their COUMADIN regimen modified; but I don't feel, based on our present data and experience at Cedars-Sinai that we can recommend anything short of the basic use of COUMADIN.

EUGENE M. BAUDET: Yes, I think for most of the mitral valve patients, COUMADIN treatment is recommended. My only exception has been a child with a ST. JUDE MEDICAL valve in the mitral position who has been on aspirin and PERSANTINE for 60 months. Aortic valve patients, are systematically anticoagulated. However, for certain cases, I don't give anticoagulant therapy. These cases are: patients who are over 70 years of age or very young, women who want a child, patients in whom I think the valve size is correct and those patients who have no problem with the subaortic channel. We have a 31-year-old woman who wanted aortic arch replacement with a ST. JUDE MEDICAL valve and she had never had a child. Now she has been without anticoagulation for almost 2 years and she became pregnant quite recently. I think it is important for her and for the child to continue without COUMADIN.

HENRI DUPON: During my presentation I gave our protocol for anticoagulant treatment. All patients are placed on anticoagulant treatment. If there is a contraindication to that treatment, we use a bioprosthesis, except, certainly, in infants.

SHAHBUDIN RAHIMTOOLA: I think there is, therefore, unanimity among the panel that patients with ST. JUDE MEDICAL valves should receive anticoagulation with COUMADIN-type drugs when there is no contraindication.

CORONARY ARTERY BYPASS

DEMETRE NICOLOFF: I want to ask Dr. LeClerc and Dr. Baudet a question. It seemed that there were very few coronary artery bypass procedures done in your patient groups. I think one of you had 38 out of 500 or 600 patients and the other one also had a small number. In contrast, here in the United States it seems that we are doing bypasses in about 50% of the patients with aortic and mitral valves. Is this because you don't see the coronary disease or is it because you exclude such patients from your selection for surgical therapy?

JEAN-LOUIS LECLERC: No, no. They are not precluded because of coronary disease. In fact, all patients above 40 years old have a coronary study and if there is significant stenosis, a coronary bypass is performed. But the population of patients that I showed you was patients operated on between 1978 and 1981; and in more recent years, we have seen more and more coronary disease, and more coronary bypasses are done at the same time as the valve surgery. There is probably still a difference with the United States. As it was said several times, the mean age of patients operated on in our experience was about 55 years; in the United States it was 61 and more.

EUGENE M. BAUDET: As was said by Dr. LeClerc, in each patient over 40 to 45 years of age for mitral valve or aortic valve disease, catheterization is performed concomitantly with cineangiocardiography. Every time there is a significant stenosis, we perform a bypass. But as you observed in our slides, the mean age of patients with mitral and double valves was about 50 and for Dr. Dupon it was 55.

SHAHBUDIN RAHIMTOOLA: Let me take that one step further. The question is whether routine coronary angiography should be done in patients undergoing valve replacement, and I would like to have a feeling from those present as to what they think ought to be done. I'll pick the arbitrary figure out of my head of age 40. At my own institution, I have instituted a policy that everybody over 35 should have coronary angiography. I would like to know from the people in the audience, would they raise their hands, if they feel that patients about to undergo valve surgery should have routine coronary arteriography if patients are age 40 and above? I think the overwhelming majority have indicated "yes." Let me ask it the other way around. Are there people in the audience who feel that such patients should not undergo routine coronary angiography? No one feels that it should not be done.

THROMBOLYTIC AGENTS

ROBERT M. SADE: I would like to ask Dr. Rahimtoola if you would survey the panel, as well as the audience, in regard to the question of the use of the thrombolytic agents, streptokinase or urokinase, in the treatment of thrombosed valves on the left side of the heart, on the right side of the heart, and the occurrence of emboli during the course of such treatment, either on the right or the left side, and the survival or nonsurvival of patients who had such treatment. I think this an important issue because it may save some patients the experience of reoperations.

SHAHBUDIN RAHIMTOOLA: That is an excellent question. Let me first ask the panelists, and I am going to try and question them separately. I would like to ask the panelists if they have used thrombolytic therapy for any thrombosed valves in the left side of the heart?

RICHARD J. GRAY: As I explained during my presentation, we have had one patient who presented 6 or 8 weeks ago with a thrombosed aortic valve. The principal problem in this patient was that the two valve leaflets opened to an included angle of approximately 60° but closed completely. We gave streptokinase based on our local hospital-wide pulmonary embolism protocol, which consists of 250,000 International Units infused rapidly over 30 to 60 minutes, followed by 100,000 Units given intravenously per hour. We wound up giving streptokinase for a total of 4 days to this patient.

There were no complications that we would even remotely construe as being thromboembolic or hemorrhagic during the streptokinase infusion. This was a 76-year-old woman who 5 years after the valve replacement had this complication during a time when her prothrombin level was near normal. She had significant unrepaired mitral disease and two coronary grafts in place and for those reasons and her age, she was thought to be a somewhat poorer risk for surgery.

This gave us further impetus for the use of streptokinase. The other impetus was that because she was less critically symptomatic, we felt we had more time. As we later found out, the opposite may be true. In the most critically affected patients, streptokinase may be more effective, more rapidly than if you take the patient to surgery. With this patient, there was an improvement in the physical exam, in other words, the intensity of the murmur and the carotid upstroke improved within an hour or two after starting the streptokinase.

We monitored the patient with an experimental heart sound spectral analysis device, which showed concomitant change in the spectrum of the heart sounds, indicating that something had changed. We didn't do the first cinefluroscopy exam for 12 hours, but at that time there was an increase in the valve opening to 28°. Subsequent, there has been improvement to 22°. The valve has not entirely normalized in its function.

We have chosen to continue conservative treatment with this patient and have added aspirin to the COUMADIN therapy. We hope that the patient will continue to do well, recognizing that there may be pannus or some untreated or unremoved material that caused the valve to initially thrombose. So, we have this experience that leads us to think that streptokinase on the left side of the heart appears to be safe, at least in one patient. After making several phone calls around the country, it appears to me this is the experience of others as well. This treatment appears to work rather rapidly and may be an important adjunct, even if surgery is eventually necessary, for the patient over the first hour or two of a very difficult symptomatic period.

SHAHBUDIN RAHIMTOOLA: Have any other panelists had a personal experience with streptokinase or urokinase?

EUGENE M. BAUDET: Five years ago I asked our cardiologists to perform the first fibrinolysis on a patient who had developed mitral thrombosis in double valve replacement. During this period they used fibrinolysis for valve thrombosis of ST. JUDE MEDICAL, OMNISCIENCE® and BJÖRK-SHILEY valves in 16 or 17 patients. However, I cannot tell you the protocol because it is the cardiologists that use it. But I can say that we have never reoperated in an emergency for thrombosis since using this approach; and there was no cerebral accident after fibrinolysis on the left side of the heart for valve thrombosis.

SHAHBUDIN RAHIMTOOLA: Has anyone in the audience successfully or unsuccessfully tried thrombolytic therapy for thrombus on the left side of the heart? One additional individual. Let me ask the panelists if they have tried it in the right side of the heart? None of the panelists. Has anyone in the audience tried it successfully or unsuccessfully in the right side of the heart? I see two physicians indicating they tried it successfully in the right side of the heart.

I would also like to add a couple of my own comments. I think the doses mentioned by Dr. Gray were much lower than what his medical center, Cedars-Sinai, uses for thrombolytic therapy in acute myocardial infarction. I would just like to emphasize that to you. The second thing is that I worry about the fact that many so-called thrombi on prostheses are, in fact, not clots or recent thrombosis but pannus on old valves; and I wonder, therefore, what a true success rate would be. If there is fibrosis and thickening on a thrombus base, then one must be concerned in fact, that fibrillolytic therapy may set these off into the circulation.

RICHARD J. GRAY: We have a modest experience in operating on patients who have failed our so-called streptokinase acute myocardial infarction protocol. As Dr. Rahimtoola mentioned, the doses used in these patients, especially when given intravenously are much larger than we used in our single valve experience. And we have had good results. That is, we have had no serious or heightened bleeding risk when these patients are operated on really quite soon after the streptokinase experience. It turns out that there is a reason for that which is that the half-life of streptokinase is actually quite short—about 4 hours. These patients have a heightened bleeding occurrence early, for the first couple of hours, but by the time the surgery is over, the streptokinase will be inactivated. Other factors may predominate. If the patient was given streptokinase for a long period of time or had debilitated liver function, fibrinogen levels might be quite low. These may be complicated patients for a number of other reasons as well. But, as was pointed out by several people I had talked to on the phone regarding this, these patients are less ill than those with a pulmonary embolus or myocardial infarction in respect to these factors and other bleeding sites.

QUESTION: I would like to say one thing. We had a young girl with an apparent thrombosed BJÖRK-SHILEY valve to whom we gave streptokinase and she subsequently had an embolic stroke that was fairly dense. So I don't think this treatment is necessarily a panacea.

SHAHBUDIN RAHIMTOOLA: A lot of the pictures we saw of the thrombosed ST. JUDE MEDICAL valve were not terribly different from the material that you get on the BJÖRK-SHILEY. But I think what you are saying is correct: that you can have a small clot at the top of the hinge mechanism that will produce disastrous effects and that small clot would be very accessible to therapy with thrombolytics.

SEWING CUFF FAILURE

RICHARD J. GRAY: I would like to ask about the problem Dr. Gielchinsky mentioned with the sewing cuff of the ST. JUDE MEDICAL valve. Perhaps, someone from St. Jude Medical, Inc. would comment on what happened.

DAVID THOMAS, VICE PRESIDENT OF REGULATORY AFFAIRS AT ST. JUDE MEDICAL, INC.: The case in question appears to have been an isolated event. The valve was examined and no defect in the cuff or its attachment were identified. We did tests for cuff retention on valves of the same size made at the same time as Dr. Gielchinsky's valve and found these to meet our design specifications in their resistance to cuff separation. At no point did we recall valves from hospitals because of a defect.

RICHARD J. GRAY: Maybe Richard Kramp, Vice President of Sales and Marketing for St. Jude Medical, Inc. can shed some more light on this particular event.

RICHARD KRAMP: The "pull test" of the remaining size 19 mm valves in that lot were within specification. We did not find that the cuff came off more easily in those valves than in others. As Mr. Thomas said, we would have to look at this as an isolated event.

QUESTION: Dr. Gielchinsky, was there anything unusual about the needles and suture material that were used in that case?

ISAAC GIELCHINSKY: The needles that were used in this case were the same type of needles used in our other cases. As a matter of fact, we tried to put the sutures in the periphery of the sewing ring to avoid the suture tails from going into the housing. So I think it was a unique case.

SHABUDIN RAHIMTOOLA: I would like to thank the panel discussants and audience for a stimulating and informative session.

VI. CLINICAL EXPERIENCE WITH CURRENT CARDIAC VALVE SUBSTITUTES: COMPARATIVE OBSERVATIONS

28. LATE COMPLICATIONS IN PATIENTS WITH BJÖRK-SHILEY® AND ST. JUDE MEDICAL® PROSTHESES

DIETER HORSTKOTTE

It is uncontested that heart valve replacement leads to both a prolongation and a better quality of life in the majority of patients with severe heart valve lesions. However, late complications still limit the long-term success of valve replacement. Thromboembolism and hemorrhage are the major problems of mechanical prostheses, the latter due to the necessity for anticoagulant therapy. Bioprostheses were introduced to try to minimize these complications; but questionable longevity, calcification and the possible need for reoperation often complicate the follow-up of bioprostheses.

Besides operative risk, these late complications must be taken into account when evaluating the advantages and disadvantages of prosthetic heart valve replacement. Also, durability, frequency of valve-related complications, risks of anticoagulation and reoperation for failed prostheses must be considered when selecting a heart valve prosthesis for an individual patient.

The frequency of these complications differs between mechanical and biological valves, as well as between the various types of mechanical valves or xenografts.

STUDY PARAMETERS

We studied 1318 consecutive patients with BJÖRK-SHILEY® or ST. JUDE MEDICAL® prostheses. The BJÖRK-SHILEY valves had been implanted between 1974 and 1982 and the ST. JUDE MEDICAL prostheses implanted between 1978 and 1983. Isolated aortic valve replacement (AVR) took place in 540 patients and isolated mitral valve replacement (MVR) was performed in 609 patients. Double valve replacement (AVR + MVR) was done in 169 patients.

RESULTS

Thromboembolism

Thrombogenicity of all prostheses is primarily due to an activation of platelets, which is indicated by reduced platelet survival time. Platelet survival was shown to be significantly reduced in patients with MVR and AVR + MVR and less so in patients with AVR. This indicates that the basic risk of thromboembolism is higher after MVR and AVR + MVR than after AVR.

Although anticoagulation was started routinely after operation, 50 thromboembolic complications occurred within a mean follow-up of 2 years. More than 50% were cerebral embolisms. Six BJÖRK-SHILEY valves were replaced because of valve thrombosis (table 28-1).

Frequency of thromboembolic events for patients with BJÖRK-SHILEY prostheses per 100 patient-years was: AVR = 1.9%; MVR = 2.8%; and AVR + MVR = 3.2%. After ST. JUDE MEDICAL valve implantation major thromboembolic episodes were significantly less: AVR = .7%; MVR = .9%; and AVR + MVR = .9%. The frequency of fatal thromboembolic events with BJÖRK-SHILEY valves was: AVR = .3%; MVR = .5%; and AVR + MVR = .5%. No patient with a ST. JUDE MEDICAL heart valve died from thromboembolic complications (figure 28-1).

When cumulative thromboembolic rates for both valves are compared, the higher rate of thromboembolism for the BJÖRK-SHILEY valve group is striking. However, the small number of patients in the ST. JUDE MEDICAL valve group who were followed up for more than 34 months limits the validity of this direct comparison.

The majority of thromboembolic episodes occurred when anticoagulant treatment was not within the therapeutic range (table 28-2). However, ineffective anticoagulation resulted in more thromboembolic events in the BJÖRK-SHILEY valve patients than in the ST. JUDE MEDICAL valve patients.

Hemorrhage

Hemorrhages account for the majority of complications after heart valve replacement, irrespective of valve type. Minor hemorrhages, mostly epistaxis or hematoma, were reported by 34% of our patients. Sixty-six major hemorrhagic complications occurred within a mean follow-up time of approximately 22 months. Thirteen of these complications were fatal (table 28-3). The hemorrhagic rate in 100 patient-years was not significantly different between AVR, MVR, AVR + MVR, BJÖRK-SHILEY or ST. JUDE MEDICAL (figure 28-2). We found major hemorrhages three times more frequent than thromboembolic events in the ST. JUDE MEDICAL valve group; after BJÖRK-SHILEY valve implantation, the frequency of hemorrhages and thromboembolic complications were identical.

Table 28-1. Late complications after heart valve replacement in 1318 patients—thromboembolic complications

	MVR		AVR		DVR	
	BSM	SJM	BSA	SJA	BSM + BSA	SJM + SJA
n =	442	167	393	147	105	64
mean follow-up (months)	23.1 ± 10.2	23.2 ± 10.3	22.1 ± 10.1	22.2 ± 1	21.4 ± 10.4	21.4 ± 10.7
cerebral	13 (2)*	2	6 (1)	1	4 (1)	1
peripheral	5	1	3		1	
abdominal, renal and others	3 (2)		2 (1)	1	1	
valve thrombosis	3		3			
Σ	24 (4)	3	14 (2)	2	6 (1)	1
TE/100 patient-years	2.82 (0.47)	0.93	1.93 (0.28)	0.73	3.20 (0.53)	0.88

*( ) fatal complications

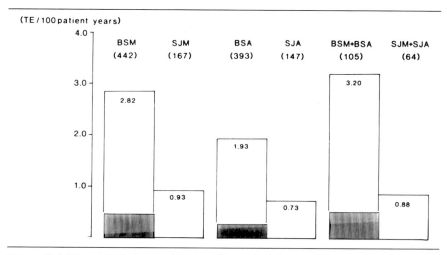

Figure 28-1. Thromboembolic complications after Björk-Shiley and St. Jude Medical heart valve replacement. The shaded areas represent fatal thromboembolic complications.

Reoperations

Reoperations were necessary because of paravalvular leaks in 29 patients (1.9%), because of prosthetic valve endocarditis with consequent severe valve dysfunction in 6 patients, and because of valve thrombosis in 6 patients with BJÖRK-SHILEY valves. One mitral prosthesis was replaced as an emergency because of fracture of the outlet strut of a BJÖRK-SHILEY Convexo-Concave valve, 11 months postoperatively. There was no instance of structural failure of a ST. JUDE MEDICAL valve.

Table 28-2. Late complications after heart valve replacement in 1318 patients—effectiveness of anticoagulant treatment in patients with thromboembolism

		MVR		AVR		DVR	
		BSM	SJM	BSA	SJA	BSM+ BSA	SJM + SJA
n =	1318	442	167	393	147	105	64
within the therapeutic range	8 11.8%	4	0	3	0	1	0
above the therapeutic range	36 52.9%	18	1	10	2	5	0
prothrombin time unknown	24 35.3%	11	2	6	0	4	1
Total	68 100%	36 52.9%		21 30.9%		11 16.2%	

Table 28-3. Late complications after heart valve replacement in 1318 patients—hemorrhage due to anticoagulant treatment

	MVR		AVR		DVR	
	BSM	SJM	BSA	SJA	BSM+BSA	SJM+SJA
n =	442	167	393	147	105	64
mean follow-up (months)	23.1 ± 10.2	23.2 ± 10.3	22.1 ± 10.1	22.2 ± 9.4	21.4 ± 10.4	21.4 ± 10.7
intracranial	6 (3)*	3 (2)	5 (3)	2	3 (1)	1
gastrointestinal	11 (1)	3	5 (1)	4 (1)	2 (1)	3
retroperitoneal	3	1	1	1	1	
others	5	2	2		1	1
Σ	25 (4)	9 (2)	13 (4)	7 (1)	7 (2)	5
Hemorrhage/100 patient-years	2.94 (0.47)	2.79 (0.62)	1.80 (0.55)	2.57 (0.37)	3.74 (1.07)	4.38

*( ) fatal complictions

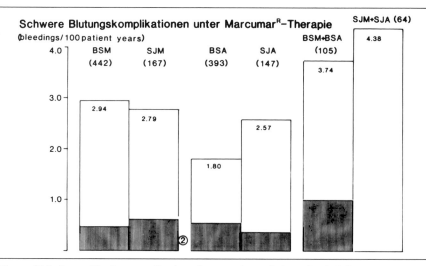

Figure 28-2. Severe bleeding complications due to anticoagulation. The shaded areas represent fatal bleeding complications.

Event-free curves

Event-free curves of complications in AVR (figure 28-3) and MVR (figure 28-4) due to severe hemorrhage, thromboembolic complications, reoperations, valve thrombosis or mechanical failure, favor the ST. JUDE MEDICAL valve. Opera-

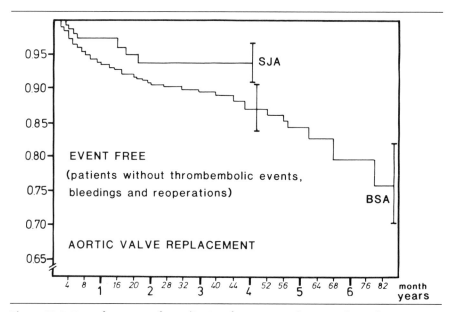

Figure 28-3. Event-free curves of complications for patients with aortic valve replacement.

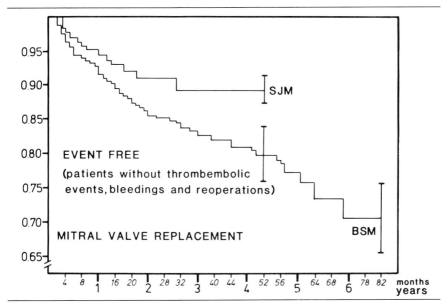

Figure 28-4. Event-free curves of complications for patients with mitral valve replacement.

tive mortality was not included in the construction of these curves. Event free curves for BJÖRK-SHILEY valve and ST. JUDE MEDICAL valve patients are significantly different because of the lower thromboembolic rates with the ST. JUDE MEDICAL valve.

CONCLUSION

Despite past and continuing improvements in prosthetic heart valve design, complications of valve replacement remain a substantial source of late morbidity and mortality. Until now, no available prosthetic heart valve meets the requirements of an ideal substitute for the human heart valve. However, concerning complication rates, the ST. JUDE MEDICAL heart valve may be a definite advancement toward this goal.

29. EXPERIENCE WITH THE ST. JUDE MEDICAL® VALVE AND THE IONESCU-SHILEY® BOVINE PERICARDIAL VALVE AT THE TEXAS HEART INSTITUTE

J. MICHAEL DUNCAN, DENTON A. COOLEY, GEORGE J. REUL, DAVID A. OTT, JAMES J. LIVESAY, O. H. FRAZIER, WILLIAM E. WALKER, PHILLIP R. ADAMS

Abstract. Over the past 6 years surgeons at the Texas Heart Institute have implanted the IONESCU-SHILEY® bovine pericardial valve and the ST. JUDE MEDI-CAL® mechanical heart valve. Between July 1978 and September 1983, 2680 patients had valve replacement with the IONESCU-SHILEY® valve with a mean follow-up of 24.6 months and a maximum follow-up of 73.8 months. Between November 1978 and October 1983, 615 patients underwent valve replacement with the ST. JUDE MEDI-CAL valve with a mean follow-up of less than 10 months and a maximum of 60 months. Both prostheses are suitable choices for a valve substitute. Each has a low profile, can be implanted easily, has favorable hemodynamic characteristics and a low incidence of thromboembolism. While the incidence of failure of the IONESCU-SHILEY bioprosthesis is still low to 5 years, we are concerned that this incidence may increase with longer follow-up. In our experience with ST. JUDE MEDICAL valves, structural failure has not occurred up to 5 years after implantation. We currently favor using the ST. JUDE MEDICAL valve in all patients requiring valve replacement except in those who cannot take warfarin anticoagulation.

INTRODUCTION

The design, fabrication and function of all cardiac valve prostheses have been directed at achieving the characteristics of the ideal valve substitute. These characteristics include: good hemodynamics, in that it should be nonobstructive and competent; it is biocompatible and is not thrombogenic; it does not degenerate or fail structurally; it can be easily inserted; it does not cause hemolysis; and it is not audible, so it does not disturb the patient. After over 20 years of experience with more than 50 different cardiac valve substitutes, surgeons are still searching for a valve substitute that will provide all of these ideal characteristics.

For the past 6 years, the ST. JUDE MEDICAL mechanical valve and the IONESCU-SHILEY bovine pericardial valve have been used by surgeons at the Texas Heart Institute. An analysis of the results of our experience with each of these valve substitutes forms the basis of this report.

OPERATIVE TECHNIQUE

All patients underwent valve replacement utilizing standard extracorporeal techniques with bubble oxygenators. Mild systemic hypothermia (30°C) was used in most cases except those in which concomitant arch replacement was performed; in these cases, hypothermia to 20–22°C with a brief period of circulatory arrest was used. Cold chemical cardioplegia was used in all cases to arrest the heart and aid in myocardial preservation during the period of ischemia. Interrupted pledget-supported everting mattress sutures were used to seat the valves.

IONESCU-SHILEY BOVINE PERICARDIAL VALVE

Between July 1978 and September 1983, 2680 patients underwent valve replacement with the IONESCU-SHILEY bovine pericardial valve at the Texas Heart Institute. The number of patients undergoing valve replacement according to position is shown in table 29-1.

Isolated aortic valve replacement (AVR) was performed in 745 patients (table 29-2). Aortic valve replacement was combined with other procedures in 598 patients. The most common procedures combined with AVR were coronary artery bypass (476 patients) and ascending thoracic aortic aneurysm resection (53 patients). Table 29-3 shows the distribution of associated procedures.

Isolated mitral valve replacement (MVR) was performed in 538 patients, while 229 patients had combined procedures (table 29-4). Reoperation, either alone or combined with another procedure, was more common with MVR than with AVR. Double valve replacement (AVR and MVR) was done in 258 patients (table

Table 29-1. Position and mortality of Ionescu-Shiley bovine pericardial valve replacements

Procedure	No. of patients	% Early mortality
AVR	1427	7.0
MVR	982	13.8
MVR + AVR	258	15.1
TVR	13	38.5
Total	2680	10.4

AVR = aortic valve replacement; MVR = mitral valve replacement; TVR = tricuspid valve replacement

Table 29-2. Aortic valve replacement of Ionescu-Shiley bovine pericardial valves

	No. of patients	% Early mortality
AVR (alone)	745	3.2
AVR (with other)	598	10.2
Reoperation		
AVR (alone)	53	18.9
AVR (with other)	31	16.1
Total	1427	7.0

AVR = aortic valve replacement

Table 29-3. Associated operations of Ionescu-Shiley valves

Operation	AVR	MVR	A/MVR
AATA	53	3	0
ADTA	3	0	0
AARC	0	1	0
ASD repair	2	12	1
ASV repair	2	0	0
VSD repair	15	5	0
Mitral valve annuloplasty	16	16	0
Tricuspid valve annuloplasty	3	52	10
Mitral valve commissurotomy	34	3	1
Tricuspid valve commissurotomy	1	4	1
Valvulotomy	1	3	0
Coronary artery bypass	476	176	33

AATA = aneurysm ascending thoracic aorta ADTA = aneurysm descending thoracic aorta
AARC = aneurysm aortic arch ASD = atrial septal defect
ASV = aneurysm, sinus of Valsalva VSD = ventricular septal defect.

Table 29-4. Ionescu-Shiley bovine pericardial valves used for mitral valve replacement

	No. of patients	% Early mortality
MVR (alone)	538	8.2
MVR (with other)	229	20.0
Reoperation		
MVR (alone)	159	18.2
MVR (with other)	56	30.3
Total	982	13.8

MVR = mitral valve replacement

29-5). Fifty-two patients underwent concomitant procedures, the most common being coronary artery bypass (33 patients).

The preoperative New York Heart Association (NYHA) Classification was known in 82% of the patients. Patients Class III or IV (71%) were fairly evenly distributed among the different types of valve procedures. Sixteen percent of patients undergoing AVR, 24% of patients undergoing MVR and 32% of patients undergoing double valve replacements were in Class IV preoperatively.

Follow-up information was obtained either by direct contact with the patient or referring physician through biannual questionnaires (table 29-6). Patients lost to follow-up were 455 (17%). The mean follow-up for the remaining 2,192 survivors was 21.6 months, with a range from 6 to 73.8 months (table 29-7). All data were computer-based at the time of discharge and at follow-up. Actuarial curves were generated using the Kaplan-Meyer method, and standard errors were calculated.

RESULTS

Actuarial survival

The early (30-day and hospital) mortality is shown in tables 29-1, 29-2, 29-4 and 29-5. Early mortality was higher in patients undergoing combined procedures and those in NYHA Class IV (table 29-7). There were no deaths in patients in Class I, and no deaths in 170 patients in Class II who had aortic valve replacement whether alone, combined or at reoperation.

Table 29-5. AVR and MVR for the Ionescu-Shiley bovine pericardial valve

	No. of patients	% Early mortality
AVR + MVR (alone)	169	10.7
AVR + MVR (with other)	52	15.4
Reoperation		
AVR + MVR (alone)	28	32.0
AVR + MVR (with other)	9	44.4
Total	258	15.1

AVR = aortic valve replacement; MVR = mitral valve replacement

Table 29-6. Follow-up for the Ionescu-Shiley bovine pericardial valve

Current survivors	2192 (81.8%)
Lost to follow-Up	455 (17.0%)
Total patient-years	4834.9
Range (months)	6–73.8
Mean (months)	21.6

Table 29-7. NYHA functional class and early mortality of patients with Ionescu-Shiley bovine pericardial valves

NYHA functional class	% Early mortality
I	0
II	2.4
III	6.8
IV	22.3
Unknown	11.3
Total	10.3

The 5-year actuarial survival, including early mortality, was 76.7% in aortic valve replacement, with 23 patients available for follow-up at 5 years (figure 29-1). For mitral valve replacement, the survival was 70.1% at 5 years with 31 patients available for follow-up. Although the number of patients undergoing double valve replacement was small, the actuarial survival at 3 years was 69.9%.

Thromboembolism

All suspected or confirmed thromboembolic episodes were counted as events and occurred in 88 patients (table 29-8). Anticoagulation therapy was continued in 29.7% of aortic valve replacements, 63% of mitral valve replacements and 70% of double valve replacements. Although 45% of all patients were continued on

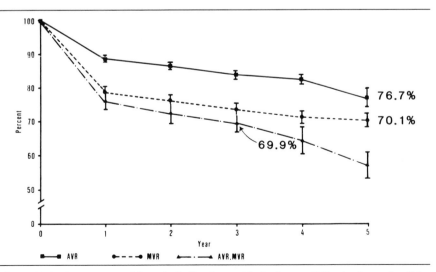

Figure 29-1. Five-year actuarial survival of patients with the Ionescu-Shiley bovine pericardial valve. Curves are shown for aortic valve replacement, mitral valve replacement and double valve replacement.

Table 29-8. Thromboembolism in patients with Ionescu-Shiley bovine pericardial valves

	Patients	Simple %	% per patient-year
AVR	40	2.8	1.4
MVR	40	4.0	2.76
AVR + MVR	8	3.1	1.95
Total	88*	3.3	1.87

*48% on anticoagulants

long-term anticoagulation, there was no significant difference in terms of thromboembolic events between patients who were taking anticoagulants and those who were not.

The linearized incidence of thromboembolism was highest in MVR patients and was 2.76% per patient-year. For patients with AVR, the incidence was only 1.4% per patient-year. Patients who had double valve replacement had an incidence of thromboembolism of 1.95% per patient-year.

Causes for reoperation

Eighty-five patients underwent reoperation during the 5-year follow-up period. The reasons for reoperation are shown in table 29-9. Tissue leaflet disruption and/or calcification were the two most important causes of valve failure. Leaflet disruption occurred in 11 patients (0.23% per patient-year), 7 with MVR and 4 with AVR. It occurred later in AVR patients (range, 50 to 58 months) than in MVR patients (range, 1.5 to 60 months). In most patients the disruption occurred in the midportion of the leaflet, where it joined the DACRON® sewing ring.

Valve calcification was the most common cause of valve failure, occurring in 33 patients and resulting in a linearized incidence of 0.68% per patient-year. It occurred more commonly in the aortic position (26 patients). The gross pathology of the valves removed revealed exuberant calcified nodules over both the free

Table 29-9. Causes for reoperation in patients with Ionescu-Shiley bovine pericardial valves

	Patients	Simple %	% Per patient-year
Valve calcification	33*	1.2	0.68
Leaflet disruption	11*	0.4	0.23
Endocarditis	31	1.2	0.64
Perivalvular leak	10	0.4	0.21
Total	85	3.2	1.76

*2.3% reoperation mortality

margins and the attached margins of the cusps. The valve leaflets were thickened and stiff and usually resulted in severe obstruction.

Age at the time of valve replacement was an important determining factor in calcification of the pericardial valve. Of the 75 patients who had AVR under the age of 30, 18.7% (14) developed significant calcification requiring reoperation. Of the 61 patients who had MVR under the age of 30 years, 8.2% (5) developed calcification. In contrast, only 12 of the 1352 AVR and 1 of the 921 MVR patients over the age of 30 years developed significant calcification requiring reoperation.

Another factor related to valve calcification was valve size. An increased incidence of calcification was noted in smaller sizes 17 through 25 mm in all patients regardless of age.

Endocarditis as a cause of reoperation occurred in 31 patients. Forty-four patients had endocarditis prior to the first operation, and only 4 of those patients had recurrent endocarditis requiring reoperation. The remainder of the patients developed endocarditis after valve replacement.

The probability of actuarial freedom from valve failure at 5 years was 85.6% for AVR, 90.9% for MVR and 97.3% for double valve replacement (figure 29-2).

DISCUSSION

The excellent hemodynamic and hydraulic characteristics of the IONESCU-SHI-LEY pericardial valve are well known and have been reported [1–7]. The transvalvular gradients are lower than other available bioprostheses, and it was believed that because of the higher content of collagen in bovine pericardium compared with that found in porcine valves, that this valve would prove more durable than

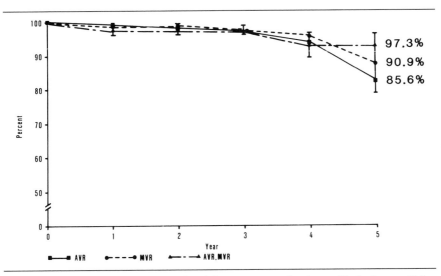

Figure 29-2. Actuarial freedom from valve failure at 5 years of patients with the Ionescu-Shiley bovine pericardial valve. The rate of reoperation increases between four and five years.

other bioprostheses. Early reports of the use of the IONESCU-SHILEY pericardial valve also confirmed the low incidence of thromboembolism similar to other bioprostheses [8–9].

The early mortality in our series of patients was high in those who required reoperation or who underwent combined procedures. Mortality was also high in patients in NYHA Class IV. Of the 745 patients who underwent isolated AVR, the early mortality was only 3.2%. Early mortality for isolated MVR was 8.2%; however, 24% of all patients undergoing MVR were in Class IV, which we believe resulted in the higher mortality.

The incidence of thromboembolism for bioprostheses has been reported for porcine and pericardial valves [10–12]. The overall linearized incidence of thromboembolism was 1.87% per patient-year. Patients maintained on anticoagulation were 48%. While our incidence of thromboembolism compares favorably with that of others with the IONESCU-SHILEY valve, it is higher than the 0.58% per patient-year reported by Ionescu in 1982 for his series of patients [13].

Valve failure, as measured by the need for reoperation, resulted in a linearized incidence of 1.76% per patient-year (85 failures in 2680 patients). This incidence is comparable to porcine valves and appears to progress at a linear rate. The failure rate seen in the porcine valves begins to increase after 5 years [14]. Since our mean follow-up is only 24.6 months, we expect to see more valve failures as more patients approach the 5-year follow-up period.

Valve calcification has been reported for both bovine pericardial and porcine valves, and a higher incidence of leaflet calcification has been observed in young patients. In our series, the highest rate of valve calcification requiring reoperation occurred in patients under the age of 30 years who underwent aortic valve replacement. Of this group, 14 patients or 18.7% required reoperation at a mean interval of 40.8 months postoperatively.

ST. JUDE MEDICAL VALVE

Between October 1978 and November 1983, 615 patients underwent valve replacement with the ST. JUDE MEDICAL bileaflet pyrolytic carbon valve at the Texas Heart Institute. Table 29-10 shows the number of patients undergoing valve replacement by position and the age range of patients in each group.

Table 29-10. Clinical Data for St. Jude Medical valves

	AVR	MVR	AVR/MVR	Total
No. of patients	412	153	50	615
male	327	71	26	424
female	85	82	24	191
Age (in years)				
range	78 (4–82)	74 (4–78)	60 (15–75)	78 (4–82)
mean	45.8	47.5	48.2	47.2

AVR = aortic valve replacement; MVR = mitral valve replacement

In patients with isolated AVR or MVR, the early mortality was 3% (table 29-11). The early mortality for double valve replacement was 11.4%. Patients who underwent concomitant procedures, in either group, had an increased early mortality, as did those patients undergoing reoperation for valve repair or replacement.

The preoperative NYHA Classification of all patients undergoing AVR was known in 412 patients, and 70.3% were in Class III or IV. Of the 153 patients undergoing MVR, 92% were in Class III or IV preoperatively (table 29-12). The postoperative Classification is shown in table 29-13. Ninety-three percent of AVR patients and 90% of MVR patients were in Class I or II following surgery.

Follow-up information was available for 72% of the patients and was obtained by direct patient contact or from questionnaires sent to the patient or referring physician (table 29-14).

While the maximum follow-up of both AVR and MVR patients was almost 60 months, the mean follow-up period for each group was slightly less than 10

Table 29-11. Early mortality of patients with St. Jude Medical valves

	No. patients	No. expired (%)
AVR	212	7 (3.30)
AVR + concomitant	113	9 (7.96)
AVR redo*	87	11 (12.64)
MVR	65	2 (3.08)
MVR + concomitant	25	4 (16.00)
MVR redo*	63	9 (14.28)
AVR/MVR	35	4 (11.43)
AVR/MVR + concomitant	7	1 (14.28)
AVR/MVR redo*	8	2 (25.00)
Total	615	49 (7.97)

*With or without concomitant procedure
AVR = aortic valve replacement; MVR = mitral valve replacement

Table 29-12. Preoperative NYHA class of patients with St. Jude Medical valves

	NYAA class				
	I	II	III	IV	Total
AVR	16 (3.88)	106 (25.73)	217 (52.67)	73 (17.72)	412
MVR	1 (0.65)	11 (7.19)	97 (63.40)	44 (28.76)	153
AVR/MVR	0 (0.00)	5 (10.00)	24 (48.00)	21 (42.00)	50
Total	17 (2.76)	122 (19.84)	338 (54.96)	138 (22.44)	615

AVR = aortic valve replacement; MVR = mitral valve replacement

Table 29-13. Postoperative NYHA class of patients with St. Jude Medical valves.

	NYHA class				
	I	II	III	IV	Total
AVR	289 (70.14)	97 (23.54)	0 (0.00)	0 (0.00)	412
MVR	79 (51.63)	59 (38.56)	0 (0.00)	0 (0.00)	153
AVR/MVR	19 (38.00)	23 (46.00)	1 (2.00)	0 (0.00)	50
Total	387 (62.93)	179 (29.11)	1 (0.16)	0 (0.00)	615

AVR = aortic valve replacement; MVR = mitral valve replacement

Table 29-14. Follow-up data for St. Jude Medical valves

	AVR	MVR	AVR/MVR	TVR
No. of patients	412.00	153.00	50.00	4.00
Total follow-up (pt.-years)	333.89	126.73	58.10	3.47
Maximum follow-up (mo.)	57.73	54.54	52.27	21.04
Mean follow-up (mo.)	9.72	9.94	13.94	10.42
Range of follow-up (mo.)	57.70	54.51	52.24	21.00
Current survivors	375.00	134.00	43.00	2.00
Lost to follow-up (%)	26.70	35.29	20.00	0.00

AVR = aortic valve replacement; MVR = mitral valve replacement; TVR = tricuspid valve replacement

months, reflecting that most of the St. Jude Medical valves used have been implanted during the past 2 years.

The calculated linearized incidence of complications and late mortality are shown in table 29-15. Six patients who had AVR, had suspected or confirmed thromboembolism, for an incidence of 1.8% per patient-year. There was one embolic episode in the MVR group for an incidence of 0.81% per patient-year. The actuarial freedom from thromboembolism for each valve position is shown

Table 29-15. Linearized morbidity and mortality rates* for St. Jude Medical valves

	AVR	MVR	AVR/MVR
Late mortality	2.99 (10)	3.15 (4)	0.00 (0)
Thromboembolism	1.80 (6)	0.81 (1)	1.72 (1)
Infective endocarditis	1.20 (4)	0.00 (0)	0.00 (0)
Paravalvular leak	—	—	—
Anticoagulant complication	1.82 (6)	0.00 (0)	0.00 (0)
Valve dysfunction	—	—	—
Valve calcification	—	—	—

*% per Patient-year
AVR = aortic valve replacement; MVR = mitral valve replacement

in figure 29-3. At 5 years, 98% percent of MVR, 95% of AVR and 94% of double valve patients were free from thromboembolism.

In the AVR group, 4 patients developed prosthetic endocarditis requiring valve replacement. Prior to the initial valve replacement, 2 of the 4 had active infection. There were only 6 minor bleeding episodes from anticoagulation, none of which was fatal. There were no cases of valve dysfunction.

Actuarial survival for all patients by valve position is shown in figure 29-4. At 5 years 80% of AVR patients were alive, as were 81% of MVR patients.

SUMMARY

The 5-year follow-up of the IONESCU-SHILEY pericardial valve indicates that the valve is performing satisfactorily with regard to thromboembolism, endocarditis, paravalvular leak and hemodynamics. Because of a much higher incidence of leaflet calcification and degeneration in children and young adults, the valve probably should not be used in patients under 30 years of age unless specifically indicated. Of concern to us is the number of valves demonstrating intrinsic failure. For example, leaflet tear or dehiscence seems to be time related, with a mean occurrence rate of 37 to 58 months and a late occurrence in the aortic position (50 to 58 months). Leaflet disruption or dehiscence added to calcification may result in a failure rate that is unacceptable at longer follow-up.

The medium-term results with the ST. JUDE MEDICAL valve are encouraging. The valve has good hemodynamic characteristics, has a low incidence of thromboembolism and is durable, with no instances of valve failure or thrombosis

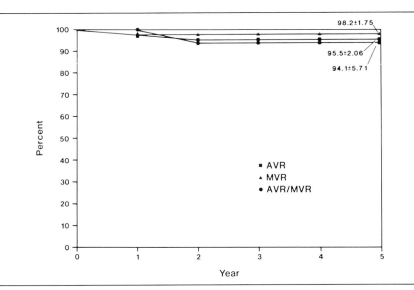

Figure 29-3. Actuarial freedom from thromboembolism at 5 years by valve position of patients with the St. Jude Medical valve.

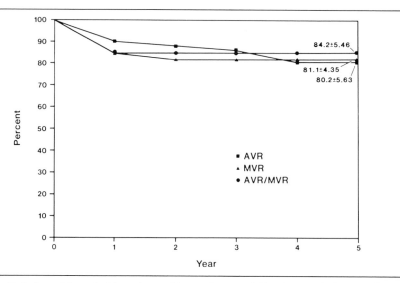

Figure 29-4. Actuarial survival by valve position at 5 years of all patients with the St. Jude Medical valve.

recorded in our series of patients. It has a low profile and is easily inserted even in the small aortic root. We currently favor this valve in all patients unless there is a specific contraindication to long-term anticoaguation.

REFERENCES

1. Ionescu MI, Tandon AP, Mary DAS, et al: Heart valve replacement with the Ionescu-Shiley pericardial xenograft. J Thorac Cardiovasc Surg 1977; 73:31–42.
2. Ionescu MI, Tandon AP, Saunders NR, et al: Clinical durability of the pericardial xenograft valve: 11 years' experience. In Cohn LH, Gallucci V, eds. *Cardiac Bioprostheses.* New York: Yorke Medical Books, 1982; 42–60.
3. Becker RM, Sandor L, Tindel M, et al: Medium term follow-up of the Ionescu-Shiley heterograft valve. Ann Thorac Surg 1981; 32:120–126.
4. Ott DA, Coelho AT, Cooley DA, et al: Ionescu-Shiley pericardial xenograft valve: Hemodynamic evaluation and early clinical follow-up of 326 patients. Cardiovasc Dis Bull Tex Heart Inst 1980; 7:137–148.
5. Smith DR, Tandon AP, Hassan SS, et al: Long-term and sequential hemodynamic investigations in patients with Ionescu-Shiley pericardial xenograft. In Bircks W, Ostermeyer J, Schulte HD, eds. *Cardiovasc Surg 1980.* Berlin: Springer Verlag, 1981; 43–49.
6. Tandon AP, Smith DR, Ionescu MI: Sequential hemodynamic studies of the Ionescu-Shiley pericardial xenograft valve up to six years after implantation. Cardiovasc Dis Bull Tex Heart Inst 1979; 6:271–282.
7. Wright JTM: Hydrodynamic evaluation of tissue valves. In Ionescu MI, ed. *Tissue Heart Valves.* London: Butterworths, 1979; 29.
8. Gonzalez-Lavin L, Tandon AP, Chi S, et al: The risk of thromboembolism and hemorrhage following mitral valve replacement. J Thorac Cardiovasc Surg 1984; 87:340–351.
9. Edmunds LH Jr: Thromboembolic complications of current cardiac valvular prostheses. Ann Thorac Surg 1982; 34:96–106.
10. Jamieson WRE, Janusz MT, Miyagishima RT, et al: Embolic complications of porcine heterograft cardiac valves. J Thorac Cardiovasc Surg 1981; 81:826–631.

11. Edmiston WA, Harrison EC, Duick GF, et al: Thromboembolism in mitral porcine valve recipients. Am J Cardiol 1978; 41:508–411.
12. Geha AS, Hammond GL, Laks H, et al: Factors affecting performance and thromboembolism after porcine xenograft cardiac valve replacement. J Thorac Cardiovasc Surg 1982; 83:377–384.
13. Ionescu MI, Smith DR, Hassan SS, et al: Clinical durability of the pericardial xenograft valve. Ten years' experience with mitral valve replacement. Ann Thorac Surg 1982; 34:265–277.
14. Gallo I, Ruiz B, Nistal F, et al: Degeneration of porcine bioprosthetic cardiac valves: Incidence of primary tissue failure among 938 bioprostheses at risk. Am J Cardiol 1984; 53:1061–1065.

30. COMPARATIVE ASSESSMENT OF SINGLE BJÖRK-SHILEY®, HANCOCK® AND ST. JUDE MEDICAL® VALVES AT 43 MONTHS AFTER OPERATION

LESTER R. SAUVAGE AND MARY A. O'BRIEN

Abstract. The value of a new cardiac valve prosthesis must be determined by comparing its performance to other prostheses. Hydraulic data, both in vivo and in vitro, provide valuable information on mechanical efficiency. However, the final assessment of the worth of a valve must be determined by its performance in vivo. The ideal protocol for comparative in vivo assessment of different valves would involve four criteria: a) alternate implantation, b) implantation by a single surgeon, c) similar diagnosis and d) equivalent implant and follow-up times. This ideal is not feasible in most practices. The greatest discrepancy is perhaps that of implant date. In our practice, the BJÖRK-SHILEY® Spherical was the mechanical prosthesis of choice from 1973 until July 1979 when we began using the ST. JUDE MEDICAL® valve. The HANCOCK® porcine was the biologic prosthesis of choice during that time but was used in smaller numbers than the mechanical valves.

INTRODUCTION

To avoid overemphasis on remembered late complications in prostheses with which we have considerable long-term experience, we compared the early results of the ST. JUDE MEDICAL valve with the *early* experience of the BJÖRK-SHILEY Spherical and the HANCOCK valves. We elected to look at the single aortic and single mitral valve replacements, with or without concomitant coronary artery bypass grafting. The total cases included 189 ST. JUDE MEDICAL single aortic or mitral implantations, 191 BJÖRK-SHILEY and 54 HANCOCK single aortic or mitral implantations. The most recent, of course, were the ST. JUDE MEDICAL and some of these had very short follow-up. We had earlier selected the first

247

65 of these to compare with our BJÖRK-SHILEY and HANCOCK prostheses; they consisted of 44 aortic valve replacements (AVR) and 21 mitral valve replacements (MVR), implanted between July 1979 and August 1980.

For comparison, we took the most recent 44 AVR and 21 MVR patients with BJÖRK-SHILEY valves, who had implant dates ranging from July 1977 to May 1979 (these prostheses all predate the Convexo-Concave model). Since equivalent numbers of HANCOCK porcine valves did not exist, all cases prior to August 1980 were reviewed: 33 AVR (implanted between April 1975 and July 1980) and 16 MVR (October 1975 to June 1979) (figure 30-1).

All 179 cases were performed by the same surgeon, with comparable numbers of BJÖRK-SHILEY and ST. JUDE MEDICAL prostheses, and enough HANCOCK porcine prostheses to make an interesting comparison. We were also able to remove follow-up time as a variable, by limiting the length of follow-up to that of the most recent ST. JUDE MEDICAL implant in the series: 43 months. For all 179 valves in the study, we considered only events that occurred within the first 43 months postimplant (figure 30-2). We previously reported the results of this same group of patients at 12 months [1] and again at 24 months [2]. As the follow-up period lengthens, the value of the observations increases.

Results are compared in terms of operative and late mortality, valve thrombosis, thromboembolism, attachment complications (paravalvular leak and valve dehiscence), infection, component failure and clinical hemolysis.

PATIENT POPULATION
Patients were not matched for sex, age or diagnosis. To some degree, older patients had been selected for HANCOCK porcine valves in an attempt to avoid warfarin.

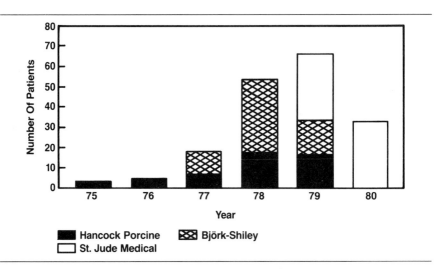

Figure 30-1. Year of implantation of the 179 single aortic and single mitral valve replacement prostheses in the study.

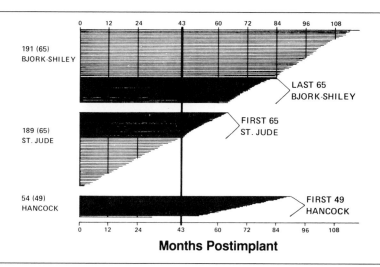

Figure 30-2. Valves selected for study (dark lines) compared at 43 months postimplantation.

In recent years, however, mean patient age for valve surgery has risen, and the patients with ST. JUDE MEDICAL valves were found to be among the oldest. Although mean ages were similar, only 11% of the patients receiving BJÖRK-SHILEY aortic prostheses were at least 70 years of age, whereas 30% of the ST. JUDE MEDICAL valves and 39% of the HANCOCK valves were in their 70s. The difference was even more marked in the mitral replacement group, where only 10% of patients receiving BJÖRK-SHILEY valves and 6% of patients receiving HANCOCK prostheses were in their 70s compared with 33% of patients with ST. JUDE MEDICAL valves. These age differences may have contributed to the differences in late death rates in the mitral replacement group. The number and timing of late deaths has created some additional variance in the number of patient-years of follow-up. See the patient-year follow-up figures in table 30-1 and the causes and times of late deaths discussed below.

Concomitant coronary artery bypass grafting (CABG) was performed in 33% of the aortic replacement surgeries and 21% of the mitral. Again, CABG has been more likely to be performed in recent years and therefore, patients with ST. JUDE MEDICAL implants had a higher incidence of CABG. In the aortic replacements, CABG was performed with 43% of ST. JUDE MEDICAL valve cases, 32% of BJÖRK-SHILEY valves and 21% of HANCOCK valves. In the mitral cases, CABG was done in 29% of ST. JUDE MEDICAL valves, 14% of BJÖRK-SHILEY valves and 19% of HANCOCK valve surgeries.

Our policy for warfarin administration is to attain a level of 1.5 times control. Patients receiving BJÖRK-SHILEY or ST. JUDE MEDICAL prostheses were typically discharged and maintained on warfarin unless contraindicated by bleeding problems.

Table 30-1. Implantation periods for 179 patients

Valve type	No. of patients	Period implanted	No. patient-years completed in this study*
Isolated aortic valve replacement			
Björk-Shiley	44	7/77–5/79	149
St. Jude Medical	44	7/79–8/80	139
Hancock	33	4/75–7/80	101
Isolated mitral valve replacement			
Björk-Shiley	21	9/77–4/79	62
St. Jude Medical	21	7/79–7/80	52
Hancock	16	10/75–6/79	55

*All patients discharged from hospital were followed for 43 months. Differences in patient-months between groups were caused by differences in group size or in number and time of late deaths.

MORTALITY

By 43 months postimplantation, 19 of 121 patients with aortic prostheses had died, as had 13 of 58 with mitral prostheses. (table 30-2)

The causes of hospital deaths are detailed in table 30-3 The only hospital death related to the prosthetic valve was one patient with a BJÖRK-SHILEY mitral prosthesis. On the second day postoperative, the patient experienced acute valve dehiscence, resulting in brain damage and death.

Causes of late deaths through the forty-third month postimplant are given in table 30-4. Late deaths due in any way to the valve prosthesis will be discussed under the appropriate complication sections below (see summary of valve-related deaths, table 30-5). The most striking observation is that all 5 patients with HANCOCK porcine prostheses who died in the first two years after discharge, died of valve-related complications (4 aortic, 1 mitral). This amounts to 10% of the patients who received HANCOCK prostheses.

THROMBOEMBOLIC COMPLICATIONS

No valve prosthesis in this series has thrombosed. The thromboembolic complications observed through 43 months are shown in table 30-6. See also tables 30-7 and 30-8 for summaries of all complications by prosthesis type. In this study, we define thromboembolic complication as a major event, not clearing within 24 hours.

The incidence of thromboembolic complications was similar in the 116 patients discharged after AVR and the 54 discharged after MVR (7 of 116 and 3 of 54). Table 30-6 separates the patients into two groups according to anticoagulation status. Patients receiving BJÖRK-SHILEY or ST. JUDE MEDICAL prostheses were usually discharged from the hospital on warfarin (1.5 times control) but several discontinued use during the first year, usually due to bleeding problems.

Table 30-2. Mortality associated with the valves

Valve type	No. of patients	Hospital		12 months		24 months		43 months		Total deaths	
		No.	%	No.	%	No.	%	No.	%	No.	%
Isolated aortic valve replacement											
Björk-Shiley	44	2	4.5	0		0		3	6.8	5	11.3
St. Jude Medical	44	2	4.5	1	2.3	3	6.8	2	4.5	8	18.1
Hancock	33	1	3.0	3	9.1	1	3.0	1	3.0	6	18.1
Isolated mitral valve replacement											
Björk-Shiley	21	2	9.5	1*	4.8	0		1	4.8	4	19.1
St. Jude Medical	21	2	9.5	3	14.3	3	14.3	0		8	38.1
Hancock	16	0		1	6.3	0		0		1	6.3

*Valve prosthesis had been explanted and replaced with Hancock prosthesis 9 months prior to death.

Table 30-3. Hospital deaths

AORTIC
  Björk-Shiley
  • Low output; 6 hours postoperative. Valve clean.
  • Triple coronary bypass graft; infarct in operating room. Valve clean.
  St. Jude Medical
  • 35 days; cerebrovascular accident in operating room; luetic aortitis. Valve clean.
  • Low output; death in operating room. Valve clean.
  Hancock
  • Hemorrhage from back of aortic root, in operating room. Valve clean.

MITRAL
  Björk-Shiley
  • Low output; unrecognized coronary disease. Valve clean.
  • 22 days; cardiac rupture second day, brain damage. Valve clean.
  St. Jude Medical
  • 84 days; metabolic encephalopathy. Valve clean.
  • Low output; 3 hours. Valve clean.
  Hancock
  • None

Aortic prostheses

The 116 patients discharged from the hospital suffered 8 cerebrovascular accidents (CVA) in 7 patients: 5 nonfatal events, one of which was followed several months later by a fatal CVA, and 2 additional fatal events. The CVA's occurred between 10 months and 39 months postimplant. One fatal event occurred in each prosthetic group. In each of the BJÖRK-SHILEY and ST. JUDE MEDICAL valve groups, a single nonfatal CVA occurred, and 2 occurred in the smaller HANCOCK population.

The patients with BJÖRK-SHILEY aortic prostheses were followed a total of 149 patient-years with 2 thromboembolic episodes (1.4% per patient-year). The patients with ST. JUDE MEDICAL aortic prostheses were followed 139 patient-years with 2 events (1.4% per patient-year). The patients with HANCOCK porcine prostheses were followed 101 patient-years with 3 events (3% per patient-year).

Mitral prostheses

The 54 patients discharged from the hospital following mitral prosthetic implant suffered 3 thromboembolic events by 43 months. These all occurred in the 16 HANCOCK patients. The CVA occurring in year one was fatal (at 11 months); the patient had already undergone removal for dehiscence of a BJÖRK-SHILEY mitral prosthesis 9 months earlier and was being maintained on warfarin when she died. The other two events were nonfatal: an embolus to the leg at 27 months (patient not anticoagulated, although she was initially discharged on warfarin) and a nonfatal CVA at 30 months (patient not on warfarin). The latter patient had a carotid aneurysm that may have been the actual source of the embolus.

Table 30-4. Late mortality at 43 months

Valve type	No. of deaths	Age at surgery	Months valve implanted	Cause of death
Aortic				
Björk-Shiley	3	70	33	Congestive heart failure
		81	34	Pneumonia
		71	39	Cerebrovascular accident (on warfarin)
St. Jude Medical	6	59	3	Infarct, coronary heart disease
		68	14	Cerebrovascular accident (off warfarin)
		65	16	Carcinoma
		61	21	Carcinoma
		38	25	Arrhythmia
		70	41	Cardiac arrest
Hancock	5	55	5	Dehiscence
		70	10	Cerebrovascular accident (off warfarin)
		58	11	Dehiscence
		63	20	Bacterial endocarditis
		61	31	Dissecting aortic aneurysm
Mitral				
Björk-Shiley	2	62	5	Trauma
		62	41	Sudden coronary death
St. Jude Medical	6	73	4	Congestive heart failure, carcinoma
		68	6	Congestive heart failure
		62	7	Congestive heart failure
		62	15	Unknown (found dead, no post)
		77	16	Carcinoma
		73	17	Congestive heart failure
Hancock	1	63	11	Cerebrovascular accident (on warfarin)

The patients with BJÖRK-SHILEY mitral prostheses were thus followed a total of 62 patient-years with no occurrence of thromboembolism. The ST. JUDE MEDICAL valve patients were followed a total of 52 patient-years with no occurrence of thromboembolism. The HANCOCK valve patients experienced 3 events during 55 patient-years of follow-up, or 5.5% per patient-year.

ATTACHMENT COMPLICATIONS

The attachment complications observed through 43 months are shown in table 30-9.

Two patients with HANCOCK prostheses experienced valve dehiscence, one at 5 months and one at 11 months. Both resulted in death. This is an incidence of 2% per patient-year in the HANCOCK aortic valve group.

Table 30-5. Summary of valve-related deaths

Valve location	Björk–Shiley	St. Jude Medical	Hancock
Isolated aortic valve replacement	1 death: CVA at 39 mo, +W	1 death: CVA at 14 mo, −W	4 deaths: CVA at 10 mo, −W[1] BE at 20 mo Dehiscence, 5 mo Dehiscence, 11 mo
Isolated mitral valve replacement	1 death: Dehiscence (in hospital)	(1 death from unknown causes)	1 death: CVA at 11 mo, +W[2]

[1] −W = patient not anticoagulated with warfarin
[2] +W = patient taking warfarin

Table 30-6. Thromboembolic complications within 43 months (no valves thrombosed)

Location	Valve type	No. patients on warfarin	No. with embolic incidents	No. patients off warfarin	No. with embolic incidents
Isolated AVR	Björk–Shiley	39	2* (5%)	3	0
	St. Jude Medical	33	0	9	2* (22%)
	Hancock	2	1 (50%)	30	2* (7%)
Isolated MRV	Björk–Shiley	19	0	0	0
	St. Jude Medical	16	0	3	0
	Hancock	10	1* (10%)	6	2 (33%)

*Each asterick denotes one fatal event.
Note: One of the two patients in the St. Jude Medical AVR group had *two* embolic events, the second being fatal.

Table 30-7. Summary of complications following aortic valve replacement

Type of valve (no. and duration of study)	Embolic episodes	Attachment complications	Component failure	Infection	Explants
Björk-Shiley (44 patients followed for 149 patient-years)	2 (1 nonfatal, 19 mo, +W[1]; 1 fatal, 39 mo, +W)	0	0	1 (nonfatal, 40 mo)	0
St. Jude Medical (44 patients followed for 139 patient-years)	2 (1 nonfatal, 14 mo, −W[2]; 1 fatal, 14 mo, −W)	0	0	0	0
Hancock (33 patients followed for 101 patient-years)	3 (2 nonfatal: 15 mo, −W; 37 mo, +W; 1 fatal, 10 mo, −W)	2 (2 fatal: 5 mo; 11 mo)	1 (nonfatal, 42 mo*; 11 mo)	2 (1 nonfatal, 14 mo; 1 fatal, 20 mo)	1 (infection)**

[1] +W = patient on warfarin anticoagulation
[2] −W = patient not on warfarin anticoagulation
*actual explant occurred outside study period
**actual explant occurring at 18 mo postop

Table 30-8. Summary of complications following mitral valve replacement

Type of valve (no. and duration of study)	Embolic episodes	Attachment complications	Component failure	Infection	Explants
Björk-Shiley (21 patients followed for 62 patient-years)	0	3 (1 fatal, in hospital 2 nonfatal: 2 mo repaired 2 mo, explanted)	0	0	1 (dehiscence, 2 mo)
St. Jude Medical (21 patients followed for 52 patient-years)	0	0	0	0	0
Hancock (16 patients followed for 55 patient-years)	3 (1 fatal, 11 mo, $+W^1$ 2 nonfatal: 27 mo, $-W^2$ 30 mo, $-W$)	0	1* (calcification)	0	0

$^1 +W$ = patient on warfarin anticoagulation
$^2 -W$ = patient not on warfarin anticoagulation
*actual explant occurred outside study period

Table 30-9. Attachment complications within 43 months

Location	Valve type	No. of patients discharged	Paravalvular leak	Valve dehiscence
Isolated AVR				
	Björk-Shiley	42	0	0
	St. Jude Medical	42	0	0
	Hancock	32	0*	2 (7%)
Isolated MVR				
	Björk-Shiley	19	1 (5%)	2 (11%)
	St. Jude Medical	19	0	0
	Hancock	16	0	0

*In previous reports (see references) of these patients, a paravalvular leak was reported in one patient with a Hancock aortic valve replacement. Since that time, the patient was reoperated and the problem demonstrated to be leaflet degeneration.

Three mitral prostheses, all BJÖRK-SHILEY valves, developed attachment problems. One dehiscence occurred 2 days postimplant, causing rupture of the cardiac wall and death of the patient. The other two events occurred during the second month postimplant. In one, the leak was successfully repaired, and in the other the valve was removed and replaced with a HANCOCK porcine prosthesis (incidence of 2% per patient-year).

OTHER COMPLICATIONS

The incidence of infection, component failure and clinical hemolysis are shown in table 30-10.

Three cases of bacterial endocarditis occurred in the 43-month period. Two were in patients with HANCOCK aortic prostheses (14 months, 20 months) and one in a patient with a BJÖRK-SHILEY aortic prosthesis (40 months). The episode at 14 months led to explant of the HANCOCK porcine prosthesis. The episode at 20 months was fatal, but the episode 40 months resulted in survival without explant.

Table 30-10. Other data within 43 months

Location	Valve type	No. patients discharged	Infection	Component failure	Clinical hemolysis
Isolated AVR					
	Björk-Shiley	42	1 (2%)	0	0
	St. Jude Medical	42	0	0	0
	Hancock	32	2 (6%)	1 (3%)	0
Isolated MVR					
	Björk-Shiley	19	0	0	0
	St. Jude Medical	19	0	0	0
	Hancock	16	0	1 (6%)	0

Late in this study, two HANCOCK valve prostheses (one aortic, one mitral) were noted to be deteriorating. Neither was actually replaced until a few months after the end of the study.

Clinical hemolysis was not detected in any patient in this study.

DISCUSSION

Summaries of complications are shown in Tables 30-7 and 30-8 (see also figures 30-3 and 30-4).

Our findings with this relatively small group of patients suggest that the BJÖRK-SHILEY Spherical and the ST. JUDE MEDICAL prostheses are probably comparable, at least through the first 43 months of implantation. No conclusion can be drawn from these data with respect to the BJÖRK-SHILEY Convexo-Concave prosthesis, since it is an entirely different valve from the Spherical model.

Warfarin anticoagulation is indicated for many patients receiving mitral valve substitutes, regardless of type, because of nonvalve-related factors such as large left atrium, history of embolism, presence of intracardiac thrombi (noted at time of operation), chronic low cardiac output and atrial fibrillation. We are encouraged by the lack of complications in our early group of patients with ST. JUDE MEDICAL mitral prostheses and feel that the use of the ST. JUDE MEDICAL valve in the mitral position is indicated if the patient can take warfarin.

Bioprosthetic valves would appear to be indicated for aortic valve replacement in elderly patients, so that anticoagulation can be avoided. In younger patients who have an absolute contraindication to anticoagulation, the bioprostheses may be implanted if the patient is also in sinus rhythm with a cardiac index above

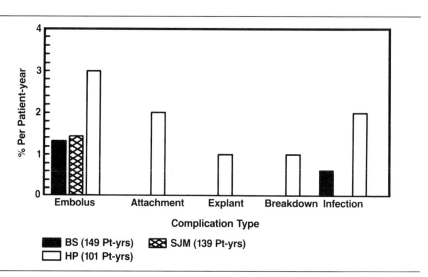

Figure 30-3. Comparative complication rates observed among the aortic valve prostheses in the study at 43 months.

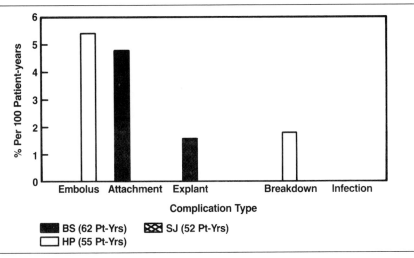

Figure 30-4. Comparative complication rates observed among the mitral valve prostheses in the study.

2 L/min/m², has a small left atrium and does not have a history of thromboembolism or intracardiac thrombus at the time of surgery. However, it is apparent from the literature that such patients would be at increased risk to experience early valve failure because of calcification.

The high incidence of attachment complications with the HANCOCK aortic series suggests that the lower tensile strength of the sewing ring may have been overcome by the high force placed on the sutures approximating the ring to the undulating configuration of the anulus. We have no explanation for the significant incidence of dehiscence complications observed with the BJÖRK-SHILEY prosthesis implanted in the mitral position.

SUMMARY

Based on this comparative study of 179 patients with ST. JUDE MEDICAL, BJÖRK-SHILEY Spherical and HANCOCK porcine prostheses from the 1975–1979 period, we draw several tentative conclusions:

1. The ST. JUDE MEDICAL prosthesis was observed through the first 43 months of implantation, in both aortic and mitral positions, to be durable, hemodynamically efficient and to have very low thrombogenicity when protected by low-dose warfarin therapy.
2. The BJÖRK-SHILEY Spherical prostheses, aortic and mitral, were also observed throughout the same period to be relatively durable, hemodynamically efficient and of very low thrombogenicity when protected by low-dose warfarin therapy.

3. The HANCOCK porcine prosthesis, in both the aortic and mitral positions, appeared during the first 43 months of implantation to be at low but definite risk of thromboembolus, making use of warfarin therapy advisable if feasible.
4. The HANCOCK aortic prosthesis appears more liable to dehiscence than the mechanical valves, perhaps due to the lower tensile strength of its sewing ring. (These were prostheses manufactured and distributed from 1975 through 1979.)

We will continue to follow this group of patients for the next few years to assess long-term performance of the prostheses.

REFERENCES

1. Sauvage LR. Comparative clinical evaluation of St. Jude, Björk-Shiley and Hancock prostheses for valve replacement. Proceedings of the Henry N. Harkins Surgical Society Annual Scientific Session, University of Washington, Seattle, Washington, September 1981.
2. Sauvage LR. A comparison of the first 24 months of 65 St. Jude, 65 Björk-Shiley, and 49 Hancock aortic and mitral valve prostheses, in DeBakey ME (ed): *Advances in Cardiac Valves: Clinical Perspectives.* New York, Yorke Medical Books, 1983, pp 108–114.

PART VI. DISCUSSION

DEMETRE M. NICOLOFF, MODERATOR

DEMETRE M. NICOLOFF: Are there any questions from the floor?

ANTICOAGULATION

LAWRENCE H. COHN: I think there have been some very provocative statements made about anticoagulation and emboli, particularly by Dr. D'Angelo. There seems to be a trend. Many of the speakers have had a number of patients in whom they have advised that aspirin and PERSANTINE® is acceptable. The first question I would like to ask the panel is, which patients are placed on aspirin and PERSANTINE? The second question, which perhaps you could clarify Dr. Nicoloff is, are there FDA restrictions on the use of the ST. JUDE MEDICAL® valve, vis-a-vis the administration of COUMADIN®? In other words, is a physician who wants to use aspirin and PERSANTINE with the ST. JUDE MEDICAL valve at medical or legal risk for doing so in regard to FDA restrictions on the use of the ST. JUDE MEDICAL valve?

DEMETRE M. NICOLOFF: I don't know if I can answer that. At the time the valve was approved, it was proposed that it be used with standard methods of anticoagulation that were being used for other prostheses. Whether that means you must use COUMADIN or not, I can't tell you. That is a vague but provocative issue. The point was to use the same recommended procedures as for other prosthetic valves.

LAWRENCE H. COHN: I think we need absolute clarification of this point at this meeting. I would also like to find out if there is data about the incidence of thrombosis when you switch patients with ST. JUDE MEDICAL valves from COUMADIN to aspirin and PERSANTINE. This is a very critical point of information. Perhaps someone from the company could expound on this for us.

DEMETRE M. NICOLOFF: If I may expand on Dr. Cohn's concerns, this question could be asked of every valve substitute. Look at the bioprosthesis; you have physicians using it with no anticoagulation, and the incidence of thromboembolism definitely varies between reporting groups. You have some groups that place all patients on aspirin or PERSANTINE. Other cardiologists say that if patients are in atrial fibrillation or have cardiomegaly, they should be anticoagulated with a warfarin product. The point is there are varying regimens, not always clear in their intent; and the same applies for mechanical prostheses. These are the vagaries that exist in every institution as far as anticoagulation is concerned, no matter what type valve substitute is being used. It would be nice to know what the incidence of thromboembolism is with every valve substitute according to these three or four methods of management.

In our group we have anticoagulated every patient except 12; and those patients came off anticoagulation because of some postoperative complicating factor. In those 12 patients there have been no emboli.

LAWRENCE H. COHN: I would like to ask a representative of St. Jude Medical, Inc. if they know the current status of Dr. Litwak's series of 100 patients who had aortic valve replacement and were placed on aspirin, only. He presented his data at about 1 year follow-up. I have heard no more of this series, and I would be interested to see if he has changed his mind because of certain events that may have occurred thereafter. Is there anyone from St. Jude Medical who can tell us if there are any restrictions on use of the valve as well?

DAVE THOMAS, VICE PRESIDENT OF REGULATORY AFFAIRS, ST. JUDE MEDICAL, INC.: In response to Dr. Cohn's questions regarding restrictions FDA has placed on the use of COUMADIN with the ST. JUDE MEDICAL valve, I would call your attention to the following statement in the physician's manual shipped with each valve:

Caution: Currently most patients implanted with prosthetic cardiac valves are routinely maintained on anticoagulants. As there are insufficient data to indicate otherwise, St. Jude Medical recommends this therapy unless, for other reasons, it is not medically indicated.

This is the same caution which FDA is asking all mechanical valve manufacturers to include in their labeling. In our case, we have recently completed a clinical trial with over 5500 patients followed with the SJM valve implanted. However, as more than 90% of patients were maintained on COUMADIN and the remainder on a variety of regimens for numerous reasons, a valid comparison of the effects of different anticoagulation regimens is not possible. We are aware of various findings regarding ST. JUDE MEDICAL valve recipients who are managed without COUMADIN, including the results presented at this symposium, but currently we have no basis for recommendations beyond calling your attention to the caution in the manual.

MANUEL R. ESTIOKO, NEW YORK, NEW YORK: Dr. Nicoloff, I just want to clarify that there were a number of cases in our series treated without anticoagulation. In the report that Dr. Litwak and I gave last year, we had 21 cases where the patients were primarily on aspirin and some were on aspirin and PERSANTINE. There was one incidence of TIA (transient ischemic attack) and the rest of the patients are doing well. Our indications for aspirin or aspirin and PERSANTINE therapy are children and those who have some contraindication to COUMADIN. We still prefer to treat anticoagulate patients with warfarin or COUMADIN.

RICHARD J. GRAY: I have a comment about this issue of thromboembolism and anticoagulation. Several presenters here, including our group from Cedars-Sinai, have a small cohort on no COUMADIN or aspirin or dipridamole therapy. Several groups here have reported a heightened incidence of thromboembolism in such patients. To a certain extent, these patients, although not randomly assigned, act as control patients, because the reason they are taken off aspirin, dipridamole and/or COUMADIN is because they have a higher incidence of complications with anticoagulant therapy.

My feeling is that heightened incidences of thromboembolism are not to be disregarded. The apparent benignancy of the situation regarding the experience of a few investigators using aspirin and dipridamole, rather than COUMADIN is just that, an *apparent benignancy*.

I would like to ask the discussants here, what is their thinking about thrombosis versus thromboembolism? Is there a difference in the pathophysiology? Is pannus formation involved in one or the other to a certain extent? Can pannus formation be prevented by COUMADIN or other therapy? Is aspirin better than COUMADIN, in that regard? I think an important distinction has to be made here between the very serious occurrence of thrombosis and, in many cases, the relatively more benign occurrence of thromboembolic events. We have been particularly impressed that the sequelae of the valve thrombosis can be catastrophic, whereas thromboembolic sequelae do seem to be transient.

C. WALTON LILLEHEI, M.D., ST. PAUL, MINNESOTA: I would like to make several comments on this question of anticoagulation and the ST. JUDE MEDICAL valve. Several centers have reported that mortality and morbidity, from COUMADIN has been greater than their mortality and morbidity from thromboembolism. This is a legitimate basis for a controlled study; and I don't think there is anything in FDA regulations that would prevent such a study based on good medical judgment. In fact, I think the Dusseldorf group has proposed starting such a study.

If some physicians are not going to use COUMADIN, presumably they will be using aspirin. In all the discussions yesterday and today, the dose of aspirin was not mentioned. Aspirin has been around for over 100 years, yet still new uses for it are being discovered; and, in fact, most of these uses are extremely dose dependent. Dosage is very important when you are using aspirin as a platelet anti-aggregate because when platelets adhere to an injured area in the endothelium or to a foreign body, such as a prosthesis, thromboxane A2 is released, which is the most potent vasoconstrictor and platelet aggregator that has been identified in the human system. The release of thromboxane A2 is inhibited by very small doses of aspirin and the inhibition is permanent for the life of the platelet which is about 7 to 13 days. Another mechanism that is also important involves prostacyclin E2, a normal constituent of the cells of the vascular endothelium, which is normally secreted into the plasma. It is a potent vasodilator and inhibitor of platelet aggregation. Larger doses of aspirin inhibit this obviously desirable mechanism that prevents platelet aggregates. So, it is extremely important to use the optimum dose of aspirin to inhibit thromboxane A2, but not to interfere with the prostacyclin E2 secretion. A large amount of information has accumulated in the last few years on the use of aspirin to prevent strokes and to prevent coronary artery obstructions. In these studies, the lower the doses have gotten, the better the clinical results have become. The most recent data that I have seen suggests that a good dose is 1 mg aspirin per kg per day. All evidence would suggest we are dealing with the same mechanisms in our efforts to inhibit thromboembolism from prostheses. Obviously, if you use a larger dose, you are going to inhibit the desirable production of prostacyclin

E2. So I suggest you scrutinize the dose you use very carefully. In most patients, you will need to go to baby aspirin (80 mg per tablet). Another option that has not been studied enough to provide information on its effectiveness is the theoretical possibility that a larger dose of aspirin could be given several times a week (thromboxane inhibition is permanent for the life of the platelet).

One of the significant problems for clinicians working in this field is the fact that there are, to my knowledge, no readily available tests for assessing in vivo these aspirin effects. Thus, all information on dosage has had to be accumulated by the painstaking process of clinical observation of patients over relatively long time periods. However, I believe that the future for this type of therapy appears bright.

LESTER R. SAUVAGE: I would like to offer some additional thoughts on your comments. I thought the same thing until we had actually done a lot of experiments in the laboratory. I do many patients with peripheral arterial reconstructions, and I was putting my patients on one pediatric aspirin twice a day. I thought it would be good to have them get this aspirin every 12 hours and catch the platelets as they were coming out of the bone marrow. We did studies on dogs and people and found that people are more sensitive to aspirin. We have tested .50 mg/kg to 30 mg/kg and there is absolutely no difference in the impact on thromboxane A2 or prostacyclin. There isn't 10% variation in the data. In a dog, thromboxane A2 or prostacyclin formation is completely inhibited at 3 mg/kg. From this I realized that having patients on the pediatric aspirin didn't make sense. A new thromboxane synthetase inhibitor from Burroughs-Wellcome actually has a very weak influence on thromboxane A2 formation. It has to be given every 6 hours; but it has a profound and prolonged impact on prostacyclin. The drug should be named prostacyclin stimulater. If you combine aspirin and the so-called thromboxane synthetase inhibitor, thromboxane formation drops and prostacyclin elevates simultaneously. We thought it would be important to give thromboxane synthetase inhibitor a couple of hours before aspirin, but in the dog, it doesn't make any difference. You can give them at the same time and get an elevation of prostacyclin. Giving 6 mg/kg of thromboxane synthetase inhibitor and 3 mg/kg aspirin will reduce the thromboxane essentially to zero and elevate the prostacyclin at least 100% —and it will last for days. There will be more information coming within the next year on thromboxane synthetase inhibitors and their effects.

QUESTION: How much aspirin do you give?

LESTER R. SAUVAGE: I've stopped telling my patients to take half an adult aspirin or one pediatric aspirin a day. The reason we had them taking half an aspirin or one pediatric aspirin was we thought there was a difference between the duration of effects with respect to thromboxane and prostacyclin. We can't demonstrate this and we've really looked for it.

QUESTION: What are you using?

LESTER R. SAUVAGE: In valve patients I'm using COUMADIN with no aspirin. I keep the patients who also have peripheral arterial surgery on aspirin. I used to keep them on low dose aspirin or pediatric aspirin. I now keep them on one adult aspirin a day and for other reasons I also give them vitamins B_6 and E.

JOSEPH LOCICERO, III: Later on this morning I'll be presenting 23 patients with ST. JUDE MEDICAL valves in the aortic position whom we intentionally placed on aspirin and PERSANTINE. We now have an average follow-up of 22 months. The longest is 44 months and we have no thromboembolism in this group. I just wanted to add this to Dr. Nicoloff's comments.

I would also like to ask Dr. Sauvage about the 9 patients who were not on COUMADIN. Are those patients on anything at all now?

LESTER R. SAUVAGE: Those patients were taken off of COUMADIN because of complications with COUMADIN. As a result, 2 had major emboli and 7 did not. All are now on aspirin.

DEMETRE M. NICOLOFF: Are there other questions? Yes, sir.

WILBERT J. KEON, M.D., OTTAWA, CANADA: I am deeply concerned that someone is suggesting aspirin and PERSANTINE offer protection in patients with either mechanical or bioprosthetic valves. We've had 500 patients with IONESCU-SHILEY® valves in the mitral and aortic positions. For patients on aspirin and PERSANTINE who have aortic valves, the incidence of thromboembolic events is 1.5% per patient-year and in the mitral position it is 4.5% per patient-year. This is just not adequate protection. Any clinical trial would have to look at the biochemistry of this very carefully. This discussion is a *deja vu* of the discussion that I hear at the hematological conferences on the mechanisms of aspirin and PERSANTINE, in particular, and I don't think they offer any protection at all to patients with valves.

PATIENT SELECTION

SHAHBUDIN RAHIMTOOLA: Dr. Horstkotte, with regard to your paper, what was the basis of selection of the two prostheses in your patients? Was this a random selection?

DIETER HORSTKOTTE: It was not a random selection. It was all patients operated on during the time frame I mentioned. All patients were listed in the paper and were re-examined despite the 2% of patients we could not follow-up.

SHAHBUDIN RAHIMTOOLA: The time frame you gave us overlaps, so all patients in that particular time frame could have received one of the other prostheses. Was there a basis for selection of these two valves?

DIETER HORSTKOTTE: No, there was no special selection criteria. All prostheses implanted in this time period have been analyzed for this paper.

PROFESSOR MARKO TURINA, ZURICH, SWITZERLAND: I have two questions for Dr. Horstkotte. The first is, who makes the decision if the patient gets a BJÖRK-SHILEY or ST. JUDE MEDICAL valve and what are the criteria for this decision? The second question is, how do you explain the large difference in the incidences of paravalvular leak between the BJÖRK-SHILEY valve and the ST. JUDE MEDICAL valve groups? You reported an incidence about 5 times higher in the aortic position, and the sewing rings on the two valves are apparently not that different.

DIETER HORSTKOTTE: Your last comment is not quite correct. The number is higher, but the number of implanted valves is also higher. You have to relate these facts to each other. The percentage of paravalvular leaks was quite similar in both groups.

MARKO TURINO: And the decision for the type of valve?

DIETER HORSTKOTTE: This is a retrospective study, which means we followed-up 98% of patients in 1981, 1982 and 1983. As to the decision of which valve would be implanted, until 1978 the BJÖRK-SHILEY valve was the valve of choice in Dusseldorf and since that time the number of patients receiving ST. JUDE MEDICAL valves has increased. I am a cardiologist, so you will have to direct that question to the surgeons in Dusseldorf.

DEMETRE NICOLOFF: I'd like to make one comment. We have studied these issues of anticoagulation. We looked at curves from the STARR-EDWARDS® valve in 1969 through 1970, and the mode of anticoagulation at that time was probably very different than it is now. When you compare thromboembolism rates reported then with those reported now, you must remember that physicians then kept the protime at 2.0 and 2.5 times control. Today the therapeutic level is 1.5, 1.8 or 2.0 times control. This variety of rates is going to show differences in bleeding complications and thromboembolic rates over the last 5 years. The ideal would be a prosthesis for which we could keep the protime at 1.5 times control and the thromboembolic rate and bleeding complications would be low. Then we wouldn't have the concern about having a patient on warfarin anticoagulation. It's the excessive use of warfarin or COUMADIN that causes the bleeding, which then leads us to shy away from using either of them and go to aspirin or PERSANTINE.

LAWRENCE H. COHN: I was going to make that exact point. As we discussed yesterday, we don't know the exact level at which COUMADIN is effective. A third protocol to a study of COUMADIN vs. aspirin and/or PERSANTINE would be to put patients on COUMADIN at a much reduced dose level. I believe such a protocol would find virtually no complications related to the COUMADIN, but what would happen with thromboembolism would have to be determined. We currently use only 1.5 to 1.7 times the control value for patients with the ST. JUDE MEDICAL or BJÖRK-SHILEY valves and we have virtually erased the hemorrhagic complications. The effect this will have on late valve thrombosis, I don't know.

EDGAR CABEZAS SOLERA, SAN JOSE, COSTA RICA: I'd like to ask Dr. Sauvage about his work. Are the complications you have seen in your series the same at 12, 36 and 43 months?

LESTER R. SAUVAGE: There has been increasing incidence of thromboembolism in time, but not with the patients on Coumadin with ST. JUDE MEDICAL or BJÖRK-SHILEY valves. The patients on COUMADIN have been remarkably free. We've had 2 patients that have developed component failure, 1 in the aortic position and 1 in the mitral position. Earlier we had no component failure with the HANCOCK valve.

DEMETRE NICOLOFF: We are over our time limit. I want to thank you all for a very lively discussion.

VII. CLINICAL FORUM

31. NONINVASIVE ASSESSMENT OF PROSTHETIC HEART VALVE FUNCTION BY CONTINUOUS-WAVE DOPPLER ULTRASOUND

ANDREAS HOFFMANN, PETER STULZ, ERICH GRADEL, DIETER BURCKHARDT

Abstract. Ten patients with prosthetic heart valve dysfunction, subsequently verified by invasive methods, were examined by a noninvasive continuous-wave Doppler ultrasound technique. Two cases of obstruction (one mitral, one tricuspid) were identified by either abnormal atrioventricular pressure half-time or by an abnormal flow pattern. Nine of 10 suspected paraprosthetic leaks in aortic, mitral and tricuspid prostheses were correctly diagnosed by detection of regurgitant flow. Experimental obstruction and regurgitation of aortic prostheses in two dogs was also detected by the Doppler method and a close correlation ($r = 0.97$) was found between pressure gradients measured directly and those calculated from Doppler data. Normal values of flow measurements in physiological and in three different types of prosthetic valves were established in 91 patients. All mean values were slightly, but significantly higher in prosthetic than in normal valves ($p < 0.05$). Our data suggest that Doppler ultrasound is a valuable method for noninvasive assessment of prosthetic heart valve function.

INTRODUCTION

Heart valve replacement is routinely performed in most major medical centers. Therefore a great deal of interest arose in noninvasive methods for the postoperative assessment of prosthetic valve function. Besides basic clinical examination, combined echophonocardiography is used for the timing of valve opening and closing as well as for measurement of the velocity of poppet motion [1,2]. Doppler ultrasound enables the assessment of direction, velocity and duration of intracardiac blood flow [3,4]. This method, therefore, would seem a suitable additional tool for use in patients with suspected prosthetic valve dysfunction.

This report summarizes the clinical experience with a relatively simple Doppler ultrasound technique in patients with correctly functioning prostheses and in 10 patients with prosthetic valve dysfunction. Validation of the method for the assessment of pressure gradients and regurgitation was documented in dog experiments.

METHODS
Patients

The patients studied had a mean age of 61 years (range 23 to 76 years) and included:

- 28 controls in whom left heart catheterization was performed for the evaluation of coronary artery disease and in whom no valve abnormalities were found.
- 6 groups of 10 patients each with ST. JUDE MEDICAL®, BJÖRK-SHI-LEY® and STARR-EDWARDS® prostheses in aortic and mitral positions (table 31-1).
- 3 patients with normally functioning tricuspid valve prostheses.
- 10 patients with clinically suspected prosthetic valve dysfunction were studied prior to catheterization, surgery or necropsy.

Table 31-1. Doppler measurements in normal heart valves and correctly functioning cardiac valves prostheses (mean values $\pm$ SEM)

Type	(n)	Size	V_{max} (m/s)	t/2 (msec)
Aortic				
Normal	(10)	—	0.9 ± 0.03	—
SJM	(10)	$24 \pm .7$	$1.5 \pm 0.2**$	—
BS	(10)	$24 \pm .7$	$2.1 \pm 0.2**$	—
SE	(10)	$26 \pm .6$	$1.8 \pm 0.2**$	—
Mitral				
Normal	(10)	—	0.8 ± 0.1	44 ± 4
SJM	(10)	$29 \pm .7$	$1.1 \pm 0.1**$	$70 \pm 3**$
BS	(10)	$28 \pm .4$	$1.4 \pm 0.1**$	$81 \pm 7**$
SE	(10)	$30 \pm .5$	$1.5 \pm 0.1**$	$64 \pm 5**$
Tricuspid				
Normal	(8)		0.6 ± 0.04	49 ± 4
Prostheses	(3)		$1.3 \pm 0.2**$	$83 \pm 20*$

V_{max} = maximum flow velocity across valve (forward flow)
t/2 = atrioventricular pressure half-time
SJM = St Jude Medical, BS = Björk-Shiley, SE = Starr-Edwards
prosthesis = BS (n = 1) + SE (n = 2)
** = p < 0.005 vs normal
* = p < 0.05 vs normal

The patients with heart valve prostheses were carefully examined by physical examination, by chest X-ray, by 12-lead resting ECG, by phonechocardiography and by determination of hemoglobin, reticulocytes, bilirubin and LDH. Correct prosthesis function was assumed from the results of these investigations.

Doppler technique

A 2 mHz Doppler instrument (Pedof, Vingmed AS) was used [3]. Analog outputs of estimated maximum flow velocity (V_{max}) and mean velocity (V_{mean}) were recorded simultaneously with the electrocardiogram and the audio-Doppler signals at 50 mm/sec paper speed. The instrument can be used both in the pulsed wave mode with the possibility of range resolution and in the continuous wave mode allowing measurement of V_{max} up to 6 m/sec.

The direction of flow was determined by the directional V_{mean} signal, where deflections are positive if flow is directed towards the transducer and deflections are negative if flow is directed away from the transducer. The transducer was placed in the suprasternal notch, along the left sternal border or over the apex, with the patient in a supine position, aiming by acoustical guidance at a longitudinal alignment of the ultrasound beam with the blood jet.

The following evaluations were made from continuous wave mode recordings:

- Timing of valve sounds.
- Assessment of forward flow through the valve by measurement of V_{max} and calculation of pressure gradients (Δp). Pressure gradients were calculated in mm Hg from V_{max} (m/sec) as $\Delta p = 4 \times V_{max}^2$, using a simplified version of Bernoulli's law of the pressure-velocity relationship [3,5,6].
- Calculation of atrioventricular pressure half-time (t/2). This is defined as the interval from peak of V_{max} (A) to peak of $V_{max} : \sqrt{2}$ (B) in diastole (figure 31-1) [7].
- Assessment of para- or transvalvular regurgitation. Mitral regurgitation [MR]: flow-signal directed from apex towards the left atrium, lasting beyond S_2, as shown in figure 31-2. Aortic regurgitation [AR]: decrescendo flow-signal directed towards the apex, beginning with aortic valve closure as shown in figure 31-3. Tricuspid regurgitation [TR]: flow-signal directed from the lower left sternal border towards the right atrium, lasting beyond S_2.

The diagnoses were verified by angiography in 6 patients, at operation in 3 or at postmortem examination in 1.

Dog experiment

Two mongrel dogs of 30 kg were operated on under general anesthesia during cardiopulmonary bypass. Myocardial protection was accomplished by cold potassium cardioplegia. The iliac artery and vena cava were cannulated for this purpose and a Shiley oxygenator was used. A BJÖRK-SHILEY and a ST. JUDE MEDICAL 19 mm aortic valve each were implanted using standard interrupted suture

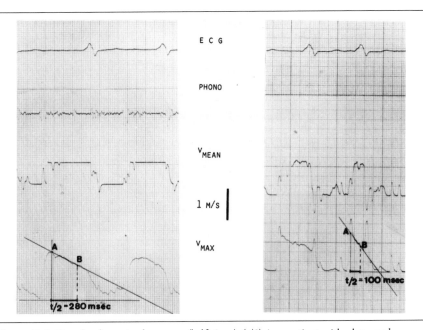

Figure 31-1. Doppler determined pressure (half-times) (t/2) in a patient with obstructed Björk-Shiley prosthesis in tricuspid position, obtained from the lower left sternal border, before (left) and after (right) fibrinolytic therapy.

technique. After closure of the ascending aorta and warming, the heart was brought back to sinus rhythm by a DC-countershock and cardiopulmonary bypass was then stopped.

Pressure data obtained from the aorta and the left ventricle were continuously recorded on a multichannel recorder. A continuous-wave Doppler transducer placed over the aortic arch was aimed at the aortic orifice. V_{max} and V_{mean} were recorded at several points during artificial inhibition producing either valve obstruction or prevention of valve closure. Statistical analysis was made using Student's t-test.

RESULTS

Normal intrinsic valves and normally functioning prostheses (table 31-1)

Mean values of maximum forward flow velocity through physiologic and prosthetic aortic valves ranged from 0.9 to 2.1 m/s depending on type of valve. Mean values of prosthetic valves were slightly but significantly higher than those of normal physiological valves.

Mean values of V_{max} through physiologic and prosthetic atrioventricular valves ranged from 0.6 to 1.5 m/s. The values in prosthetic valves again were significantly higher than in normal valves.

Regurgitant flow was not observed in any of the normal intrinsic valves and

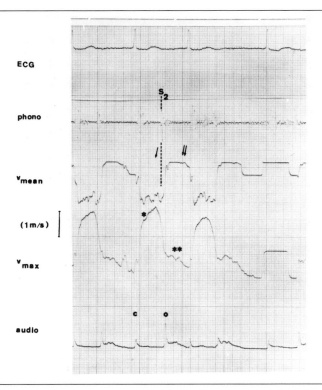

ECG

phono

v mean

(1 m/s)

v max

audio

Figure 31-2. Doppler tracing from the apical area of a patient with mitral regurgitation due to paravalvular leak in a St. Jude Medical prosthesis. Mean velocity recording shows a holosystolic negative deflection away from the probe (↙) together with high velocity flow seen in the maximum velocity tracing (*). In diastole normal flow across the prosthesis is present (↙↙,**). Opening (o) and closing (c) sounds of the prosthesis are clearly detectable in the audio signal.

only in 2 of 63 correctly functioning prostheses, which were ST. JUDE MEDICAL valves in the aortic position.

Paraprosthetic leaks (table 31-2)

A total of 10 paraprosthetic leaks were suspected clinically in 8 patients. These included 3 cases of aortic, 2 cases of mitral, 2 cases of combined mitral and aortic, and one case of tricuspid paraprosthetic regurgitation (figures 31-2 and 31-3). Regurgitant flow was demonstrated by the Doppler examination in all instances, and all but one of the lesions were confirmed subsequently by angiography, operation or necropsy. Concomitant aortic regurgitation was suspected in one of these patients but was not confirmed at operation.

Prosthetic valve obstruction

Intermittent obstruction of a BJÖRK-SHILEY mitral prosthesis was suspected clinically because of irregular prosthetic sounds. The Doppler examination re-

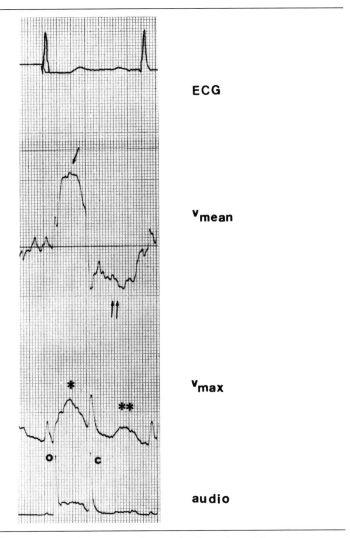

Figure 31-3. Doppler tracing using the suprasternal approach of a patient with aortic regurgitation in a St. Jude Medical prosthesis due to paravalvular leak. Mean velocity recording shows a positive deflection during systole (↗) and a negative deflection in diastole (↗ ↗) indicating systolic flow towards and diastolic flow away from the probe. Systolic (*) and diastolic (**) flows are seen in the maximum velocity tracing. Maximum velocity and audio signal reveal both opening (o) and closing (c) events of the prosthesis.

vealed changing prosthetic valve opening and closing as well as alternating flow patterns. Pressure half-time varied from 50 to 70 ms (within normal limits). At operation, the tilting disc was found to be intermittently inhibited by pannus overgrowth.

Table 31-2. Doppler findings in patients with dysfunction of cardiac valve prostheses

Patient	Valve type/ position	Clinical finding	Doppler finding	Final diagnosis
SH	BS/M + A	MR, AR	MR, AR	MR (op)
MM	SJM/M	MR	MR	MR (cath)
BM	SE/M	MR	MR	MR (cath)
HJ	SJM/M + A	MR, AR	MR, AR	MR, AR (cath)
HH	SJM/A	AR	AR	AR (cath)
CG	SE/A	AR	AR	AR (cath)
MB	SE/A + M + T	AR	AR	AR (op)
ZS	SE/T	TR	TR	TR (necropsy)
BA	BS/M	Obs	Obs	Obs (op)
PS	BS/T	Obs	Obs	Obs (cath)

BS = Björk-Shiley, SJM = St Jude Medical, SE = Starr-Edwards
M = mitral, A = aortic, T = tricuspid
MR, AR, TR = mitral, aortic, tricuspid regurgitation
Obs = obstruction

In a second patient, obstruction of a BJÖRK-SHILEY tricuspid prosthesis was diagnosed because of a highly prolonged t/2 of 280 ms (figure 31-1). Angiography revealed virtual immobilization of the disc valve. Disc movement was restored after fibrinolysis and after fibrinolytic treatment, t/2 returned to 100 ms (figure 31-1).

Experimental prosthetic dysfunction

In our dog experiments, external inhibition of the prosthetic opening produced various pressure gradients corresponding to elevated flow velocities as recorded by the Doppler technique (figure 31-4). The peak-to-peak pressure data obtained at different degrees of obstruction (0–60 mm Hg) were correlated to the pressure gradients calculated from Doppler measurements. The correlation coefficient of the two measurements was r = .97 (n = 10) (figure 31-5). When closure of the prosthesis was externally inhibited, pressure recordings in the aorta showed marked widening of the aortic pressure amplitude and there was clear evidence of regurgitant flow on the Doppler tracings (figure 31-6).

DISCUSSION

Normal values

In patients with correctly functioning ST. JUDE MEDICAL, BJÖRK-SHILEY and STARR-EDWARDS cardiac valve prostheses in aortic, mitral and tricuspid positions, maximum forward flow velocities as well as atrioventricular pressure half-times were slightly, but significantly, elevated when compared to physiological valves. This would indicate there is minor obstruction to blood flow caused by artificial valves (table 31-1). Normal values for artificial valves have not been published previously except for BJÖRK-SHILEY valves in mitral position [8].

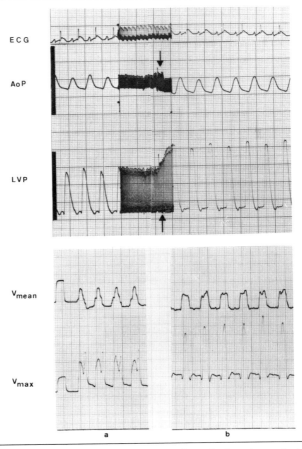

ECG

AoP

LVP

V_mean

V_max

a   b

Figure 31-4. Experimental obstruction ($\nearrow$) of a St. Jude Medical aortic prosthesis in a dog. In the top panel direct pressure recordings from the left ventricle (LVP) and the ascending aorta (AOP) are shown. Doppler flow velocity recordings (lower panel) were made before (a) and during (b) obstruction, showing a marked increase in V_{max} during obstruction. Calibration marks are 100 mm Hg (pressure recordings) and 1 m/s (Doppler recordings).

The values for physiological valves in our groups of patients are within the same range as those reported by Hatle, et al [3].

Prosthesis obstruction

Prosthetic valve obstruction in the outflow position is detected by elevated values of V_{max}. In our series no such incident was observed and the reliability of the Doppler method therefore was tested in an animal experiment revealing close correlation of calculated pressure gradients from noninvasive Doppler data and directly measured pressure gradients. It must be emphasized that the continuous-

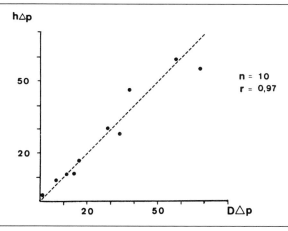

Figure 31-5. Correlation of pressure gradients measured by direct pressure recordings (h $\triangle$ p) and calculated from Doppler peak velocity measurements (D $\triangle$ p) in dog experiments.

wave Doppler technique was employed to detect velocities of several m/s such as those occurring in obstructive lesions [3]. This technique was successfully used by several groups [5,6,9,10,11] to predict pressure gradients in aortic stenosis and was recently reported to have predicted the pressure gradient in an obstructed aortic bioprosthesis [12]. High pulse repetition frequency (HPRF) for the pulsed-wave Doppler technique recently became available, making the measurement of high velocity flow in the pulsed-wave mode possible [13,14].

In the atrioventricular position, the preferable measure indicating obstruction to flow is the pressure half-time (t/2) as described for mitral stenosis [5,15]. One of our patients with tricuspid prosthetic obstruction showed marked prolongation of t/2, which reversed to near normal after successful fibrinolytic therapy. In a patient with intermittent inhibition of the tilting prosthetic disc, t/2 remained normal. The diagnosis was made by the qualitative finding of markedly alternating flow and irregular timing of valve sounds.

Paraprosthetic regurgitation

A total of 8 cases of paraprosthetic leaks were correctly identified by the Doppler method. The diagnosis is based on the finding of regurgitant flow, which is absent in most correctly functioning prostheses and physiologic valves. Difficulties may arise when a systolic signal within the left ventricular outflow tract is mistaken for mitral regurgitation. Distinction of these two flow signals, which have similar directions, should be made by their duration (mitral regurgitation lasting beyond the second heart sound). Previous experience with pulsed-wave Doppler techniques in valvular heart disease has been reported by several authors, showing good diagnostic accuracy for the assessment of aortic and mitral regurgitation [15–17].

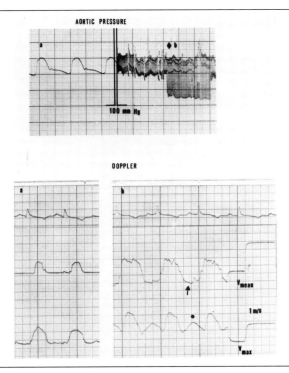

Figure 31-6. Experimental regurgitation through a Björk-Shiley prosthesis in a dog. In the top panel a direct pressure recording from the aorta shows marked widening of the pulse pressure during regurgitation (b). In the lower panel Doppler recordings from the aortic arch before (a) and during (b) regurgitation reveals diastolic flow directed away from the probe (negative deflection in V_{mean}, ↗) and diastolic V_{max}-signal (*) not present without regurgitation (a).

Trivial transvalvular regurgitant flow may be present in virtually all correctly functioning prostheses as shown by *in vitro* and angiographic studies [18,19]. In our series, such clinically silent regurgitation was detected by the Doppler technique in only 2 out of 63 cases, both ST. JUDE MEDICAL aortic prostheses. Paravalvular and transvalvular leakage may be differentiated. The former can be recorded from both sides of the prosthesis. The latter is only demonstrable within the cardiac chamber receiving the regurgitant flow, due to complete rejection of ultrasound by the prosthetic material itself. The strength of the Doppler method obviously is to confirm clinically suspected significant paravalvular leaks in the presence of difficult clinical findings such as tachycardia or multiple murmurs.

Although the combined application of two-dimensional echocardiography and Doppler ultrasound, when using the HPRF technique, may offer the advantage of easy localization of a sample volume and spectral analysis even of high Doppler frequencies, the continuous-wave technique seems to yield accurate results in clinical practice at considerably lower expense.

CONCLUSION

Continuous-wave Doppler ultrasound seems to be a valuable addition to the cardiologist's armamentarium for noninvasive evaluation of pressure gradients, obstruction and regurgitation in patients with heart valve prostheses.

REFERENCES

1. Mintz GS, Carlson EB, Kotler MN: Comparison of noninvasive techniques in evaluation of the nontissue cardiac valve prosthesis. Cardiology 1982; 49:39–44.
2. Amann FW, Burckhardt D, Hasse J, et al: Echocardiographic features of the correctly functioning St. Jude Medical valve prosthesis. Am Heart J 1981; 101:45–51.
3. Hatle L, Angelsen B: *Doppler Ultrasound in Cardiology*. Lea + Febiger, Philadelphia 1982.
4. Pearlman AS: Doppler echocardiography. Int J Cardiol 1983; 3:81–86.
5. Holen J, Aaslid R, Landmark K, et al: Determination of pressure gradient in mitral stenosis with a noninvasive ultrasound Doppler technique. Acta med scand 1976; 199:455–460.
6. Hatle L: Non-invasive assessment of differentiation of left ventricular outflow obstructions with Doppler ultrasound. Circulation 1978; 64:381–387.
7. Hatle L, Angelsen BA, Tromsdal A: Non-invasive assessment of pressure drop in mitral stenosis by Doppler ultrasound. Br Heart J 1980; 43:284–292.
8. Holen J, Simonsen S, Froysaker T: An ultrasound Doppler technique for the noninvasive determination of the pressure gradient in the Björk-Shiley mitral valve. Circulation 1979; 59:436–42.
9. Hoffmann A, Pfisterer M, Schmitt HE, et al: Non-invasive assessment of pressure gradients in valvular aortic stenosis by Doppler ultrasound. Circulation 1982; 66:II–121.
10. Hoffmann A, Amann FW, Burckhardt D: Nicht-invasive Beurteilung von Druckgradienten bei Aortenstenose mit Doppler Ultraschall. Schweiz Med Wschr 1982; 112:1597–1600.
11. Kwan OL, Waters J, Takeda P, et al: Relative value of continuous wave Doppler compared to two-dimensional echocardiography in the quantitation of valvular stenosis. Circulation 1982; 66:II–121.
12. Wilkes HS, Berger M, Gallerstein PE, et al: Left ventricular ouflow obstruction after aortic valve replacement: detection with continuous wave Doppler ultrasound recording. J Am Coll Cardiol 1983; 2:550–553.
13. Cannon SR, Richards KL, Morgann RG: Comparison of continuous wave and high pulse repetition frequency Doppler for quantifying aortic stenosis. Circulation 1983; 68:Suppl III–228.
14. Sahn DJ, Valdes-Conz LM, Scagnelli S, et al: Comparison of continuous wave and high PRF 2D-Echo Doppler for pressure gradient estimation in animal models and human patients. Circulation 1983; 68:Suppl III–228.
15. Quinones MA, Young JB, Waggoner AD, et al: Assessment of pulsed Doppler echocardiography in detection and quantification of aortic and mitral regurgitation. Br Heart J 1980; 44:612–620.
16. Blanchard D, Diebold B, Peronneau P, et al: Non-invasive diagnosis of mitral regurgitation by Doppler echocardiography. Br Heart J 1981; 45:589–593.
17. Hoffmann A, Burckhardt D: Evaluation of systolic murmurs by Doppler ultrasound. Br Heart J 1983; 50:337–42.
18. Dellsperger KC, Wieting DW, Baeler DA, et al: Regurgitation of prosthetic heart valves: Dependence on heart rate and cardiac output. Am J Cardiol 1983; 51:321–8.
19. Levang OW, Levorstad K, Haugland T: Aortic valve replacement: A randomised study comparing the Björk-Shiley and Lillehei-Kaster disc valves. Scand J Thorac Cardiovasc Surg 1980; 14:7–19.

32. POTENTIAL FOR IMMOBILIZATION OF THE VALVE OCCLUDER IN VARIOUS VALVE PROSTHESES

OSCAR BAEZA

Tilting disc valves were introduced with the LILLEHEI-KASTER® valve in 1967. These valves have experienced increasing popularity because they have achieved improved hemodynamics and durability in comparison with these characteristics in central flow tissue valves. On the other hand, the presence of mobile prosthetic valve elements introduces the potential for interference (immobilization) of the occluder by suture material or tissue, a potentially lethal complication.

During clinical evaluation of the MEDTRONIC HALL™ valve from 1979 to 1980, 56 valves were implanted in 48 patients. Two episodes of disc immobilization in the closed position were caused by impingement of suture material during aortic valve replacement. Both patients survived after reinstitution of cardiopulmonary bypass, trimming of the suture material and reorientation of the valve housing. We diagnosed a stuck aortic prosthesis because of sudden hypotension, marked dilatation of the left ventricle and the absence of valve clicks.

Two other patients died after mitral valve replacement with the MEDTRONIC HALL valve because of immobilization of the occluder. One died a few hours after surgery and autopsy showed wedged suture material between the disc and valve housing. The other patient died several days after surgery and this time the disc was immobilized by a remnant of chordae tendineae.

Another patient presented a similar complication in the tricuspid position during mitral and tricuspid valve replacement. The episode recurred twice, requiring replacement with a tissue valve. The incidence of this complication was more than a statistical coincidence, since we were aware of the potential catastrophe and tried to prevent it.

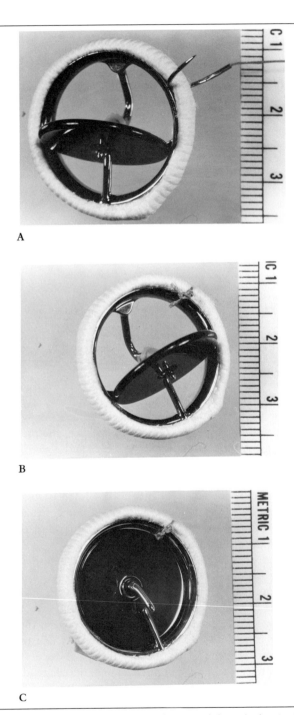

A

B

C

Figure 32-1. Sutures placed too close to the prosthetic metal frame lead to inpingement of the suture tail.

Sutures placed too close to the metal frame or cut too long, after being bathed by fluid or blood at 37°C can become flaccid and protrude between the disc and housing (figure 32-1). The result can be a "stuck" occluder. Prevention requires that sutures be placed at least 1.5 mm from the metal housing and knots be tied toward the side of the patient anulus (figure 32-2).

Recently, another stuck valve occurred during mitral valve replacement with a BJÖRK-SHILEY® prosthesis due to the interference from the endocardial surface of a small, hypertrophied left ventricle. Sudden hypotension, associated with dilatation of the right ventricle, acute left atrial hypertension and absence of valve clicks, prompted reinstitution of bypass and reorientation of the valve housing.

This potentially lethal complication happens more frequently, in our experience, with valves in which the occluder enters the valve housing like a door fitting into its frame. The MEDTRONIC HALL and the BJÖRK-SHILEY belong to this

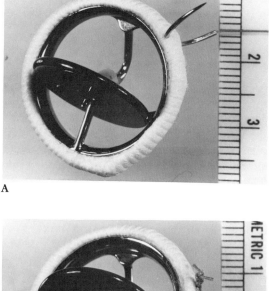

A

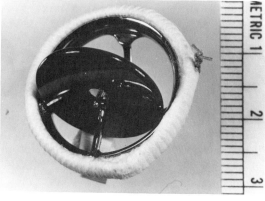

B

Figures 32-2. Correct technique for placement of the sutures through the sewing cuff (1–2 mm from the metal frame).

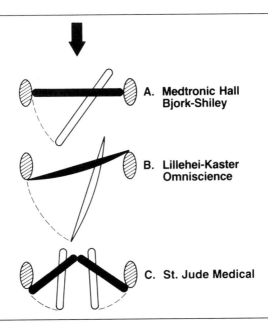

Figure 32-3. Closure angle of occluder to valve housing.

category (Figure 32-3A). Long sutures or residual tissue could immobilize the occluder at any location of the valve circumference [1].

Occluders of the LILLEHEI-KASTER and OMNISCIENCE® valves do not completely enter the valve housing during closure. Therefore, immobilization of the disc will be produced only when the foreign material is interposed near the retaining struts (Figure 32-3B).

The two leaflets of the ST. JUDE MEDICAL valve close with an angle to the frontal plane of the valve (Figure 32-3C). This peculiar design makes it virtually impossible for the occluders to be immobilized by sutures or foreign material. Moreover, the ST. JUDE MEDICAL valve is the only true low profile, tilting disc valve and, therefore, interference by a small left ventricle or by papillary muscles is theoretically improbable in the mitral position.

CONCLUSION

In summary, tilting disc immobilization is a potentially lethal complication. Its prevention requires an awareness by the surgeon who must place the sutures far from the valve housing. The MEDTRONIC HALL valve and, in a lesser degree, the BJÖRK-SHILEY valve have a certain predilection for this complication compared with other tilting disc valves. The ST. JUDE MEDICAL valve is the least prone to this complication.

REFERENCE

1. Starek PJK: Immobilization of disc heart valves by unraveled sutures, Ann Thorac Surg 1981; 31(1):66–69.

33. ESCAPE OF A LEAFLET FROM A ST. JUDE MEDICAL®
PROSTHESIS IN THE MITRAL POSITION

E. HJELMS

Abstract. Twenty-three months after mitral valve replacement for mitral stenosis with a *ST. JUDE MEDICAL®* heart valve prosthesis size 31, a 29-year-old man suddenly went into a profound cardiogenic shock and pulmonary edema due to escape of one of the leaflets from the prosthesis. At emergency operation the valve was replaced with another type of prosthesis. The escaped leaflet was retrieved from the abdominal aorta and was found to be intact. The cause of the escape was found to be a fracture in the pivot area. Further examination with optic and scanning electron microscopy (SEM) revealed an old fracture in the base of the pivot, covered with organic material, and another fracture at the top of the pivot area, not covered with organic material, and therefore probably very recent and responsible for the break-off of part of the area and subsequent escape of the leaflet. The cause of the primary fracture is unknown.

INTRODUCTION

The ST. JUDE MEDICAL heart valve prosthesis has been used clinically since 1977. It has demonstrated excellent hemodynamics *in vitro* [1] as well as *in vivo* [2], a very low incidence of thromboembolic complications compared with other mechanical valve prostheses and a low degree of hemolysis [3].

Lately, however, there have been reports of valve thrombosis in both the tricuspid [4] and mitral positions [2]. Furthermore, a case of mechanical dysfunction without thrombosis in a ST. JUDE MEDICAL prosthesis in the mitral position has recently been reported [5].

Reprinted with permission from Thorac Cardiovasc Surgeon 1983;31:310–312. Georg Thieme Verlag, Stuttgart, New York.

This chapter presents a previously unreported complication of the ST. JUDE MEDICAL prosthesis, escape of a leaflet from the prosthesis and embolization of the leaflet to the periphery.

CASE REPORT

A 27-year-old male, who experienced symptoms of mitral stenosis (MS) at the age of 10 and had a closed valvotomy at the age of 13, was admitted with recurrent symptoms of mitral stenosis. He was in sinus rhythm and presented the usual clinical signs of MS. Echocardiography and a catheter study confirmed the diagnosis and demonstrated moderate pulmonary hypertension of 74/34 mm Hg and a calculated valve area of 0.8 cm².

The mitral valve was excised and a ST. JUDE MEDICAL mitral valve prosthesis size 31 was implanted under cardiopulmonary bypass combined with moderate hypothermia and cold cardioplegia. The prosthesis was implanted using continuous Prolene 2-0 suture.

The postoperative course was uneventful. He had a short period of atrial flutter but was discharged in sinus rhythm after digitalization.

After recovering from the operation, he started an active life including sport activities on no medication apart from anticoagulation. Twenty-three months after the operation he suddenly fell ill during a basketball match. He experienced palpitation, tachycardia and coughed up frothy pink sputum. The patient was immediately brought to the hospital, where he was found to be in cardiogenic shock with a systolic blood pressure of 80 and tachycardia of 160/min and in severe pulmonary edema.

Standard pulmonary edema treatment with digitalization, morphine and frusemide was instituted, but caused only slight improvement. He was then intubated and put on a respirator. Clinical examination revealed a systolic murmur at the apex, but stethoscopy was difficult as the heart sounds were obscured by the persistent pulmonary edema. However, several examiners were quite certain that a prosthetic opening and closing sound could be heard. A 2-D echocardiography (ECG) was inconclusive. The ECG showed supraventricular tachycardia. Because of persistent cardiogenic shock and intractable pulmonary edema in spite of intensive treatment, it was decided to operate immediately without further investigation, presuming that the condition was due to prosthetic malfunction. At operation the ST. JUDE MEDICAL valve was nicely healed in with no paravalvular leak, but there was only one leaflet present in the prosthesis. This remaining leaflet was moving freely. The prosthesis was explanted. The left atrium, the pulmonary veins and the left ventricular cavity were examined with great care, but the escaped leaflet could not be found. An OMNISCIENCE® mitral valve prosthesis size 29 was implanted. On inspection of the explanted valve, a fracture was found in the valve housing going through one of the butterfly pivot areas corresponding to the escaped leaflet (figure 33-1). Postoperatively, the patient needed inotropic and respiratory support for a prolonged period of time, but he subsequently recovered. The embolized leaflet was located in the abdominal aorta by 2-D echocardiography and was retrieved 28 days after

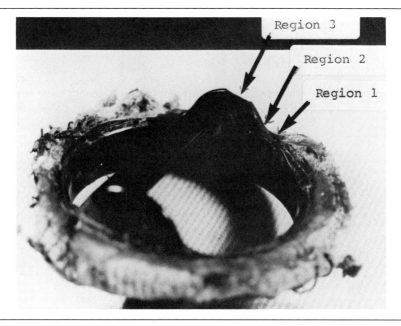

Figure 33-1. The explanted prosthesis showing one leaflet missing and the fractured pivot with three different types of surfaces: region 1 covered with organic material; region 2, a transition between regions 1 and 3; and region 3 without organic material covering the fracture surface.

the emergency operation. The escaped leaflet was found to be macroscopically intact.

The explanted prosthesis and the retrieved leaflet were examined optically and with scanning electron microscopy (performed by St. Jude Medical, Inc.). Three distinct regions were identified in the pivot area (figure 33-1). The fracture surface at the base of the pivot, closest to the orifice ring, was relatively smooth, but heavily infiltrated with organic material. In the butterfly area the fracture surface was found to be very ragged. In the third region, at the top of the pivot, the fracture surface was smooth with less adherent material. In region 2 the surface at the orifice's inside diameter was very rough and irregular, while at the outside diameter it was clean and like that of region 3 (figures 33-1 and 33-2).

On examination of the escaped leaflet with scanning electron microscopy wear marks, suggesting abnormal movements of the leaflet, were found.

Histological examination of the removed organic material on the surface of the fracture of the pivot (performed by J. E. Edwards, M.D., St. Paul, Minnesota, USA.) showed that the material consisted of old fibrin into which fibroblasts had entered and some collagen developed.

DISCUSSION
The escape of the leaflet in this case was due to a fracture through the pivot area, however, the cause of this fracture is obscure. According to preclinical testing [5]

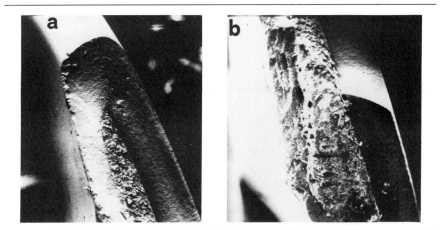

Figure 33-2. a) SEM of region 3. Note the smooth surface on the outside as well as on the inside diameter. b) SEM of region 2. The inside diameter is very rough whereas the outside part of the fracture surface is smooth like the surface in a.

of this type of valve prosthesis, the safety factor against stress fracture in the pyrolytic carbon is more than 20, which should be more than adequate even under periods of increased cardiac output and increased intracavity pressures, which occur during physical exercise. The fact that part of the fracture line as seen in region 1 (figure 33-1) was covered with organic material, which on histological examination revealed a high degree of organization in terms of fibroblast ingrowth and development of collagen (in contrast to the noncovered area at region 3) suggests that fractures have occurred at different times. These findings suggest that the first fracture had occurred before or during insertion of the valve prosthesis, taking into account the time required for organization of the organic matter on the surface of region 1. However, the insertion of the prosthesis was not difficult and was performed using continuous suture technique, which involves very little handling of the prosthesis as it is placed in the mitral orifice with the first throw of the continuous stitch and subsequently only touched at the sewing ring. The other possibility is trauma to the prosthesis during its shelf life, but certainly no dysfunction or other abnormality of the valve prosthesis was noticed at the time of insertion. The cause of the extension of the fracture line with break off of part of the pivot area and subsequent escape of the leaflet is unclear; but the abnormal wear on the leaflet, suggesting repeated leaflet trauma together with forces generated by the infiltrating tissue from region 1, could theoretically force the remainder of the cracked pivot area to fall away. It is important to notice that, with this bileaflet type of valve prosthesis, a severe and life-threatening malfunction of the prosthesis can occur without giving the traditional signs of prosthetic malfunction in terms of muffling or disappearance of opening and closing sounds, because of the preserved function of one of the leaflets.

CONCLUSION

Prosthetic malfunction not due to thrombosis or tissue interposition, although rare, can occur with the ST. JUDE MEDICAL heart valve prosthesis. It is extremely important to handle this all pyrolytic carbon valve prosthesis with great care before and during insertion. A preinsertion lesion of the prosthesis can manifest itself as malfunction very late after insertion, as in this case after almost 2 years.

The usual stethoscopic signs of prosthetic malfunction do not necessarily show in this bileaflet type of valve since preserved function of just one of the leaflets can produce normal opening and closing sounds.

REFERENCES

1. Bowen TE, Tri TB, Wortham DS: Thrombosis of a St. Jude Medical tricuspid prosthesis. J Thorac Cardiovasc Surg 1981;82:257.
2. Emery RW, Nicoloff DM: St. Jude Medical cardiac valve prosthesis. J Thorac Cardiovasc Surg 1979;78:269.
3. Hehrlein RW, Gottwik M, Fraedrich G, et al: First clinical experience with a new all-pyrolytic carbon bileaflet heart valve prosthesis. J Thorac Cardiovasc Surg 1980;79:632.
4. Nicoloff DM, Emery RW, Aron KV, et al: Clinical and hemodynamic results with St. Jude Medical cardiac valve prosthesis. J Thorac Cardiovasc Surg 1981;82:674.
5. Palmquist WE, Nicoloff DM, Emery RW, et al: St. Jude Medical all-pyrolytic carbon heart valve. Presented at the 13th Annual Meeting of the Association for Advancement of Medical Instrumentation, 1978.
6. Ziemer G, Luhmer I, Oelert H, et al: Malfunction of a St. Jude Medical heart valve in mitral position. Ann Thorac Surg 1982;33:391.

34. PROPHYLAXIS AGAINST THROMBOEMBOLISM USING ASPIRIN AND DIPYRIDAMOLE IN PATIENTS WITH THE ST. JUDE MEDICAL® AORTIC PROSTHESIS

JOSEPH LOCICERO, III

Since January 1980, 52 patients at Northwestern University in Chicago, Illinois underwent ST. JUDE MEDICAL® aortic valve replacement. Seven of these patients also had simultaneous mitral valve insertion. Five patients died in the hospital: 2 intraoperative deaths, 2 arrhythmia deaths and 1 septic death.

Of the remaining 47 patients, 24 patients were placed on COUMADIN® (COU): 13 had compelling reasons for long-term anticoagulation and 11 were treated at the surgeon's or cardiologist's request. Twenty-three patients were placed on aspirin and Dipyridamole (ASA + DIP): 7 patients left the hospital on ASA + DIP, 13 patients were switched from COU to ASA + DIP at 6 weeks, and 3 patients were switched from COU to ASA + DIP at 6 months. Dosage was 650 mg aspirin a day and 75 mg Dipyridamole three times a day.

By January 1984, 24 patients on COU accrued 422 months in follow-up. The longest follow-up was 44 months and the mean follow-up was 18.5 months. Seven patients had major complications and 2 were switched to ASA + DIP. Three patients on COU had thromboembolic complications. These patients were considered at increased risk of thromboembolism at the time of surgery.

The 23 patients on ASA + DIP, plus the 2 crossover patients, accrued 509 months of follow-up. The longest follow-up was 44 months and the mean follow-up was 21 months. Sixteen patients have been on ASA + DIP for more than 1 year. There have been no thromboembolic complications in this group. The only problem was in a patient who developed dizziness attributed to vertebrobasilar disease.

ASA + DIP patients had significantly lower complications than COU patients. We recommend that patients who receive ST. JUDE MEDICAL aortic valves and who do not require anticoagulation for other reasons may be safely treated with ASA + DIP after 6 weeks of COU. We anticoagulate patients with mitral and double valve replacements; patients with nonconvertible atrial fibrillation; patients with preoperative thrombophlebitis or thromboembolus; and patients with documented atrial or ventricular clot, whether or not we remove it at the time of surgery.

PART VII. DISCUSSION

RICHARD J. GRAY, MODERATOR

DOPPLER ULTRASOUND

RICHARD J. GRAY: I would like to start the discussion with two questions. Professor Burc-khardt, is it easier to visualize a valve in the aortic position than in the mitral or tricuspid position with your technique? Also, because the ST. JUDE MEDICAL® and other prostheses have a certain amount of regurgitation, is your technique sensitive enough to detect this regurgitation and does it lose some specificity in the process?

PROF. DIETER BURCKHARDT, BASEL, SWITZERLAND: In answer to your first question, it was equally feasible to reach the aortic, mitral and tricuspid prostheses with the Pedof equipment used in our study. The unit allows registration of flow in the pulsed and continuous wave mode, but it is not connected with echocardiographic equipment. We, therefore, explored the valve, using primarily the continuous wave mode with the audio signal, which clearly defines opening and closing events, as a guide.

In answer to your second question, in 63 patients with normally functioning prostheses we were not able to detect any degree of regurgitation when the patients were investigated by the suprasternal approach. However, 2 patients with ST. JUDE MEDICAL valves in the aortic position had some degree of regurgitation, which was seen using the apical approach. This "physiologic" regurgitant flow was not detectable when we scanned from the suprasternal notch in contrast to the patients with paravalvular aortic leakage, whose regurgitation was demonstrable using both the suprasternal and the apical approach.

RICHARD J. GRAY: Do you have any feeling what the sensitivity and specificity of this test might be in detecting leakage?

DIETER BURCKHARDT: We could detect some regurgitant flow in 2 out of 10 patients with ST. JUDE MEDICAL aortic valves, which may reduce the specificity of the method. Although it does seem possible to differentiate between transvalvular and paravalvular leakage as mentioned above. However, data on specificity and sensitivity can only be obtained from prospective studies.

DISC IMMOBILIZATION

RICHARD J. GRAY: Is there anyone in the audience who has experience with suture impingement of discs or leaflets as described by Dr. Baeza?

JOSEPH J. AMATO, M.D. NEWARK, NEW JERSEY: We had two similar experiences, one during my residency training at Presbyterian St. Luke's Hospital in Chicago with a BJÖRK-SHILEY® valve, and the other, which also involved the BJÖRK-SHILEY valve, was reported to me by one of my associates, Dr. Gielchinsky. Both of these situations could have been fatal. One patient survived only because the situation was recognized and the patient brought immediately back into the operating room.

The observations that Dr. Baeza has made are important, and I congratulate him. I think that in a residency training program especially, one has to adhere to the principles he pointed out, and that the sutures must be placed on the periphery of the cuff. The resident or attending surgeon must cut the sutures short so they won't protrude centrally into the orifice with the potential to occlude. A clue to suture problems is if the patient is in normal sinus rhythm and the clicks of the valves don't correspond to the heart beats. I think it behooves someone to pay attention to this and bring the patient back into surgery to correct this potentially fatal complication, if it happens.

RICHARD J. GRAY: Has anyone had experience with the ST. JUDE MEDICAL valve, when suture material has been documented as the cause of leaflet motion impairment in the early postoperative period?

ROBERT M. SADE: We haven't had a suture do that, but we did have a chordae tendineae in the left ventricle flip into the valve orifice. It did not produce acute and total immobilization of the valve, but it did keep the valve from closing completely and resulted in a severe hemolytic problem. When I reoperated I resected a piece of the chordae tendineae and the patient did fine, afterwards. Foreign material in a ST. JUDE MEDICAL valve can be a problem.

In our experience two patients had valve thrombosis in the aortic position; both had small aortic roots and heavily calcified aortic stenosis as the indication for surgery. We speculated noncomplete removal of small pieces of calcium might have been related to the eventual occurrence of thrombosis. This may further underscore the fact that clearances are relatively small with most tilting valves and probably with the ST. JUDE MEDICAL valve as well, especially in a small aortic root. I would appreciate any other comments in that regard.

[EDITOR'S NOTE: *Extraneous material left in or around the anulus is a matter of concern, regardless of the valve substitute being used. It is a situation that can have adverse effects, including embolism of a nonthrombotic nature; initiating thrombus formation or bacterial endocarditis; or becoming the focus for development of a parabasalar leak. To this list we can add the potential to interfere with poppet function.*

Regarding sutures, their position and their length, this is probably more of a consideration with bioprosthetic replacement of aortic valves. There are any number of experiences and reports of suture abrasions of tissue leaflets. In fact, this is why we have, in the past, favored HANCOCK® valves over other tissue valves. While the sewing ring of the HANCOCK valve is large, bulky and creates hemodynamic problems, there is a lesser chance of leaflet erosion with the HANCOCK valve than with the CARPENTIER-EDWARDS® valve where the sewing ring is smaller and the distance between suture tips and leaflets is diminished. The amazing thing, I guess, is not that suture ends can be enough of a cutting edge to injure a metallic poppet—it is a wonder the sutures have not injured tissue valves more often.

Finally, a comment about valve thrombosis. It seems there is a clear-cut propensity for valve thrombosis to occur when anticoagulants aren't given or are interrupted, or that it happens with greater frequency in the aortic position. Finally, from what we have been able to glean from our two experiences with valve thrombosis with the ST. JUDE MEDICAL valve, valve thrombosis seems to occur in small valve sizes when oversizing the prosthesis in relation to the anulus occurs. Whether this cuts down on leaflet tolerances within the aorta is a matter for conjecture, as is much of this discussion!]

ESCAPED LEAFLET

RICHARD J. GRAY: Are there any questions from the audience concerning the escaped leaflet reported by Dr. Hjelms or has anyone had similar occurrences? We should ask someone from quality control at St. Jude Medical, Inc. whether or not there is an incidence of rejected valves because of malfunctions in the way the various parts are fabricated. Does the company reject some valves because of cracks that are seen? Do some parts arrive broken? What are the other possible explanations besides inappropriate handling at the time of surgery that might explain what Dr. Hjelms reported?

RICHARD KRAMP, VICE PRESIDENT OF SALES AND MARKETING, ST. JUDE MEDICAL, INC.: There was nothing wrong with the carbon coating of the valve reported by Dr. Hjelms that either we or the people at CarboMedics, Inc. could determine. You probably are aware that all of the pyrolytic carbon parts, with the exception of the Sorin valves, come from CarboMedics, Inc. The components of the valve in question were within dimensional specifications. The valve passed various quality control checks that would insure that it went out of our company intact. In terms of the genesis of the fracture, there appears to have been a traumatic event to the orifice. We do not know how that may have happened *in vivo*. We have not seen another part or valve fail in this manner. What happened to this valve appears to be an isolated and unique event.

RICHARD J. GRAY: So parts are only rejected for being out of dimension; they are not rejected for being broken or potentially broken or having been x-rayed and found to have cracks. Is that correct?

RICHARD KRAMP: No, it is not correct. There are a variety of quality control checks. We have now entered a rather complex subject. For instance, all leaflets are stressed to a certain point. There are elaborate controls over the quality of the crystalline structure of the pyrolytic carbon, and various physical characteristics have to be met. There is nothing unusual about the valve Dr. Hjelms reported on, however; it appears to be a typical valve. There is no engineering insight into what happened to the valve. Apparently the failure had nothing to do with durability, I might add. There was no fatigue phenomenon in the pyrolytic carbon. The people who developed the valve parts at CarboMedics, Inc. looked at this valve and reported that they felt the initial fracture simply lowered the threshold at which the rest of the housing would fail in the basketball game. The initial fracture was presumably a precursor to the second fracture. So it would seem that something happened to this valve after fabrication and sometime before or during implantation which resulted in the clinical situation described by Dr. Hjelms.

RICHARD J. GRAY: Dr. Nicoloff, do you have a comment?

DEMETRE NICOLOFF: There was a case presented 2 years ago by a group from Germany in which they chipped out a piece of carbon with the needle as they were putting the stitches through the cuff. As you know, you can put a lot of force on a needle, especially if you have a Kaye needle with a very sharp point. This could conceivably have happened in the area of Region 1 when the valve was removed, there could have possibly been some force put on the pyrolytic carbon at the time the valve was being sewn in place. Is it possible, Dr. Hjelms that you got that initial fracture and then, as Mr. Kramp just mentioned, it led on to the other failures at a later time?

E. HJELMS: I can't answer that question, but the valve was sewn in with a trocar pointed needle with a prolene stitch, using a continuous suture. We did not notice any of the throws of the stitch being very close to the carbon ring.

DEMETRE NICOLOFF: The other concern here is that the leaflet as viewed through scanning electron microscopy did show some wear, which is not typical or usual with these valves when removed several months or even years later. Was there any postoperative occurrence in this patient that might have led you to suspect there was an unusual stress, hemodynamically or by stress? Did the patient sustain any injury or fall?

E. HJELMS: He had a completely uneventful postoperative course and, as I said, was very fit afterwards. He was young and very active. I don't know whether that had anything to do with the final event.

QUESTION: Have any escaped leaflets been reported to the company?

RICHARD J. GRAY: Good question. Dave Thomas, do you want to answer that?

DAVID THOMAS, VICE PRESIDENT, REGULATORY AFFAIRS, ST. JUDE MEDICAL, INC.: To date, six cases of leaflets exiting the valve orifice have been reported. These events are attributable to a variety of causes. In two cases the problem occurred when a rigid instrument was inserted across the valve. This either damaged the pivot recess enough to allow the leaflet to escape, or it applied enough force to the leaflet to distort it, causing the leaflet to come out of the valve orifice. In another case, the valve was inserted without utilizing the handle provided. Consequently, the surgeon inadvertently dislodged one leaflet while pushing the valve into the anulus with his fingers.

In addition to these intra-operative valve escapes, there were three reports of leaflets exiting the orifice postoperatively, without documented evidence of trauma to the valve. In the case reported by Dr. Hjelms, the condition of the explanted valve orifice and escaped leaflet are consistent with trauma well before the escape of the leaflet, perhaps perioperatively.

In two other cases, leaflets have escaped, but in neither case was the leaflet retrieved; therefore, we are unable to establish a cause for the the leaflet escape. It is notable that pyrolytic carbon part failures, while rare, have been reported for occulders in a number of valves of differing designs. The unusual, and apparently inexplicable, failure of a pyrolytic carbon component seems more likely to be related to how well we are currently able to control the manufacturing of these components than it is attributable to differences in prosthesis design.

[EDITOR'S NOTE: *An important point should be made here concerning all valve substitutes and, perhaps, in particular, the ST. JUDE MEDICAL valve. Because these devices do have a track* record of durability, whatever it is, or will be, we cannot assume that the valves are indestructible in man's hands. They are extremely delicate, albeit durable, and are deserving of a light, delicate touch. In our own practice, we avoid touching the valve as much as possible, even to the point of testing leaflet function with a soft, pediatric, red rubber catheter after the valve is in position, prior to tying the sutures or after the sutures have been tied, Furthermore, once the valve is seated, no attempt should be made to alter the position of the pyrolytic parts within the sewing skirt. Unlike some of the caged-ball valves where a SILASTIC® ball could be "popped" out, these valves should not be handled. And this extends to the way sutures are passed through the sewing ring.]

RICHARD J. GRAY: Are there questions or further comments about the issue of anticoagulation? Dr. LoCicero, you said three patients were placed on COUMADIN® for specific indications. What were the indications in these three people?

JOSEPH LOCICERO, III: Two of the patients had double valves. One patient with a double valve had two thromboembolic events prior to surgery. The third patient was in chronic atrial fibrillation.

RICHARD J. GRAY: Do you anticipate continuing your regimen?

JOSEPH LOCICERO, III: We feel very confident about our results in spite of the fact that it is a very small and very early series. We are currently doing a dental prophylaxis study going back to pick up additional patients, prior to 1980. Our series will total about 70 patients when we include those. I would like to join Dr. Sade, Dr. D'Angelo and everyone belonging to the rather vocal minority who support the concept that we now need a randomized prospective trial using aspirin in patients who do not require COUMADIN for other reasons, when implanting mechanical valves in the aortic position.

RICHARD J. GRAY: I would like to point out two important considerations as we think about this further. The first is that we really know very little about the clotting mechanism in relation to flow through intravascular prostheses or foreign bodies, let alone differences that exist between the right and left sides of the heart. Something has been made of the differing role that platelet aggregation may play, but this is all very rudimentary. My second point pertains to that issue. While we believe platelets are critical to the clotting mechanism, we really are just beginning to learn about their biochemistry in relation to adhesiveness and clotting. In that regard, we really are not even certain about what the supposed antiplatelet adhesive agents do, let alone how they do it. It seems to me, therefore, to be premature to suggest that a regimen of aspirin and dipridamole might be considered as a regimen of anticoagulation.

UNUSUAL EVENT WITH THE BJÖRK-SHILEY VALVE

RICHARD J. GRAY: One more comment. Dr. Pluth?

JAMES PLUTH: This has nothing to do with the ST. JUDE MEDICAL valve, but within the last year we removed a BJÖRK-SHILEY valve that had been inserted with silky Polydek. One of the knots had migrated towards the valve and a hole had been ground out after a period of 2 ½ years through the pyrolytic carbon to make a hole where the suture had been. Shiley Corporation said that they had never seen that before, but it was a definite 3 mm hole.

VIII. CLOSING OBSERVATIONS

35. SUMMARY AND CONCLUDING REMARKS

SHAHBUDIN RAHIMTOOLA

When evaluating thromboembolism, survival and complication data from different studies, we must look closely at the sampling of patients because there are going to be problems in evaluating the data. When the patient sample is small and when individuals within each sample are at varying degrees of risk, these factors will affect the results. These are the likely causes for the disparity in results that have been presented at this symposium and a comparison of data with different prosthetic brands or models, even from the same center, is going to result in some inconsistency of data.

COSTS OF INNOVATION
Another problem I see is that we view innovation with the philosophy that if a new valve looks good, we want to try it. An example of the costs of putting in these valves can be gathered from experience with use of the Braunwald-Cutter valve. An article published in *The Annals of Thoracic Surgery* stated that approximately 700 patients, all from the same centers, had to undergo reoperation because of problems with valve durability. The dollar costs of these 700 operations at $30,000 per operation would be $21,000,000.

Aside from dollars, I refuse to accept that there is no emotional or other trauma that adds to the unappreciated cost of reoperation. Even if one accepts that the operative mortality of a second operation is the same as a first operation, i.e., 5%, then 35 of those 700 patients paid with their lives for innovation.

I bring up these costs, not because I am against innovation, but to point out the

301

real costs in making a significant change. Making a change is a weighty matter that must be done with great circumspection. It is a lesson we have relearned many times in the treatment of valvular heart disease with prosthetic valves.

Before we take the next step, whether it is to new devices or changes in anticoagulation, we should look at the real costs. The next new-looking device should be accepted for experimental procedures. There is not an ideal prosthesis on the market and, clearly, we should continue the search for such a device.

THE ST. JUDE MEDICAL® VALVE

From the data presented here and other hemodynamic data available in the literature, it is clear that the ST. JUDE MEDICAL valve produces excellent hemodynamics. It unquestionably has one of the best hemodynamics of any mechanical prosthesis currently available or being experimentally evaluated in humans the present time. It certainly has better hemodynamics than many of the bioprostheses. Of course, it does not match the normal valve; no prosthetic valve does. However, one must keep in mind that hemodynamics is only *one* factor to be taken into account when choosing a valve replacement.

I view the results on the ST. JUDE MEDICAL valve that we have heard at 2 and 3 years as most satisfactory. In fact, I would say the data presented on this valve is comparable to any others that are currently available, or perhaps even better than some. Even though the studies presented are up to 5 years, the number of patients in these studies beyond 3 years is small.

I learned two things at this meeting: that the data on this valve at 3 years is as good or better than that for other valves at 3 years; and that the ST. JUDE MEDICAL valve has the usual problems of mechanical valves, namely thromboembolism and thrombosis. The incidence, however, of these are low. In fact, with appropriate anticoagulation therapy the incidence is very low. It is clear to me that no data has been presented that would suggest that we can delete anticoagulant therapy, and in fact, Professor Baudet's data are very convincing about the need for anticoagulant therapy.

DURABILITY

Because the STARR-EDWARDS® valve started first, it will always be 10 years ahead of every other valve in proven durability. The second longest implant record would be for the BJÖRK-SHILEY® Standard valve (the Convexo-Concave model has a much shorter record of durability). The bioprosthesis, at least in the United States would be next in durability. The ST. JUDE MEDICAL valve is gaining in proven durability, possibly to 5 years.

PROSTHESES SELECTION

As a cardiologist in the clinical setting, I select a mechanical prosthesis for a patient because of durability. I select bioprostheses for patients who cannot or should not take anticoagulants, women who want to have children and patients with a life expectancy of less than 7 or 8 years. Patients who should not be taking anticoagulants are those who would be at risk because of their occupation, sports participation or who have a contraindication to anticoagulant therapy because of associated medical disorders.

ANTICOAGULATION

What about anticoagulants and other drugs to modify the occurrence of thromboembolism? This is a matter that cannot be determined without considerable additional research. I am all for valve research, if done within a proper protocol. COUMADIN® should be used for all patients with mechanical valves, unless otherwise contraindicated.

Should we add dipyridamole? Possibly. I hesitate to do so in spite of data showing the advantages of adding dipyridamole, because I know how variable the natural history of the incidence of thromboembolism is.

A better plan might be to limit additional antiplatelet therapy to the high-risk group in whom platelet survival is reduced; this defect can be improved with antiplatelet therapy. Other high-risk groups would be those with atrial fibrillation or a history of thromboembolism, probably those patients with a large left atrium and certainly patients with clots in the heart. They should certainly be treated with COUMADIN, and one could make an argument for antiplatelet agents as well.

36. SUMMARY AND CONCLUDING OBSERVATIONS

JACK M. MATLOFF

It is clear that the ST. JUDE MEDICAL® valve represents a significant design change, which has achieved improved hemodynamic function and, perhaps, decreased the incidence of thromboembolism after valve replacement. However, the *hinge* design for leaflet movement remains a major concern for long-term durability. There is less concern about the materials from which the valve is made; pyrolytic carbon has been in use long enough to show durability and biocompatibility.

HEMODYNAMIC PERFORMANCE

Our group changed to this valve, initially in a limited trial of high-risk patients, because of the valve's hemodynamic performance. More recently, it has become our valve of choice for patients requiring a mechanical prosthesis. The valve's hemodynamic performance is probably why most physican's have made the change to this valve. The experience presented in this symposium indicates the valve is being used primarily in the presence of a small anulus, with restricted inflow to the left ventricle and restricted outflow from the left ventricle to the aorta. It is also being used in high-risk patients with significantly compromised left ventricular function. The valve is easy to use in these circumstances, especially when annular enlargement is not required. The supposed simplicity of enlargement procedures has to be questioned in light of the potential for reoperation, a consideration with any cardiac valve substitute.

The goal of achieving better hemodynamic function with the ST. JUDE MEDI-

CAL valve seems to have been met. Horstkotte's study [1] on late hemodynamic function, as well as the data cited by Dr. Rahimtoola, adequately support this conclusion; transvalvular gradients are very small and do not rise as much as with other valve substitutes as flows are increased.

Thus, the ST. JUDE MEDICAL valve has the potential to have a dynamic influence in patients with valvular heart disease. Improvement in clinical status as measured by the New York Heart Association Classification, while considered *soft* data, does support hemodynamic improvement with this valve. One must not lose sight of the fact that patients with valvular disease are concerned about quality of life, as well as longevity. The primary indication for valve replacement surgery remains relief of symptoms, which may be the best measure of hemodynamic improvement.

THROMBOEMBOLISM

A secondary effect of improved hemodynamic function may be reduced incidence of thromboembolism after valve replacement with the ST. JUDE MEDICAL valve. Although COUMADIN® usage is still indicated, a decreased incidence of thromboembolic events clearly contributes to improved quality of life and survival. Long-term survival, excluding the status of ventricular function during the first two years after surgery, is largely influenced by the results of thromboembolism and anticoagulation.

Clearly, this valve creates less stasis, and perhaps that is one reason it achieves the low thromboembolic rates reported at this symposium. In addition, there is the *washing effect* that Dr. Juro Wada of Tokyo was concerned about earlier. This issue, if it ever was one, is over forever.

Only one report in this book mentions asynchronous closure of the valve's leaflets. Dr. Dupon indicated that this phenomenon is a result of valve positioning in the mitral anulus and that an *anti-anatomic* orientation obviates asynchronous closure. At Cedars-Sinai we personally feel that this phenomenon has nothing to do with the hemodynamic function of the valve, nor does it have anything to do with the potential for thromboembolism.

The issue has been raised here whether the decreased incidence of thromboembolism with the ST. JUDE MEDICAL valve equals the incidence of anticoagulant complications that results from chronic COUMADIN administration. This consideration underscores the suggestion made by those who have considered stopping anticoagulation in their patients with ST. JUDE MEDICAL valves. This issue is another example of the problem of omission and commission in medicine. If the patient on anticoagulants has a problem, it is seen as an error of commission; if the patient *not* on anticoagulants has a problem, it is considered an error of omission. We cannot escape the fact that errors of omission seem more acceptable than those of commission; this is another expression of the dictum that a physician should first do no harm. This is not the issue.

The issue is that anyone who has a valve substitute, including a bioprostheses, still must be considered at increased risk for a thromboembolic event. Consistent with Dr. Fisk's presentation of nonvalvular factors that contribute to thromboembolism, at Cedars-Sinai we anticoagulate all patients with mitral bioprostheses. Rarely will we discontinue anticoagulants for some of the reasons listed by Dr. Rahimtoola. From what has been reported, especially by Dr. Sauvage, porcine aortic valve replacements should be considered for antiplatelet adhesive therapy, due to the potential for a bioprosthesis in the aortic position to also be associated with thromboembolic events. A consensus appears to have been reached here, that anticoagulant therapy is indicated in the presence of a mechanical prosthetic valve, including the ST. JUDE MEDICAL valve.

Because anticoagulant-related complications are a continuing problem with COUMADIN usage, it appears to be a promising suggestion that patients should be less anticoagulated. The guideline of a prothrombin time 1½ times control instead of 2 times control may be a direction to further explore. If so, I urge that Dr. J. Sullivan's protocol [2] for use of COUMADIN along with PERSANTINE® be followed. Sullivan's original protocol used 400 mg of PERSANTINE a day rather than 150 or 225 mg. I would urge everyone treating valve patients to refer back to that chapter once again.

The issue of an *anticoagulation* regimen of aspirin used in combination with PERSANTINE instead of warfarin sodium is an issue we should avoid, except, perhaps, in children. Aspirin plus PERSANTINE does not constitute anticoagulation therapy. While its use in children is yet to be resolved, it is obvious that their situation is different from adults. In order to arrive at a guideline for pediatric use, it may be important to collect results from many centers before considering a specific method of therapy. This data may already exist and a systematic examination of such data could be important. With the advance of DRGs and other restraints, it may be appropriate to suggest a new role for industry, including St. Jude Medical, Inc. That role would involve funding research and development of this issue in the clinical setting. Some of the studies mentioned by Dr. Rahimtoola on anticoagulation and thromboembolism would be particularly appropriate for consideration for such funding.

In response to patient-related factors in thrombogenicity as defined by Dr. Fisk, some are anatomic, some are functional, and some are probably hematologic and totally without our appreciation. There appears to be some feeling at this symposium that different clotting mechanisms are in effect on right- and left-sided circulation; and there is the issue of clotting as related to platelets and other factors. Dr. Lillehei's comments on thromboxane A2 and prostacyclin are most appropriate. Atrial fibrillation still is and probably always will be a problem. While occasional patients with long-term atrial fibrillation have surprisingly been converted to sinus rhythm after valve replacement with the ST. JUDE MEDICAL prosthesis, a significant number of patients are not converted; and all patients have the potential to later develop this rhythm. An additional consideration is *preoperative* thromboembolism and left atrial thrombus. These patient-related phenomena require careful attention and they determine the need for anticoagulation irrespective of the presence of a valve substitute.

Valve thrombosis remains an extremely serious complication. This was the primary, and perhaps the only, concern about the BJÖRK-SHILEY valves before the question of durability arose in the most recent Convexo-Concave BJÖRK-SHILEY prostheses.

With the ST. JUDE MEDICAL valve, thrombosis is also of potential concern, because of the delicacy of the hinge mechanism and its function. Although the potential for trouble is real, the problem appears, in fact, to be miniscule. Reports at this symposium show it occurs most often in relation to poor, or no, anticoagulant therapy. A point made during discussion that should be emphasized is that thrombosis with the ST. JUDE MEDICAL valve is not necessarily sudden or fatal, since it may involve only one *hinge* mechanism and one leaflet. Again, the issue of the *hinge* mechanism will really be the point on which this valve will ultimately succeed or fail.

The largest problem we see is that physicians and patients are sometimes not willing to continue with a stable situation. It is important to remember that the most dangerous time for patients with valve substitutes occurs when changes, whether planned or spontaneous, are made in anticoagulant regiments. There are no hard data, only anecdotal protocols, for how COUMADIN should be discontinued. Discontinuation of COUMADIN may expose patients to more risks than if they had not started anticoagulation. Professor Baudet and others have pointed out that the incidence of anticoagulant-related problems can be very low if appropriate care is taken in their management.

STRUCTURAL INTEGRITY

To date, the ST. JUDE MEDICAL heart valve is proving to be durable. Based on experiences with large series reported at this symposium, I believe it is appropriate to talk about 4- or 6-year durability. This is still only an intermediate follow-up, not long-term follow-up. The standard of durability (and only durability) is the STARR-EDWARDS® caged-ball valve with a silastic poppet (Model Nos. 1260 and 6120). The first Harken and STARR-EDWARDS valves were implanted 24 years ago. Given the ages of large patient populations at that time, a minimal standard for durability must be 15 to 20 years; and we are nowhere close to that with the ST. JUDE MEDICAL valve.

As Dr. Rahimtoola noted, we seem to be approaching the time when the limits of bioprosthetic durability may be defined. Dr. Duncan's report on the IONESCU-SHILEY® valve has to be placed in this perspective. As has been indicated, recent BJÖRK-SHILEY valve models do not have the durability track record of the STARR-EDWARDS caged-ball valve. Present convexo-concave valves cannot follow on the experience of the original spherical models; they are newer valves, newer even than the ST. JUDE MEDICAL valve, and the natural history of convexo-concave valves is yet to be defined. Within 2 or 3 years we will begin to have follow-up of the ST. JUDE MEDICAL valve from 8 to 10 years. One can anticipate that the issue of its durability as compared with bioprostheses will come into focus at that time.

With due respect to the Mayo Clinic experience, reoperations, for whatever indications and under what ever conditions, are to be avoided. At our institution a number of reoperations for coronary disease are done, with heightened concern each time, for the patient's condition. Reoperations are necessary, but they are never easy for the patient, family or surgeon. Since the ST. JUDE MEDICAL valve, even with anticoagulants, appears to have lower complication rates necessitating reoperation than bioprostheses, the next 2 to 3 years may tell what the primary indications for the ST. JUDE MEDICAL valve are going to be.

MORTALITY RATES

Mortality rates, particularly early operative mortality rates, have been reported here as decreased. As has been discussed, one has to be aware of sampling as a factor in such reports. The impact of improved techniques in myocardial preservation should be added to that consideration. The figures presented here are less than those seen in the literature.

Beyond experience and other factors noted, consider what the contribution of the valve's excellent hemodynamic function may be to these lessened mortality rates. When we get involved in complex pathological situations requiring multiple concommitant procedures, the issues are more difficult to ferret out and the risks go up significantly. The problem of coexisting coronary disease, as noted in my presentation, remains only for mitral valve disease. With coronary disease and mitral regurgitation, which are etiologically related, we are where we were 3 to 5 years ago with postinfarction ventricular septal defect.

The issue is not how good surgical therapy is, but rather, how can we select patients at greatest risk, so they can be treated earlier, in order to preserve both ventricular and valvular function.

A plea has to be made that early mortalities not be excluded from follow-up analyses. We have heard this view expounded and have seen analyses of survival beginning after the first 30 days postoperatively. The primary mortality from valve surgery may not occur in the first 30 days, but probably occurs in the first 7 to 12 postoperative months. Each presentation of survival including operative mortality showed additional significant mortality from 2 to 12 months. When discussing survival we have to begin with a population of patients at risk, and the analysis should focus on survival at 1, 5, 10, 15 and 20 years. This will keep operative mortality and its influence on outcome in perspective.

CONCLUSION

It is critical for all doing cardiac surgery, whether on valvular, coronary or congenital lesions, to keep precise data. Dr. Rahimtoola, in his opening presentation, indicated some patients do not realize they have a valve substitute, or if they do, what position it is in or what kind it is. There is probably more truth to that statement than any of us care to admit. Just as patient education is critical, our data must be kept in a scrupulous manner so that its validity is not in question. Furthermore, data must be collated easily and reviewed regularly so we know what we are doing for our patients. This is the prime responsibility that goes with the practice of cardiac surgery. By doing this we can identify the subtle factors that affect outcome.

In this regard, I always have been conservative about changes in cardiac surgery. The fact that we changed to the ST. JUDE MEDICAL valve may be cause to question this statement; but we made the change for specific reasons, based on prior experience. The ST. JUDE MEDICAL valve is still a new valve when compared with the STARR-EDWARDS valve; but it is becoming a less new valve all the time. When the data presented here are reviewed, individual surgeons may decide to make a change. That should not be done *a priori*. Individual results should be carefully examined and re-examined. If the results are not acceptable and it is felt that significant improvement can be achieved, then a change may be in order. If so, considerations other than the choice of a valve substitute may be involved. Thus, it is necessary to begin the process of change not with the fact that there is a new valve that shows promise but with the track record of your own experience with existing technology.

REFERENCES

1. Horstkotte D, Haerten K, Seipel L, et al: Central hemodynamics at rest and during exercise after mitral valve replacement with different prostheses. Circulation 1983;68(suppl II):II–161–II–168.
2. Sullivan J, Harken D, Gorlin R: Pharmacologic control of thromboembolic complications of cardiac valve replacement. N Engl J Med 1971;284(25):1086.